Preventive Strikes

Preventive Strikes

Women, Precancer, and Prophylactic Surgery

ILANA LÖWY

The Johns Hopkins University Press

Baltimore

The Johns Hopkins University Press
2715 North Charles Street
Baltimore, Maryland 21218-4363
www.press.jhu.edu

Library of Congress Cataloging-in-Publication Data
Löwy, Ilana
Preventive strikes : women, precancer, and prophylactic surgery / Ilana Löwy.
p. cm.
Includes bibliographical references and index.
ISBN-13: 978-0-8018-9364-3 (hardcover : alk. paper)
ISBN-10: 0-8018-9364-X (hardcover : alk. paper)
1. Cancer in women—Surgery—Social aspects. 2. Precancerous conditions—
Surgery—Social aspects. 3. Breast—Cancer—Surgery—Social aspects.
4. Ovaries—Cancer—Surgery—Social aspects. 5. Social medicine. I. Title.
[DNLM: 1. Neoplasms—prevention & control—France. 2. Neoplasms—
prevention & control—Great Britain. 3. Neoplasms—prevention & control—
United States. 4. Precancerous Conditions—surgery—France. 5. Precancerous
Conditions—surgery—Great Britain. 6. Precancerous Conditions—surgery—
United States. 7. Genetic Predisposition to Disease—France. 8. Genetic
Predisposition to Disease—Great Britain. 9. Genetic Predisposition to Disease—
United States. 10. History, 20th Century—France. 11. History, 20th Century—
Great Britain. 12. History, 20th Century—United States. 13. Women's Health—
France. 14. Women's Health—Great Britain. 15. Women's Health—United States.
QZ 204 L917p 2009]
RC281.W65L69 2009
616.99'4071—dc22   2008056007

A catalog record for this book is available from the British Library.

*Special discounts are available for bulk purchases of this book. For more information,
please contact Special Sales at 410-516-6936 or specialsales@press.jhu.edu.*

The Johns Hopkins University Press uses environmentally friendly book materials,
including recycled text paper that is composed of at least 30 percent post-consumer
waste, whenever possible. All of our book papers are acid-free, and our jackets and
covers are printed on paper with recycled content.

To Barbara Rosenkrantz

CONTENTS

∞

My first debt is to the institutions that have made this research possible. INSERM—the French Institute of Health and Medical Research—has given continual support to my atypical investigations, while my research center, CERMES, has provided excellent intellectual and material conditions for my work, a rare privilege in a time of reduced support for "useless" studies, those devoid of economic value. Additional support for this study has come from grants from the Fondation de France and the French National Cancer Institute (INCa). I was extremely lucky to able to benefit from the resources of two extraordinary institutions: The Radcliffe Institute, where I started the research on this book, and the Max Planck Institute for the History of Science (MPIWG), where I wrote large parts of it. My gratitude goes to Drew Faust and Judith Vichniac at the Radcliffe Institute and to Loraine Daston, Jürgen Renn, and Hans Jörg Rheinberger at the MPIWG, for creating a scholars' paradise.

My second—and crucial—debt is to archivists. The invisible work of librarians and archivists makes historical studies possible. While working on this book I met highly skilled, dedicated, and enthusiastic archivists. I'm very grateful to Nathalie Huchette and Laurence Leclerc at the Curie Institute, Paris; Jonathan Evans and his colleagues at the London Hospital Archives; Katie Ormerod and her colleagues at the Archives of St Bartholomew's Hospital, London; Hilary Ritchie at Addenbrooke's Hospital, Cambridge (UK); Jim Gehrlich at the Archives Service of New York Hospital; Stephen Novak and his colleagues at the Archives and Special Collections of the Health Sciences Library, Columbia University; and Jack Eckert and the staff of the Rare Books and Manuscript Department, Countway Library, Harvard University, for their essential help.

Research is a collective endeavor, and exchanges with colleagues are one of the great pleasures of that occupation. This study started as an investigation of the introduction of genetic tests for hereditary predisposition for malignant tumors. I discussed on multiple occasions ideas that led to this book with the other two participants in the project, Maurice Cassier and Jean-Paul Gaudillière. At CERMES, Isabelle Baszanger was a permanent source of stimulating reflections on cancer treatment and the meaning of this disease. Numerous other people provided data, ideas, and critiques and greatly enriched my work. An incomplete list includes Olga Amsterdamska, Robert Aronowitz, Emm Barnes, Christian Bonah, Bettina Borisch, Soraya Boudia, Pascale Bouret, Allan Brandt, Lynda Bryder, Alberto Cambrosio, David Cantor, Patrick Castel, Soraya de Chadeverian, Angela Creager, Loraine Daston, Yolanda Eraso, Gerd Gigerenzer, Jeremy Greene, Volker Hess, Nathalie Jas, Peter Keating, Nikolai Krementsov, Nancy Krieger, Gertchen Krueger, Gerald Kutcher, Margaret Lock, Harry Marks, Andrew Mendelsohn, Ornella Moscucci, Diane Paul, Naomi Pfeffer, John Pickstone, Toine Pieters, Theodore Porter, Viviane Quirke, Rayna Rapp, Hans Jörg Rheinberger, Charles Rosenberg, Helene Rouch, Naomi Sayre, Robert Sayre, Christiane Sinding, Carsten Timmermann, Elisabeth Toon, Helen Valier, and George Weisz. Many of the colleagues who helped to shape this book are part of the "cancer network"—a group of scholars involved in study of the history of malignant tumors, organized by David Cantor, John Pickstone and Carsten Timmermann. And very special thanks to Robert Aronowitz, with whom I conducted for many years an extremely fruitful dialogue about early diagnosis of malignant tumors and the management of embodied risks.

Olga Amsterdamska, Isabelle Baszanger, Jean-Paul Gaudillière, Harry Marks, John Pickstone, and Doreen Valentine provided important critiques of the manuscript and helped to eliminate some of its shortcomings. I wish I were able live up to their high standards. At the Johns Hopkins University Press, Jacqueline Wehmueller was a highly supportive, stimulating, and helpful editor; Ashleigh McKown provided crucial help with practical issues; and Michele Callaghan did wonders improving my English.

American Cancer Society, Brazilian National Cancer Institute, Bulletin du Cancer, Hospital Medicine, Hodder Education Editions, JAMA, Ligue Contre le Cancer, National Library of Medicine (USA), and Wellcome Images gave permission to reproduce images. Thanks to David Cantor, Venita Paul, and Luiz Teixeira for help with securing high-quality reproductions.

My rapidly growing family provides intellectual stimulation, new interests, moral support, food, and laughter. It helps me to keep in perspective the ups and downs of academic life and to take my own work with a grain of salt. Thank you Woody, Tamara, Rodolfo, Daniel, Shafak, Naomi, Juan Carlos, Rachel, and Arnaud.

This work is dedicated to Barbara Rosenkrantz, mentor, adviser, supporter, colleague, friend, and a wonderful human being. Barbara is living proof that the right strategic moves and the mobilization of appropriate networks are not the only ways to succeed in academia and that one can choose instead intellectual integrity, critical spirit, honesty, and courage.

Preventive Strikes

Introduction:
Embodied Risk

Radical Solutions

This study originated in a perplexing observation. For one year I observed the counseling that people with a hereditary risk of malignancies received in a major French cancer treatment center. The oncogenetics department providing this counseling combined innovative research in molecular biology with more traditional family studies and the performance of genetic tests. I was impressed by the professionalism and the humanity of the clinical geneticists who worked in the department. I was also impressed by their powerlessness. Women diagnosed with a mutation in the *BRCA* gene were told that they had a high probability of developing breast or ovarian cancer and received two recommendations: undergo intensive medical surveillance—frequent mammography, ultrasonography, and clinical examinations—and have a prophylactic removal of their ovaries (at that time, the center's doctors did not promote preventive mastectomy—the removal of healthy breasts).

The center's geneticists were not sure how efficient surveillance was, but they were persuaded that a preventive removal of healthy ovaries greatly reduced the risk of developing breast or ovarian cancer. The contrast between the sophistication of a diagnostic technology grounded in the latest developments in molecular biology and the crudeness of the solution to the diagnosed gene mutation—the mutilation of a healthy female body—bewildered me. My bewilderment led me to an interest in the history of preventive surgery for cancer, in the scientific justification of such surgery, and to the search for an explanation why this approach is mainly directed toward women.

Preventive surgery to treat cancer is a century-long practice. Its goal was to detect and treat malignant tumors as early as possible. Doctors who observed "ac-

cessible" cancers, such as skin or breast malignancies, concluded that cancer progresses in a linear and orderly way: It starts as a localized lesion, spreads to nearby
tissues, and then produces distant metastases, so-named because they are found
in different part of the body from the original lesion. These metastases probably
arise through the circulation of malignant cells in the blood or the lymphatic system. At the same time, surgeons became aware of a correspondence between the
size and the extent of spread of a malignant tumor and the success of an operation
for the tumor, with smaller and less invasive tumors' being more readily treated by
surgery. This was not an absolute rule, because not all surgeries for small and
contained tumors were successful. However, patients with extended tumors—
those that have spread beyond their place of origin—nearly always succumbed
to their disease. These two observations were made independently, but in the
early twentieth century they were joined in a single conceptual framework—
"cancer schemata." In this view the conviction that small, localized tumors were
an early stage in the development of a malignancy was linked with the idea that
cancers can be cured at that stage. The "early stage in the natural history of the
disease cancer," a description that does not define a specific time frame, was then
translated into the practical injunction "shortly after the appearance of suspicious symptoms or signs," a very different concept.[1]

The next step was a call for the early detection of malignant tumors. Cancer
experts stipulated that the only way to transform a fatal disease into a treatable
condition was to be "faster than the cancer."[2] A wish to detect malignancies as
early as possible became one of the central elements of the cancer education campaign conducted by cancer charities such as the American Society for the Control of Cancer (which in 1945 became the American Cancer Society), the British
Empire Cancer Campaign, and the Ligue Française Contre le Cancer. Prophylactic
surgery was a logical extension of this trend. In the early twentieth century, cancer experts developed the concept of "precancerous" or "premalignant" lesions
(that is, changes in cells and tissues that precede the advent of malignancy) and
proposed a preventive ablation, or surgical removal, of organs that harbor such
lesions—initially, mainly breasts. This approach was then justified by their belief
that the amputated organs were bound to become malignant very soon.

In more recent times, the notion of premalignant lesions was extended to
changes in macromolecules. Attempting to explain to their patients the meaning
of mutations that increase their chances of developing cancer, some geneticists
described such mutations as "molecular lesions." At first sight, the term *molecular lesion* is a puzzling concept. The word "lesion" comes from the Latin word
"laesio," or an attack or injury, and describes damage to organs and tissues. It was

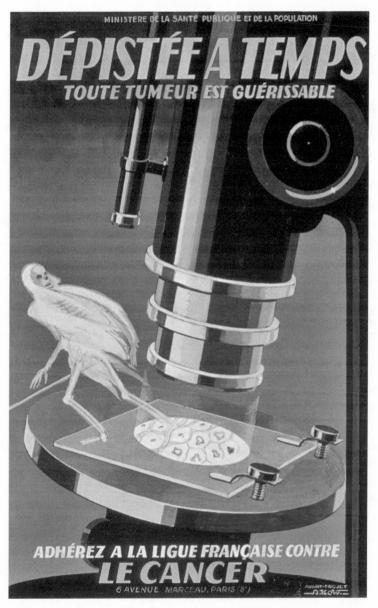

Poster supporting the early detection of cancer, put out in the 1950s by what was then known as La Ligue Française Contre le Cancer. National Library of Medicine. Used by permission of La Ligue Nationale Contre le Cancer.

introduced in the early nineteenth century in the context of efforts to correlate clinical signs with morbid changes in the body. It is not surprising that first observations of cancerous lesions were made with the naked eye (gross anatomical lesions). Later, the technology arose to view them under the microscope (histological lesions). This shift from personal observations by surgeons to verification by pathologists will be discussed in greater detail in chapter 3.

The concept of lesions, French philosopher of medicine Georges Canguilhem has proposed, is central to the distinction between the normal and the pathological.[3] Molecules belong to a different domain of study, that of chemistry. The term *molecular lesion* collapses a distinction between two levels of functioning of the organism, tissues and molecules, and two modes of explanation, the pathological and the biochemical. This "molecularization" of pathological phenomena is one of the defining traits of present-day biomedicine.[4] Researchers who studied precancerous states extended the notion of lesions to nonmorphological changes and then to genetic defects associated with an increased risk of cancer.[5] Such an extension highlights the importance of cytological diagnosis of cancer. In the early twenty-first century a diagnosis of cancer is not definitive until it is confirmed by a pathologist who examines fixed and stained preparation of suspicious tissue.

The term *molecular lesion* points also to similarities between the diagnosis of mutations that predispose one to cancer and of precancerous changes in tissues. In both cases, patients are informed that the presence of abnormal elements in their body, be they altered DNA sequences or modified cells, puts them at higher than average risk of malignancy. Consequently, they face an uncertainty whether an illness will develop (event uncertainty), when it will develop (time uncertainty), and how severe it will be (damage uncertainty). They frequently also face difficult choices.[6] In both cases a diagnosis of an "embodied risk" of cancer can put people in limbo between health and disease (becoming a "healthy ill"), change the way they feel about their dangerous body parts ("living with a ticking bomb"), and lead to a split between the self and the treacherous part of the body.[7] Having prophylactic surgery for a precancerous lesion—be it histological, cellular, or molecular—is one way of healing such a split.[8]

Diagnosis of Disease and Diagnosis of Risk

Prophylactic surgery extended the notions of early detection and early treatment from cancer to precancer. Its history is inseparably intertwined with that of the diagnosis of precancerous changes. Intervention—a preventive ablation of potentially dangerous organs and tissues—relies on the capacity to identify such threatening body parts. It is grounded in the implicit supposition that premalignant lesions are well-defined entities that can be recognized by specialists. The history of surgical (and occasionally radiological) management of cancer risk is, to an important extent, a history of diagnoses of precancerous conditions and persisting uncertainties linked with such diagnoses.

Diagnosis, the art or act of identifying and classifying diseases from their signs and symptoms, is a key organizing principle of modern medicine. Before the rise of "scientific medicine" in the nineteenth century, diseases were loosely defined entities with names like "fever" and "dropsy" that varied according to place, season, and above all the temperament and predisposition of the patient. The supposition that diseases are stable entities, historian of medicine Charles Rosenberg persuasively argues, opened the way to a rational management of sick bodies and homogenization of medical practices.[9] Diagnostic categories, in this framework, give meaning to signs sent by the body, differentiate the normal from the pathological, and define what a given complaint is, what its prognosis is, and how it should be treated. In these ways, these categories structure clinical, administrative, and patient practices.

One can propose, paraphrasing anthropologist Mary Douglas's description of commodification, that "diagnosis is a ritual activity which uses technologies and embodied skills to make firm and visible a particular set of judgments in a fluid process of classifying people and events."[10] Diagnostic categories incorporate and sum up beliefs of professionals and guide medical and administrative interventions. In parallel, they shape the subjective experience of sick people and social attitudes toward complaints of ill health. When dealing with contested "emergent illnesses"—for example, chronic fatigue syndrome—patients who have multiple, debilitating symptoms fight for a "real" diagnosis of somatic disorder to validate their experience.[11] In the case of precancer, the opposite is true. People do not face symptoms without a diagnosis but rather a frightening and often life-changing diagnosis, without distressing symptoms.

In modern medicine, diagnosis is mainly a technological endeavor. Diagnostic techniques produce specific ways of thinking about disease. When the techniques change, the definition of disease changes, too. The history of preventive treatment for cancer is the history of concepts and practices that made a diagnosis of precancerous conditions possible. It belongs to two distinct narrative strands: that of the emergence of new diagnostic categories and the reclassification of established ones and that of the management of disease risk—that is, the treatment of people who feel perfectly well but who may become ill in the future.

Today diagnostic tests may be as important for the healthy as they are for the sick. Many any such tests capitalize on the anxiety of healthy ("asymptomatic") people.[12] These tests may also produce a new kind of subjectivity. People are defined as being at higher than average risk of disease, either because they possess dangerous body parts (embodied risk) or because they have statistically abnormal readings of a laboratory test ("fear by numbers").[13] Those diagnosed as being at risk may acquire a new identity and became members of new social networks.[14] An example of this is the people calling themselves "pre-vivors," which is discussed further in chapter 4, a word coined for those determined to have a genetic likelihood for cancer and not the disease itself. The shift from diagnosis of disease to diagnosis of risk has important social and economic consequences. It produces new classes of consumers of drugs, medical technologies, and professional services and thus new markets for merchandise and services. "The politics of life itself" is also just politics.[15]

Biomedical Cancer and Lived Cancer

The biological phenomenon of malignancy probably has existed as long as the human race; "cancer"—that is a specific pathological condition, identified by physicians but recognized by lay people as well—was described in antiquity. By contrast the diagnosis of premalignant lesions does not exist without a cytology laboratory.[16] People can suspect that they harbor a malignant tumor, but they cannot feel "precancerous." They receive this information from a pathologist. The diagnostic category of precancer belongs to the universe of biomedical science, not to that of a direct, lived experience.

People who live in industrialized countries—and, in a globalized world, increasingly everywhere else, too—frequently perceive the external world through two distinct frameworks of reference: commonsensical and scientific.[17] In some areas of scientific inquiry, such as the production of geographic maps, commonsensical and scientific knowledge are closely related. The first satellite images produced a sense of wonder through their familiarity. Seen from the space, the earth looked exactly as it was depicted on an old-fashioned globe. In spite of this, the majority of images produced by science are distant from the realm of commonsensical knowledge. When asked if a virus is a live organism or part of inanimate nature, French biologist André Lwoff was reported to say, "a virus is a virus is a virus."[18] One can similarly propose that an electron microscope image of a virus is an electron microscope image of a virus, that is, a sui generis entity that cannot be fully reduced to another object. The same is true for numerous other entities produced by scientific techniques and instruments.[19]

Scientific and commonsensical frameworks produce distinct images of the body: the lived body, apprehended through the senses and experience, and the scientific body, shaped through experts' understanding of structure and functions of living organisms. Visualization methods used by scientists and doctors implicitly assume a perfect continuity between the two bodies. Techniques and instruments of science are presented as amplifying tools that allow us to perceive elements inaccessible to our senses. The exhibition Genetic Portrait by and of the photographer Gary Schneider illustrated this view. Schneider depicted his own body through the double filter of photographic art and science.[20] He exhibited imprints of his hands on a photosensitive paper, panoramic x-ray photographs of his teeth, photographs of his spermatozoids as seen under a light microscope and from a preparation of his own chromosomes, electron microscope images of his cells, and autoradiographic images of his DNA. Schneider treats all the elements of his genetic portrait as equally representative of his biological identity. Subcellular particles and DNA strands are parts of a given individual in the same way his hands or his teeth are. A microscope; an x-ray machine; a light, electronic, or scanning microscope—all these sharpen and extend our ways of seeing. Images created by scientific instruments and techniques represent nevertheless entities that are no less real than those observed by the naked eye or a magnifying glass and have the same ontological status: DNA sequences *are* Gary Schneider.

Schneider's exhibition constructs a seamless continuum that goes from a hand to a tumor-suppressing gene. Such a continuum was made plausible by a gradual education of the public to view images produced by scientific instruments and techniques as straightforward extensions of the impressions they receive through their senses. X-ray images played an important role in this education. An x-ray film is a perfect mediation tool because it lumps together images that belong to a nonscientific world, such as panoramic view of one's teeth, with those devoid of commonsensical meaning, such as shadows on x-ray images of lungs. Such shadows may represent a disease process and may therefore be linked with manifestations that belong to the world of lived experience of a patient, for example shortness of breath or pain, but there is no simple, commonsensical equivalent of a dark spot on an x-ray film of the lung. Patients can learn to decode the meaning of such a spot, but only if they leave behind their lay frame of reference and adopt a scientific one.[21] The discontinuities between x-ray images and ordinary photographs are, however, masked by iconic images produced in the early days of x-ray technology (a classic example is an image of bones of a hand wearing a ring). The straightforward decoding of such iconic images reinforces the impression that all x-ray films are nonproblematic representations of a hidden reality.

Similar impressions of a smooth transition from commonsensical to scientific images are produced through a display of continuity between entities viewed with the naked eye, a magnifying glass, and a light microscope. Such a continuity exists—sometimes. Spermatozoids are not visible to the naked eye, but to see them, it is sufficient to put a drop of a sperm fluid under a microscope. By contrast, to see chromosomes it is necessary to kill a living cell and to subject its content to complicated chemical manipulations. A slide that displays chromosomes is called "preparation," a self-explanatory term. In some sense at least, chromosomes are produced by methods that make them visible. This is even truer for observations made with an electron microscope, an instrument that records the resistance of objects to a beam of electrons. To make cells visible with this technique, they need to be sliced by a microtome, dehydrated, and fixed with salts of heavy metals. Some shapes and forms visible under an electron microscope can be related to those perceived by a light microscope, but many others cannot.[22] Finally, during an autoradiography of DNA specimen, the observed material destroys itself in the process of preparation of the radiography film. The studied object can be seen only when it does not exist anymore.[23] Microscopic preparations, and even more so DNA autoradiography plaques, may be defined as "epistemic things" or "quasi-objects"—irreducibly underdetermined entities that are at the same time material and conceptual and that came into being in the artificial world of the laboratory.[24]

In medicine, the "quasi-objects" produced by increasingly complicated medical technology construct a "quasi-reality" of scientific perception of disease or altered function. Such a perception is not entirely disconnected from a lived experience produced by signals sent by the body, but the relationship between the two may be as complex as the one between a radiographic image of DNA segments of a person and her photographic portrait.[25] Some images produced by medical technologies such as tumor-inhibiting mutation included in Schneider's self-portrait, belong exclusively to the biomedical body and have no direct equivalent in the lived one. Other images may have such an equivalent. An x-ray film of a broken bone is directly connected to pain and loss of mobility. Others still have an intermediary status. The majority of the methods used to display premalignant lesions belong to this third category. A suspicious shadow on a mammogram or a cluster of atypical cells on a microscopic slide may indicate the presence of an already existing pathology or the danger of future pathology. It may also resist interpretation, in which case doctors may attempt to extrapolate from data what can be easily correlated with clinical observations to those with a blurred or ambivalent meaning. The definition of specific changes in tissues observed in fixed and stained preparations of tissues as premalignant was often grounded in such extrapolations.

The rise of the category of precancer was related to changes in the treatment of the disease of cancer. With the adoption of cancer schemata and of the principle of early detection and prompt intervention, cancer experts dissociated the scale of the proposed treatment from the magnitude of clinical symptoms and intensity of disease-induced suffering.[26] Patients diagnosed with extended or metastatic malignancies were classified as hopeless cases and were offered palliative treatment only. Radical therapy—extensive surgery and radiotherapy—was reserved mainly for hopeful cases, that is, for patients with localized small tumors. In earlier periods, people with cancer were usually prompted to see a doctor when they experienced distressing symptoms. A newly diagnosed cancer patient was often a very sick individual. With the diffusion of information about warning signs of cancer, people who had minor symptoms (a small lump, a wound that heals slowly, a change in a mole) but otherwise felt perfectly well, were diagnosed with a malignancy and submitted to drastic and mutilating surgical or radiological treatment. The experience of cancer became increasingly that of a healthy person who becomes sick as a result of a medical intervention. From the patient's point of view, the treatment of an asymptomatic tumor was a preventive therapy.

Once established, the principle that cancer treatment is frequently dissociated from the presence of distressing symptoms was extended to treatment of candidate precancerous lesions. For example, many premalignant lesions of the breast were discovered in women who noticed suspicious symptoms and went to the doctor fearing that they had cancer. These women were already prepared for the possibility of losing a breast if diagnosed with a malignant tumor and could be persuaded that a similar, usually somewhat less drastic, surgery was needed to eliminate a premalignant lesion. The acceptance of immediate mutilation, they were told, would protect them from a worse mutilation and danger of death in the future. Consequently, some patients diagnosed with precancerous lesions followed a "cancer script," that is, a therapeutic trajectory similar to that of people diagnosed with an invasive malignancy. The similarity of patients' trajectories reinforced in turn the blurring of boundaries between cancer and precancer.

The present-day concept of cancer risk was developed after World War II. The new focus on the management of health risks reflected global changes such as the rise of the "risk society," a growing role played by health insurance, and an increased state intervention in health care. It also mirrored specific developments within medicine, such as studies on the danger of cardiovascular disease or debates about links between smoking and lung cancer.[27] The shift from a lived cancer, experienced by the patient as suffering and disruption of vital functions, to biomedical cancer, an entity diagnosed through the use of medical techniques and dissociated from a subjective experience of sickness was not, I propose in this book, a recent development. It was linked with the development of surgical pathology in early twentieth century and was closely associated with the history of diagnosis and treatment of two female cancers—those of the breast and of the uterus.

Women and Malignancies

Today cancer is a unisex disease. Some cancers are strictly sex-specific. Thus a man cannot have an ovarian tumor and a woman cannot have a prostate tumor. Other malignancies are much more prevalent in one sex, e.g., breast cancer for anatomical and physiological reasons or lung cancer for social ones. The overall rates of cancer deaths are nevertheless similar in both sexes. Until the mid-twentieth century, however, cancer was perceived mainly as a female pathology. This view probably reflected a greater facility of diagnosing cancer in women. Before the generalization of cytological analyses and medical imagery techniques, the differential diagnosis of cancers of internal organs was often difficult. However, the main female cancers, breast and uterus, produce typical symptoms. Together with head and neck tumors, another group of malignancies easily recognizable through their clinical signs, they symbolized the horror of "dread disease"—a gradual decomposition of the flesh, increased suffering, a slow and painful death.[28] Breast and cervical cancers played a key role in the establishment of cancer schemata. Thanks to their relative accessibility to medical gaze, physicians were able to observe different stages of growth of these tumors, from small lesions to extended ones. These observations were then employed to construct a general view of natural history of the disease of cancer. In a parallel development, treatment of female malignancies favored the development of cutting-edge therapies of cancer: radical surgery and radiotherapy. The role of female cancers as model tumors was reflected in the importance attributed to these malignancies in scientific literature. For example, among the 130 working papers published by the Cancer Commission of the League of Nations between 1923 and 1939, twenty-two were dedicated to tumors of the breast and uterus. Four additional papers discussed malignancies induced by work conditions (two described lung cancer among miners and the other two skin cancer among workers in the chemical industry). All the remaining articles discussed "cancer" in general; they mainly provided statistics on the prevalence of malignant tumors and mortality from this disease.[29]

The visibility of female cancers helps to explain why these pathologies first became targets of efforts to eliminate cancer danger through a preventive surgery. Another, and perhaps even more important factor in the development of preventive operations, was the existence of a long tradition of surgical excision of women's reproductive organs, both diseased and healthy. The medical discourse, Ella Shohat explains, figures the female body, and especially female reproductive organs, as "a walking pathological laboratory."[30] Hysterectomy (ablation of the uterus) and oophorectomy (ablation of the ovaries) were employed to treat numerous "female complaints," including psychological ones but also to reduce the danger of gynecological malignancies.[31] Feminist activists, from those who participated in the struggle against the Contagious Diseases Act for its unfairness in blaming prostitutes for the spread of venereal disease in the United Kingdom in the 1860s and 1870s to those who a century later founded the Women's Health Movement and criticized doctors' lack of sensitivity to women's needs and their wish to control female reproductive functions. Activists described surgical ablation of ovaries ("the castration of women") and unnecessary hysterectomies as typical expressions of a brutal treatment of women by the medical profession.[32] During the controversy on radical mastectomy for breast cancer, some activists similarly attributed the enthusiasm for this mutilating operation to surgeons' misogyny and their perception of breast, uterus, and ovaries of women past their reproductive age as "useless organs."[33]

Other researchers proposed, however, that in the latter case surgical radicalism was directed against tumors, not against women. Cultural critic Erin O'Connor argued that the nineteenth-century discourse about breast cancer was about the advanced malignancies, the women who died painful, ugly deaths, and the doctors who watched them and desperately tried to do something to prevent such deaths. Moreover, the biological traits of breast cancer—its visibility, its variability—transformed it into an especially telling example of the disease of cancer. When thinking about female malignancies, O'Connor concluded, doctors did not think "female," they thought "malignancy."[34] Barbara Rothman—who in her previous work had strongly criticized misogynistic trends among U.S. gynecologists—arrived at a similar conclusion. Recent controversies on conservative versus radical surgery for breast cancer, Rothman proposed, were driven by surgeons' aspiration to do the best (in their understanding) for their patients, while avoiding medical mistakes. The treatment for breast cancer was not very different from the treatment for testicular cancer. In the latter malignancy, too, doctors readily eliminated "suspicious" sexual glands: "It is not that medicine is not misogynistic: it is that this is irrelevant in this instance. It was a statement about cancer, not about breasts and not about women."[35]

O'Connor and Rothman are probably right. Attitudes toward radical surgical treatment of already existing malignancies were similar in both sexes. Men had their full share of "heroic surgeries." The treatment of head and neck tumors, cancers linked to consumption of alcohol and tobacco and therefore less common in women, often included disfiguring and mutilating attempts to eliminate all of the tumor and the regional lymph nodes. The dramatic consequences of such surgeries contributed to a low visibility of head and neck tumors in the public discourse on cancer. These pathologies were too horrid to contemplate.[36] One should distinguish, however, between a surgical treatment of cancer and cancer risk. Until recently, the latter was proposed nearly exclusively to women. One notable exception was the management of a rare hereditary form of colon cancer, familial adenomatous polyposis (FAP), treated by a prophylactic removal of the colon (colectomy). Such surgery was proposed to people who developed numerous intestinal polyps. Men and women with the FAP mutation (a dominant hereditary trait, unrelated to gender) develop colon cancer in early or midlife and the excision of the polyp carrying colon was—and is—the only way to prevent malignancy.

In contrast to what evolved to be the case with breast and uterine cancers, the preventive ablation of the colon in people with FAP was proposed only to people who had nearly 100 percent chance of developing colon cancer. A preventive surgery for female tumors was proposed to healthy women, when the chance of developing cancer was unknown. It is reasonable to assume that the preventive ablation of healthy breasts, ovaries, and uteruses was facilitated by the—gendered—tradition of surgical excision of female reproductive organs. The recent development of preventive mastectomy can be also related to the history of cosmetic surgery. Cosmetic surgery is at the same time a genderless transformative technology (men seek cosmetic surgery, too) and a strongly gendered approach. In spite of a flurry of publications that claim that men have become as interested as women in the surgical enhancement of their bodies, the data on users of cosmetic surgery continue to show a strong gender bias. Women's greater readiness to use surgery to eliminate a perceived source of unhappiness and psychological suffering, and the popularity of techniques such as breast augmenta-

tion, might have helped to decrease controversy about employing surgery to reduce disease risk.[37]

A recent emphasis on preventive medicine may put an end to gender imbal-
ance in the uses of preventive surgery to reduce the danger of malignancy. The
introduction of mammography led to an increase in the diagnosis of premalignant changes in the breast and to a parallel increase in the number of women who
faced difficult therapeutic dilemmas. Men may face similar dilemmas. From the
1990s on, the diffusion of PSA (prostate specific antigen) screening, especially in
the United States, led to a rise in surgical treatments for localized prostate cancer.
Men with high PSA levels are encouraged to undergo blind needle biopsies and,
if such biopsies uncover limited malignant changes, to undergo a risky prostate
surgery, in spite of the fact that in many cases localized malignant changes in the
prostate will never produce a clinical disease.[38]

Treatment of localized prostate cancer (an invasive, that is, "true" malignancy)
continues, nevertheless, to be a controversial issue. Some experts advocate more
aggressive surgical and therapeutic approaches; others stress the value of watchful waiting.[39] The treatment of ductal carcinoma in situ (DCIS) of the breast (an
abnormal proliferation of cells, limited to the milk ducts), a condition with an
unknown potential to become malignant, is less controversial. Women diagnosed
with DCIS undergo as a rule partial or complete ablation of the breast, often followed by radiotherapy or drugs such as tamoxifen. Watchful observation is rarely
presented as an acceptable therapeutic option for this condition.[40] Moreover,
women were and continue to be seen as responsible for future generations, a self-
perception that shapes their attitudes towards prophylactic elimination of breasts
and ovaries.[41] In the early twenty-first century, too, gender produces differences
in management of precancerous conditions and cancer risk, although the mechanisms that create such a difference cannot be reduced to the misogyny of the
medical profession.

Following Preventive Surgery over Time

The diagnostic category of precancer and the practice of prophylactic surgery,
this work proposes, are entities that are "good to think with" because they display
the rationality—or rather the multiple rationalities—that guided cancer diagnosis, prevention, and treatment in the twentieth century.[42] Thinking about precancer forces us to reflect what cancer is and how experts differentiate the normal
from the pathological, while study of the uses of prophylactic surgery illuminates
the ways doctors deal with diagnostic uncertainty and manage cancer risk.

The century-long history of precancer and preventive surgery interrogates in parallel patterns of stabilization and diffusion of debatable diagnostic and therapeutic practices. The identification of precancerous lesions, and treatment of such lesions through prophylactic excision of suspicious body parts, was and remains problematic. Detection and treatment of these lesions, nevertheless, played an important role in the efforts to prevent and cure malignancies in the twentieth century. In this book, I focus on two female tumors—breast and cervix—and on three Western countries—France, the United States, and the United Kingdom. Grounded in the examination of selected case studies, the book does not provide an exhaustive overview but rather a series of snapshots.[43] These snapshots unfold a story shared by all the developed nations: the one of diagnosis of precancerous lesions and the rise of preventive surgery. Along the way they also reveal national, regional, and local differences in diagnosis and management of precancerous lesions. Such differences reflect structural variables (organization of health care, health insurance, patterns of specialization, division of medical labor), but they also reflect the contingent development of medical cultures and local traditions. Both similarities and differences are important. Similarities display the existence of a major trend in Western medicine, namely, the increased role of screening, risk management, and prophylactic treatment and the consequence of this increased role: the blurring of boundaries between disease and disease risk.[44] Differences indicate that professional practices are historically and geographically situated and, therefore, open to questioning and change.

One of the elements open to such questioning is the role of schemata in the understanding of human diseases. Professional and lay understating of cancer was and continues to be shaped by the aspiration of identifying and eliminating precancerous lesions. The extraordinary viability of this idea reflects its plausibility, its ability to address well-entrenched fears, and its capacity to channel activities of multiple constituencies. It also points to risks of excessive simplification of complex phenomena. Present-time medicine, political scientist Louise Russell points out, aspires to detect pathological conditions before they produce symptoms: "A common theme runs through the articles, programs, and waiting room brochures: Catch it early, treat it early and live longer . . . That common theme, played out in its many variants, is simple, direct and misleading." The recommendations presented in publications that promote early detection, Russell explains, are pseudo-truths that, like the pseudo-elements of the physical sciences, bear a deceptively close resemblance to the real thing: "They convey the rules of the thumb developed by experts and leave out the complexities and the tradeoffs, a mixture of solid information and educated guesses, that have gone into their development."[45] A historical study displays such discarded complexities and trade-offs and can therefore provide a glimpse of the "real thing" behind powerful, plausible, and oversimplified images.

The first chapter of this book focuses on the consequences of the growing role of histological analysis—and therefore of biopsy—in cancer diagnosis. In the late nineteenth century, diagnosis of cancer was made exclusively by surgeons on the basis of gross anatomical observations. This chapter describes the gradual transformation of cancer into a "pathologist's disease," diagnosed in the laboratory. The new focus on the microscopic definition of cancer favored in turn the rise of the concept of premalignant lesion, an intermediary stage between a normal tissue and a fully malignant one.

The redefinition of cancer as a disease of cells and tissues modified diagnostic categories. At the same time, the rise of radiotherapy (the destruction of cancer cells with x-rays) and radium therapy (the destruction of cancer cells with radiation from radium) of malignant tumors in the 1910s and 1920s led to controversies about the relative efficacy of "knife versus rays." Both terms have since been replaced with radiation therapy. To compare treatments, experts elaborated a homogenous classification of stages in progress of the clinical disease cancer ("staging"). Data collected using such classification, explained in the second chapter, confirmed that small tumors that did not spread to nearby tissues and lymph nodes had the best chances of being cured. Staging and the development of cancer registries favored the promotion of early detection of malignancies, and by extension, a striving to identify and eliminate surgically the "earlier than early" precancerous lesions.

Before World War II, efforts to eliminate very early malignant lesions were focused on breast cancer. The third chapter follows the diagnosis of borderline lesions of the breast at that period and it is focused on cystic mastitis, a usually benign but painful swelling in the breasts. This condition was at once time classified as precancerous, but doctors provided widely divergent estimates of its danger. Consequently, the treatments for cystic mastitis varied from watchful observation to radical mastectomy. An intermediary solution was a "diagnostic mastectomy," the removal of a breast to examine it in the pathology laboratory, a surgery seen as qualitatively different from a true—that is, radical—mastectomy, in which the chest muscles and lymph nodes were removed as well.

Mastectomies for cystic mastitis became less frequent in the 1930s. After World War II other proliferative lesions—carcinoma in situ and atypia, or atypical cells—replaced cystic mastitis as typical precancerous lesions of the breast. The fourth chapter discusses diagnosis and treatment of in situ cancers of the cervix and the breast. The two conditions had a different fate. In situ cervical cancers were at first treated by hysterectomy, like fully invasive tumors are, but later doctors switched to conservative methods of elimination of cervical lesions. By contrast in situ tumors of the breast, especially DCIS, continued to be treated with the same methods as invasive breast cancer, and women diagnosed with this condition follow a "cancer script."

The development of the Pap smear—a test that looks for the presence of abnormal cells in vaginal secretions—made possible mass campaigns for the detection of cervical cancer. These campaigns, the fifth chapter argues, were a success story with a twist. Lobbying by cancer experts, cancer charities, and activists led to the general use of Pap smears. Experts failed, however, to achieve a consensus over the classification of proliferative lesions of the cervix and the interpretation of cervical smears. This difficulty was circumvented through the transformation of the Pap smear from a definitive diagnostic test to an indication of a need for further investigation and through a parallel development of conservative methods of elimination of all the suspicious cervical lesions.

The practical success of screening for cervical cancer was in turn an important incentive for the development of other screening campaigns, especially for breast cancer. The sixth chapter studies the rise of mammographic screening and compares it briefly with the fate of screening for other malignancies. Public debates that accompanied the introduction of mammography screening focused on dangers of radiation and on the problem of false negative mammograms. They seldom discussed other major drawbacks of this technology: large number of false positive tests, diagnosis of "nondisease" (lesions that look like invasive cancer but will not produce a clinical disease in the woman's lifetime), and a steep increase in diagnosis and in treatment of precancerous changes in tissues. Similar dilemmas appear in screening for prostate cancer and, to some extent, for colon and lung malignancies.

In the 1990s, diagnosis of cancer risk, until then mainly limited to the investigation of changes in tissues and cells, was extended to a search for mutations that increase the probability of developing cancer in the future. The seventh chapter looks briefly on links between heredity and cancer before the era of molecular biology and then examines the effects of the introduction of genetic tests for susceptibility to cancer. A comparison between the use of such tests in France, the United States, and the United Kingdom highlights the role of variables such as intellectual property rules, the price of genetic tests, and the organization of health care and professional cultures of geneticists, oncologists, and surgeons in the definition of a hereditary risk of cancer and the management of such a risk.

Genetic tests were initially seen as a first step in the development of more efficient cancer prevention and cure. However, as the eighth chapter explains, between 1995 and 2007, the main consequence of the introduction of testing for hereditary susceptibility to breast and ovarian cancer was a large increase in surgical excision of danger-laden body parts: ovaries and breasts. Both operations, especially prophylactic mastectomy, remain controversial. Nevertheless, many women diagnosed with mutations that predispose them for tumors feel that they cannot accept life at risk and are compelled to undergo such surgeries. For people diagnosed with a hereditary risk of cancer, a true alternative to preventive surgery is often not surveillance, that is, life under intensive medical gaze, but a gradual loss of interest in their risk ("noncompliance" and "denial" in the professionals' terminology).

The key role of the diagnostic category of precancer in the modern edifice of cancer prevention and treatment, the concluding chapter proposes, led to its integration in a dense network of scientific, medical, and public health practices: education campaigns and mass screening, biopsies, biochemical and genetic tests, and surveillance and preventive surgeries. The heuristic success of this diagnostic category had, however, a price—a systematic overlooking of problematic links between premalignant lesions and the clinical disease of cancer. The uncertain status of such lesions—and today also of molecular lesions—continues to be at the origin of many dilemmas faced by people who live with a permanent threat of cancer.

A note on terminology: The argument developed in this work is that the terms *premalignant lesion* (or *precancerous lesion*) and *early tumor* were nearly always indeterminate. Scientists who artificially induce tumors in laboratory animals usually can estimate how early or late these tumors are on an absolute time scale and can compare tissues before and after exposure to a tumor-inducing stimulus, such as radiation (although even tumors that appear after irradiation may be the result of an acceleration of growth of an already existing malignancy). Clinicians do not have access to similar information. It is difficult to determine if a recently diagnosed small tumor represents a newly formed cancer or a slow-growing one and to predict whether observed changes in tissues will progress to malignancy, regress, or remain stable. However, it is very hard to contest the claim that cancer can be cured if it is caught "early enough." A successful cure of a tumor is seen as a proof that the intervention was made sufficiently early; a failure to cure is evidence that the tumor was treated too late.

The faith in the efficacy of early treatment of malignant growths appeared in the early nineteenth century, along with the rise of surgery for cancer. It was consolidated through the development of new diagnostic methods such as biopsy, new treatments such as radiotherapy, and new social practices, such as the "do not delay" campaigns of cancer charities. The diffusion of the early detection paradigm was also strengthened by the conviction that beyond a certain point in a cancer's trajectory, the patient cannot escape any more a painful, protracted death. Until very recently, cancer was seen as an "all or nothing event"—a disease that is either cured or leads to an inevitable demise.[46] This image of cancer, quite different from images of other, potentially fatal pathologies such as cardiovascular diseases or diabetes, helps to explain people's willingness to undergo drastic preventive treatments. The two claims behind the "early detection and early intervention" principle are accurate. A localized small cancer is indeed easier to treat, and from some point in their trajectory on, malignant tumors can be, at best, partly controlled but not cured. These correct observations led, however, to a more problematic step: the transformation of the "precancer" hypothesis into an absolute, rigid rule that has organized thinking about cancer and preventive interventions.[47]

The practical difficulty of differentiating between a tumor that is small and localized because it is not very aggressive and one that is small and localized because it just started its growth is the origin of much of the prognostic uncertainty in oncology.[48] Keeping this in mind, it is more accurate to speak about "presumed premalignant lesion," "supposedly early tumor," "suspected precancerous changes" or "alleged early detection of cancer." Alas, systematically including qualifying adjectives is cumbersome, as is a frequent utilization of quotation marks. I elected therefore to employ the actors' vocabulary and to speak about precancer or early detection of cancer. This stylistic choice mirrors a broader reality: the rhetorical power of cancer schemata, the credibility of the diagnostic category of precancer, and the tenacity of the belief that one can cut down the risk of cancer by cutting it out.

CHAPTER ONE

Biopsy

The Redefinition of Cancer as a Pathologist's Disease

The rise of the concept of precancer and of the aspiration to physically eliminate precancerous lesions is directly linked with the definition of cancer as "pathologist's disease," that is, an ailment diagnosed in the pathology laboratory. Even people who present symptoms that strongly indicate the presence of a malignant growth are "officially" classified as cancer patients only when their diagnosis is confirmed by a pathologist. This rule, established in the early twentieth century, is still valid a century later.[1] The maintenance of pathologists' quasi-absolute control over diagnosis and monitoring of malignancies is unusual. The decades after World War II were a period of an intensive "molecularization" of biology and medicine, a process driven by the rapid expansion of biological and biomedical research and accelerated by introduction of instruments that automatically performed laboratory tests.[2] Standardized tests, often performed by machines, play an increasingly large role in the definition and follow-up of human diseases. Diagnosis of cancer continues, however, to be grounded in the very specialized realm of the pathologist. Tests that reveal abnormal levels of biological markers linked with cancerous growths (e.g., PSA for prostate cancer, C-125 for ovarian cancer) are seen mainly as indications to start a search for transformed cells or, alternatively, to refine a diagnosis of cancer, not to establish one. In 2010, too, a patient has cancer because a pathology report said so. A pathologist's verdict is indispensable in obtaining access to treatments in a national health system, reimbursement of medical expenses by health insurance, or a leave of absence from work. It is also the point at which an individual acquires a new identity as a "cancer patient"—and then, if he or she is lucky and enters a long-term remission—becomes a "cancer survivor."

Pathologists obtained control over cancer diagnosis roughly between 1910 and 1930. Before it became a pathologist's domain, cancer diagnosis was made by surgeons, and before that, by general practitioners. Until the second half of the nineteenth century, surgeons rarely operated on cancer patients. Physicians and lay persons alike believed that cancer was hereditary and incurable. Moreover, surgical operations for cancer were dangerous, and their success rate was very low. Even if the patient survived the operation, he or she usually died promptly when the disease returned.[3] The success of Fanny Burney's surgery for breast cancer in 1811 was later seen as a proof that she probably had a benign tumor of the breast. (She provided a gruesome description of her ordeal of surgery without anesthesia.)[4] The advent of anesthesia in the 1840s and then the development of aseptic techniques beginning in the 1860s made some surgeries for malignancies more acceptable. Those included hysterectomies (surgical ablation of the uterus) and oophorectomies (surgical ablation of ovaries) and dissection of tumors in other parts of the body.[5] It also made the development of radical surgery possible— large and often mutilating excisions of malignant growths.

The term *radical surgery* was proposed in 1906 by U.S. surgeon George Washington Crile, who developed a new technique of dissection of lymph nodes of the head and the neck in patients with cancers of this region and introduced in the discussion of this technique a distinction between radical and less radical surgical approaches. Only the former, he argued, could lead to a cure.[6] Crile coined a new term but not a new concept. Many surgeons of his time had already adopted the principle of extensive excision of malignant growth together with the surrounding tissues, an approach usually linked with the development of the "complete surgery" for breast cancer by Johns Hopkins surgeon William Steward Halsted.[7]

Radicalism in breast cancer surgery preceded, however, the development of Halsted's mastectomy. Halsted followed ideas developed by surgeon Charles Hewitt Moore from Middlesex Hospital, London, while Moore was inspired by German surgeons Lothar Heindenhain and Richard von Volkman. Volkman added the dissection of axillary lymph nodes to the ablation of the breast. Moore proposed in 1867 that every surgery for malignant tumors of the breast, even a very small one, should be as extended as far as technically possible and should include the ablation of axillary lymph nodes. Halsted's main innovation was to add the systematic removal of both pectoral muscles and large portions of the skin.[8] The surgeons' standard recommendation was that "too much rather than too little skin should be removed, and not infrequently skin grafting will have to be resorted to."[9] The skin necessary to cover the breast was usually taken from the thigh. Skin grafts often induce pain and discomfort and might have been fol-

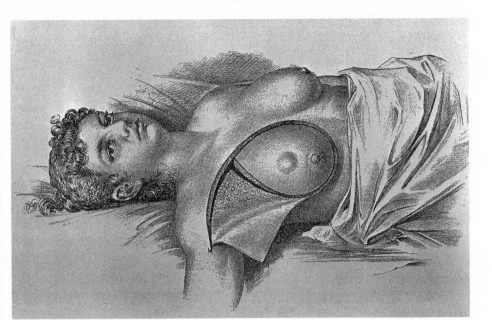

A depiction of a mastectomy from Halsted's surgical papers. Wellcome Images.

lowed by infection, especially in the preantibiotic era. However textbook and articles that describe radical mastectomy seldom mention such complications, perhaps because they were seen as unavoidable consequence of this surgical intervention, and as negligible, compared with consequences of untreated cancer.[10] Halsted's surgery became later identified with extreme forms of surgical radicalism, but in his time Halsted was seen as a conservative surgeon. He was an adept of a "physiological approach" that carefully took into account the effects of surgery on the body and put the accent on safety in the operating room.

Halsted was persuaded that the diagnosis of cancer belonged to the jurisdiction of surgeons. Thirty years later, such a diagnosis became mainly the province of pathologists. The shift to pathological diagnosis of cancer changed its nature. A diagnosis of a tumor by surgeons was made very rapidly, on the basis of their impressions in the operating room. It relied on several senses, above all sight and touch. When cutting through a tumor, a surgeon was able to feel resistance and texture, elements that helped to define a growth as malignant or benign. Decisions to perform a conservative or more extended operation were therefore grounded in evidence that could not be reproduced or controlled from the outside.

The nature of pathologists' knowledge was different. Their main source of information was a careful observation of preparations of fixed and stained slices of tissue. Pathologists occasionally attempted to reconstitute the surgeon's impressions. Accounts provided by the pathology laboratory of the London Hospital included detailed description of the gross aspect of the sample provided by the surgeons, but also of the impressions generated when cutting through this sample: smooth, gritty, elastic, resistant, grained, hard to cut, and so on.[11] Tactile sensations provided nevertheless only supportive clues. Pathologists rely nearly exclusively on sight, and their main skill is the ability to recognize specific forms and link them with diseases.[12] This ability is perfected through debates among professionals on the diagnosis of difficult cases and sustained by the circulation of slides: stained, paraffin-fixed slices of tissue and, to a lesser extent, photographs and drawings. Sharing of slides and images favored professional control over diagnosis and a collective production of knowledge.

Surgeons and pathologists made diagnoses grounded in the transmissible knowledge of the expert. The justification of their respective moral right to make decisions that may have dramatic consequences for the patient was, however, different. Surgeons were proud of their capacity to take risks and to make rapid decisions, a heroism akin to the one exercised in a battlefield. The moral right of the pathologists to make a decision that may change the patient's life was grounded in a different kind of heroism: the one that, as Loraine Daston and Peter Galison put it, "requires painstaking care and exactitude, infinite patience, unflagging perseverance, and an insatiable appetite for work."[13] Between 1910 and 1930, the latter moral attitude became increasingly perceived by medical elites as the only one that makes reliable diagnosis of a malignant tumor possible. The main area in which this change took place was the diagnosis and the treatment of breast cancer and, to a lesser degree, of cancer of the uterus.

Malignant and Benign Changes in the Breast, 1880–1910

In the late nineteenth century, cancer was redefined as a disease produced by abnormal proliferation of cells. At first, the new view of cancer did not modify medical practices.[14] From the 1880s on, experimental studies of malignant tumors in laboratory animals included detailed microscopic observations, but knowledge generated in these studies was not incorporated into a routine diagnosis of malignant growths.[15] At that time, diagnosis of cancer was made by surgeons who were persuaded that they were able to recognize malignant tumors, either when they examined the patient or during an exploratory surgery. The pathologist was mainly "the Keeper of the Dead," and his main job was to dissect cadavers.[16]

Stephan Jacyna has shown that in late nineteenth century, surgeons were familiar with cytological diagnosis of malignancies and occasionally asked for a
pathologist's opinion before undertaking an extended surgery for cancer, especially of the breast. This was, however, a rare event. In the majority of cases, the
pathologist's role—if any—was limited to analysis of tissues excised by the surgeon and the confirmation of a diagnosis of cancer.[17]

In the late nineteenth century, the term *cancerous growth* covered a wide spec-
trum of pathological changes. For example, notes made by British surgeon and
cancer specialist William Sampson Handley during his training at St. Guys
Hospital, London, in 1894, included malignant tumors in a wider category of
"lesions which fail to heal." Handley described a great variety of advanced, often
necrotic, lesions that could be treated only through surgical removal, such as tuberculous cysts, lupus of the buttock, enlarged tuberculous glands, sebaceous
cysts of the scalp, syphilitic changes of the skin, papilloma of the anus, a melan-
otic sarcoma that originated in a mole, an extended Paget's disease of the nipple,
and cysts of the scrotum. He stressed the similarities among these lesions and
the difficulties of differential diagnosis, while focusing exclusively on their gross
anatomy.[18]

The reliance on clinical signs and gross anatomy to recognize malignant
tumors and the definition of such tumors as a pathology that belongs to the
surgeon's jurisdiction, affected the nature of the disease called "cancer." In the
nineteenth and early twentieth century, women often consulted doctors only
when they suffered from painful, and sometimes necrotic, lesions of the breast.
This tendency favored the observation of slow-growing breast tumors. Very aggressive breast tumors that spread rapidly often killed the patient before she was
able to see a physician. When a person presented an extensive breast disease, a
surgical extirpation of cancerous lesions alleviated an already existing suffering.
However, this extirpation rarely produced long-term cures. Halsted initially legitimated a radical surgery for breast cancer with the wish to prevent a local spread
of a tumor. His primary goal was to save the patient from suffering induced by
the extension of a malignant growth or the agony of an additional surgery, not to
save the patient's life.[19] Other surgeons also noticed that a successful radical mastectomy (when the women recovered, while the surgeon was certain he removed
all the malignant tissue) usually failed to protect the patient from death: many
operated women succumbed shortly after their surgery to a metastatic disease.[20]

Surgeons also noticed that women diagnosed with a small, localized breast
tumor had a better chance of achieving a cancer-free survival.[21] This observation
was in agreement with a view of cancer as a disease that starts in a single site and

later spreads to other tissues and organs. The "local to general" view of breast malignancies was consolidated in the early twentieth century by the adoption of the view, initially propagated by Handley, that breast cancer spreads through the lymphatic system. Handley claimed that cancer of the breast migrates from one lymph node to another and then to adjacent tissues.[22] The lymphatic-spread hypothesis replaced an earlier "embolic theory," which stressed the role of blood circulation in the genesis of metastases. In Handley's descriptions, extended breast cancer had a quasi-anatomical continuity with the primary tumor, and the main issue was how to completely eliminate the cancer of the breast, with all its microscopic ramifications.[23] Radical surgery for breast tumors was named (especially by American authors) "the complete operation," a term that strongly hinted that all the other forms of surgery were incomplete and therefore dangerous. The adoption of radical mastectomy consolidated in turn the "local to general" view of the natural history of breast cancer. Long-term remissions were attributed to a successful extirpation of all the malignant tissue and were seen confirmation of the view that breast cancer always starts as a localized disease.[24]

The next step was to persuade women to consult their physicians without delay for suspicious symptoms.[25] One of the most enthusiastic promoters of the early detection paradigm, Johns Hopkins surgeon Joseph Colt Bloodgood, claimed that early detection would lead to cures of 90 percent of breast malignancies.[26] The principle of early detection was transposed to uterine tumors, too. Writing in 1906, French surgeon Ledoux Lebard explained that the success of treatment of early cases of breast cancer should stimulate physicians to similar efforts in the treatment of cervical malignancies. He proposed to open "examination stations for 'cancer suspects'. . . if possible directed by the most competent specialists, and endowed with the most perfect diagnostic apparatus necessary for a rapid diagnosis of cancerous lesions." [27] The main focus of surgeons remained, however, breast cancer. The "do not delay" message, spread by doctors and by cancer charities, convinced women with small and painless tumors of the breast to see a physician. According to Bloodgood, in the early twentieth century, only 10 percent of women treated for breast cancer were early cases (women with small, localized tumors and no lymph node involvement), but their number had risen to 25 percent under the influence of local and national education programs.[28] With the diffusion of the injunction to focus on early stages of malignancy and the strong encouragement of women to see a doctor as soon as they notice any suspicious changes in their breast, surgeons started to see more women with borderline breast lesions and more often faced difficulties deciding if a given lesion was malignant or benign.

Circa 1900, the majority of women who consulted a physician for breast cancer suffered from an advanced disease, sometimes with dramatic manifestations such as suppurating, painful abscesses, tumors that covered the entire chest wall (cancer en curaisse), or a breast that appeared to be "eaten by the crab." Surgery textbooks from that period enumerated the typical clinical signs of breast cancer: the puckering and dimpling of the skin, reversal of the nipple, tumors that adhere to the skin and the chest wall, immobility of the tumor, and enlarged lymph nodes.[29] In such cases, surgeons were confidently able to make the diagnosis of breast malignancy on the basis of clinical signs alone. However, they increasingly realized that their ability to diagnose breast cancer was inversely proportional to their chances to treat it successfully. Typical (that is, advanced) breast tumors were nearly always fatal, whereas while when a differential diagnostic of cancer was difficult, the patient had a chance to be cured.[30] For example, at the Johns Hopkins Hospital, 80 percent of women who were definitively diagnosed with breast cancer only during a surgery survived for five years after the radical operation. By contrast, among those diagnosed with cancer on the basis of clinical signs, only 25 percent survived for a similar length of time.[31]

The improvement of results of the treatment of breast cancer, some specialists accordingly proposed, did not come from the perfection of surgical techniques but from the improvement of diagnostic ones. "It is monumental," British surgeon Edred Corner explained in 1908, "that, as matter of fact, of the late years, every improvement in treatment has been done in the way of extending our operations, while little or nothing has been done in the way of improving our powers of diagnosis."[32] Ideally, Corner proposed, cancer should be diagnosed at a microscopic stage, before the development of a fully formed tumor. James Ewing, one of the leading U.S. cancer experts of the time, shared this view. He proposed concentrating doctors' effort on treatment of very early and, if possible, borderline cases. Such cases, Ewing argued in 1913, are the only ones that offer real chances of a surgical cure.[33] The key for therapeutic success was to treat malignant lesions very early. And, the specialists increasingly agreed, such lesions could be diagnosed only under the microscope.

Precancer: The Beginnings

In the nineteenth century, experts believed that cancer was a local manifestation of a constitutional disorder and were persuaded that a predisposition (diathesis) to develop cancer ran in families, like a predisposition to tuberculosis or insanity. When cancer was seen as a systemic disorder, many physicians believed that a surgical elimination of malignant growths would only exacerbate a person's suffering. When performed, surgery for cancer aimed mainly at the reduction of distressing symptoms. The systemic perception of cancer was challenged by the advent of cytology. Pathologists, such as Rudolf Virchow and Julius Cohenheim, defined cancer as specific changes in tissues.[34] The development of the original cancerous lesion was attributed to a persisting irritation of tissues, usually by a chemical or chemicals or by physical means. Such irritation, it was assumed, induced chronic inflammation ("tumor," that is, swelling), an abnormal proliferation of cells (hyperplasia), and finally, in some people, a malignant degeneration. The initial cellular changes were seen as a local reaction. Accordingly, such surgeons as William de Morgan and Charles Moore proposed that cancer can be cured surgically if treated early.[35]

The irritation theory of carcinogenesis partly derived from the observation of occupational cancers. The classical examples were Percival Pott's determining the incidence of carcinoma of the scrotum among chimney sweepers, Volkman and Bell's determining the high rates of cancer of the anus and the scrotum among workmen employed in distillation plants, and the observation of a high frequency of malignancy among people who worked with tar or mineral oil. Such cancers, doctors noted, often started as a simple wart or a lesion that failed to heal. If left untreated, the local lesion was transformed into a true cancer, which then led to a generalized disease.[36] The idea that cancer starts as a local irritation was then extended to all malignancies. Breast cancer was presented as an exemplary case of a transition from a "chronic tumor," an inflammatory state induced by an irritating stimulus such as the blocking of the milk ducts, to a true malignancy.[37] Carcinogenesis was seen as a very slow process. For example breast cancer was linked with the blocking of milk ducts during lactation and a consecutive accumulation of "*materia morbi*" in the breast, while the disease itself was usually observed in women well past their reproductive years.[38] The conviction that many years separate the initiating event from the development of a malignant growth led to a hope that the identification and elimination of precursor lesions can prevent cancer. The conviction that cancer always starts as a localized event had important practical consequences. Such theory—cancer schemata—included not only the logical supposition that fully developed malignancies are preceded by an earlier, intermediary stage but also the less straightforward assumptions that such an intermediary stage can be reliably identified by doctors and that its removal offers a unique opportunity for a cure.

Proliferative changes in the breast were seen as the first step in the road to malignancy. Not all such changes were equally prone to malignant degeneration.

The first aim of a differential diagnosis of proliferative changes in the breast—usually a suspicious lump—was to decide if a given lesion was dangerous at that time. An additional and equally important goal was to decide if such a lesion would become dangerous later. The differential diagnosis of breast lesions was, however, a difficult task. Surgery textbooks provided descriptions of numerous noncancerous breast lesions, such as cystadenoma, hyperplasia, hypertrophy, papillary adenoma, periductal fibroma, periductal sarcoma, fibromata, myxomata, abnormal involution, keloid tumors, and chronic inflammation. The precise differences among all these lesions were not always clear and estimates of their potential to become malignant in the future varied greatly.[39] Textbooks pointed to the indeterminacy of cytological classifications and difficulties of differential diagnosis of breast lesions, especially when dealing with small, localized tumors. As British surgeon C. B. Lockwood warned his colleagues in 1905: "You will remember when confronted with a young an ambitious tumor to assume an attitude of intelligent humility and carefully eschew diagnostic omniscience and infallibility."[40] Other experts agreed. "In no department of surgery," Boston surgeon Collins Warren explained in the same year, "has the classification of the diseases of an organ or the pathological nomenclature been more confusing than it is in the diseases of the mammary gland. . . . In this case national and even local systems have added again to the confusion."[41]

Facing a difficulty to provide an accurate diagnosis, some surgeons energetically promoted radical surgery for all the suspicious lesions of the breast, especially in women nearing or past menopause. A practitioner who usually sees breast cancer cases, William Rodman explained, needs to be taught that 80 percent of all the mammary tumors are malignant.[42] Historians of medicine like to quote the statement, made in 1903 by Bloodgood: "in regard to tumors, lynch law is by far the better procedure than 'due process.' "[43] Bloodgood liked to employ strong language, but his description as the spokesman of the most extreme branch of surgical activism may be unfair. His proposal to act promptly when facing a suspicious lesion reflected a generally held opinion. Moreover, Johns Hopkins surgeons were seen as more cautious than the majority of their peers and were criticized for their reluctance to perform radical mastectomies.[44]

George Herbert Fink used the term *precancerous* in 1903 to describe tumors that have a high probability of becoming malignant.[45] He argued that nearly all noninvasive breast tumors, especially in women over 40, belong to the latter category and should be treated by surgical removal of the breast.[46] This view was extended to other pathological conditions of the breast. Dr. Clark Stewart recommended radical mastectomy for women who had chronic inflammation of the breast, because in the great majority of the cases, he said, such inflammation leads to the development of adenocarcinoma.[47] Dr. William Jepson similarly proposed that a large number of benign growths are only temporarily benign. A growth in at least nine out of ten "involuted" breasts (those that undergo age-related degeneration) must be looked at as malignant, and the right treatment for such breasts is therefore an "entire extirpation," that is, a radical surgery.[48]

Decisions concerning patients treated for breast cancer in St Bartholomew's Hospital, London, in the early twentieth century were grounded exclusively in the surgeon's diagnostic skills. The main role of the—rare—microscopic diagnosis was to validate or invalidate the surgeon's diagnosis. Following is a typical case:

> A 36-year-old woman was admitted to St Barts in June, 1907 with a tumor in the breast. She gave birth 6 months ago, then noticed swelling in the right breast since, then a small hard tumor. She also had blood stained discharge from the nipple. Clinical examination revealed palpable lymph nodes in right and left axilla. Operation made by M. Warning: removal of the right breast and the pectoral fascia. The glands in the axilla were not removed. Note in the file: "no complete microscopic evidence that it is carcinomatous, but probably a duct carcinoma."[49]

In another case, a woman with an inflammatory condition of the breast underwent a radical mastectomy:

> A 34-year-old woman, admitted in June 1907 with a complaint of a mass in the breast noticed 4 weeks ago. The mass was slightly adherent, nipple slightly retracted, and the patient had palpable glands in the axilla. The tumor looked inflammatory. She underwent complete removal of the breast with pectoral fascia and part of the pectoral muscle, all in one piece. Some glands were also removed. Pathological examination of the excised tissue showed no signs of malignancy. Pathologist's report, "chronic inflammation of the breast, nothing in the gland." Final diagnosis, "acute mastitis."[50]

Confronted with surgeons who assumed that every suspect lesion of the breast should be treated by radical mastectomy, women had an excellent reason to hesitate to see a doctor when they discovered such a lesion. Bloodgood realized that excessive surgical activism was a major obstacle for efforts to convince women to rapidly consult a physician for suspicious changes in the breast. Accordingly he replaced his earlier "lynch" approach with the advocacy of more accurate diagno-

sis of breast lesions.[51] A more precise diagnosis will reduce the number of unnecessary radical surgeries and will lessen women's fear of seeking medical help, he
said. This in turn should lead not only to an increase in number of cures but also
to the prevention of malignant tumors. In 1913, Bloodgood emphasized the need
to diagnose precancerous lesions and proposed a new approach—a preventive
surgery for cancer: "In every location that we encounter cancer, we also meet
lesions that, histologically, are not cancer. When these lesions are radically removed, we never observe recurrence or death from cancer which could be attributed to the removed tumor. . . . These lesions, which histologically are not cancer, and which are curable up to 100 percent by radical removal, may be called
precancerous. . . . The hope for almost complete eradication of cancer rests on
the recognition and the complete eradication of the pre-cancerous lesion, whatever this may be."[52]

The key word here was "recognition." Early tumors did not produce distinct
clinical symptoms. Many surgeons were nevertheless confident in their ability to
diagnose a true breast malignancy during a surgery, especially when they related
gross anatomical finding to previous clinical observations. One of the leading
British cancer experts, Sir Harold Stiles, declared in 1908 that "a knowledge of
the histological structure of a lump in the breast is of little value for the patient
unless the surgeon can associate it with a correct life-history. With this knowledge at his command, it will be very rarely necessary for the surgeon to be supported in the operating theatre by an expert pathologist armed with a freezing
microtome." [53]

Other surgeons however noticed that in many cases observation of the tumor
during surgery was not sufficient to provide an accurate diagnosis.[54] For Sampson Handley, "The future of breast surgery rests as much with the early diagnosis of doubtful swellings by means of exploratory incision and microscopic
examination, as with improved methods for the extirpation of fully developed,
clinical carcinoma."[55] Exploratory incisions, a precondition of a microscopic diagnosis of cancer, were, however, problematic. The removal of a suspicious lump
or a part of it without a wide excision of surrounding tissues, surgeons feared,
might lead to rapid spread of malignant cells through the bloodstream, precisely
the effect they wanted to prevent through surgery.

Biopsy and the Rise of the Frozen Section

A microscopic examination of tumor cells was perceived as a reasonably safe procedure, if the suspected lesion was superficial or if it secreted a cell-containing

liquid. By contrast a breast biopsy was seen as a dangerous procedure, because of the need to cut through tissues and the delay before diagnosis and surgery. In a typical biopsy, the excised tissue is embedded in a paraffin block (hence the name "paraffin section"), cut by a microtome into thin slices, fixed and stained for several days, then examined by a pathologist.[56]A delay of several days between a biopsy (that is, excision) of a breast tumor and a mastectomy (if this tumor was found to be malignant) was seen as extremely dangerous. A woman who has a small, curable tumor and who undergoes such a "two stage procedure," Bloodgood affirmed in 1913, will be almost surely condemned to death.[57] This was a circular argument. Only a careful microscopic diagnosis could spare women unnecessary radical mastectomies, but such a diagnosis was viewed as too dangerous if not followed immediately by a radical surgery. The answer to this dilemma was the adoption of a technique that made a very rapid examination of suspicious tissues possible: the frozen section. In this method, tissue is frozen and cut by a chilled microtome (hence the name "frozen section") then fixed in formaldehyde and rapidly stained. This process only takes a few minutes and can be done while the patient is on the operating table.[58] If malignancy were to be found, the surgeon would change his instruments, redrape the patient, and proceed immediately to radical mastectomy.

The frozen section technique was developed in the late nineteenth century. Stiles's allusion, in 1908, to the presence of a microscopist with his microtome in the operating room, indicates that this approach was employed by some surgeons. In the early twentieth century, it was, however, a rare event because frozen section was seen as a questionable technique.[59] During a heated controversy on this topic in New York in 1917, adversaries of frozen section argued that diagnosis made on the basis of a frozen section was not sufficiently reliable. Many tumors are mixed (are composed of malignant and nonmalignant parts), and a rapid examination of a single section of the tumor may fail to reveal malignancy. Moreover, biopsy during surgery greatly increased the danger of dissemination of malignancies. Advocates of the new technique in the United States, among them James Ewing, affirmed in contrast that when carefully executed, this method was an invaluable aid for diagnosis. "Would anyone," Ewing rhetorically asked, "like to have his tongue cut off for a small indurated ulcer without knowing positively that it was cancer?"[60]

In spite of early opposition, the frozen section became gradually integrated into routine surgical diagnosis of breast cancer in the United States.[61] In the 1920s, an increasing proportion of patients (at least in the big cities) consulted physicians for tumors that could not be diagnosed with certainty without a microscopic examination.[62] Summing up the Johns Hopkins experience, Blood-good stressed the dramatic effects of education of the public on the kind of tumors seen in the clinics: "As more and more women are correctly informed, and there is less delay in seeking advice after a warning symptom, the number of patients in the benign group has increased rapidly. Records before the writer show an increase from a single case in 1897, to almost 100 in 1930. The clinical group in which operation has been decided against, and in which malignancy can be excluded with practically no risk, has in thirty three years increased from less than one to more than seventy percent."[63]

In the 1920s, even doctors who worked in small hospitals and clinics were occasionally confronted with doubtful or borderline tumors. The shift in the population of people seeking surgery for tumors increased the need for arrangements for a frozen section in all the operating rooms. It also increased the demand for pathologists trained in this technique and favored the development of a new subspecialty: surgical pathology.[64] The generalization of frozen section favored close interactions between surgeons and pathologists. Surgeons' initial resistance to microscopic diagnosis of cancer reflected, among other things, a fear of loss of an essential skill, namely the ability to differentiate benign and malignant growths, and the transfer of this skill to distant, anonymous experts. Early critiques of the "biopsy dogma" protested against sending biopsy samples to central pathology laboratories. They argued that pathologists in such a laboratory had no clue how the sample was obtained and could not judge if the diagnosis corresponded to clinical data. The development of frozen section favored direct contacts between surgeons and pathologists and a better coordination between the laboratory and the clinics.[65] With the development of this technique, the pathologist became a direct collaborator of the surgeon and worked under the surgeon's orders in the operating room. This arrangement benefited pathologists, too. Their presence during surgeries allowed them to take a part in the surgeons' activities and to view themselves as experts involved in the care of living patients, no longer as only guardians of dead flesh.

Bloodgood became convinced that frozen section should not be reserved exclusively for the diagnosis of borderline breast tumors. Every operation for breast cancer, he proposed, should include a rapid microscopic examination of excised tissues. His conversion to the principle of cytological diagnosis of cancer reflected his growing conviction that even skilled and highly experienced surgeons like himself might be unable to judge during a surgical operation whether a given tumor was benign or malignant. In 1915, Bloodgood operated on a woman for a breast tumor that was clinically evaluated as benign because it was present in the breast for ten years. However, during the surgery the tumor showed every sign of malignancy: "When I bisected this tumor, I was surprised to find that it had the appearance of cancer. It felt and cut like cancer; it cupped on section; there were the fine dots and lines so characteristic of a carcinoma of the breast." The patient underwent a radical mastectomy, but microscopic examination of this tumor did not reveal malignancy. This was, Bloodgood explained, a particularly unsettling experience, as was an opposite case: a tumor that macroscopically looked perfectly benign but was found to be malignant in a paraffin section. Bloodgood's conclusion was that only pathologists can provide truly reliable knowledge about the nature of a breast tumor.[66] This conclusion can be read as confirmation of the reversal of hierarchy of proof. In the early twentieth century, pathologist's diagnosis was seen mainly as a confirmation of surgeon's observations. Thirty years later, surgeon's impressions were seen as secondary to final verdict provided by observation of stained slice of tissue under the microscope.

In the late 1920s, frozen section became a "state of the art" technique in the treatment of breast tumors in the United States. Frozen and fixed sections were seen as complementary techniques. Frozen sections made a rapid diagnosis and an appropriate intervention possible. Fixed sections were then systematically used to confirm and refine the initial diagnosis. The latter technique favored exchanges among experts, the establishment of libraries of reference slides, and homogenization of microscopic diagnoses of cancer. The status of frozen section as an indispensable diagnostic tool was made official by guidelines issued in 1930 by the committee for the treatment of malignant diseases of the American College of Surgeons, which stated that, "the diagnosis of cancer in its early stages is extremely difficult and it may be impossible without an exploratory operation. In order for the patient's possibility of cure to not be jeopardized, such exploratory operations should be conducted only under such conditions that the appropriate treatment, whether by surgery or by radiation, may be carried immediately when the diagnosis is established by the pathologist by the means of frozen section."[67]

Biopsy and Frozen Section at the New York Hospital, 1914–39

Analysis of records of patients treated for cancer at the New York Hospital from 1914 to 1939 illustrates the penetration of frozen section into routine cancer surgery. In 1914, few patients were examined during surgery; but in some cases a frozen section made a difference.

M.A., a 47-year-old house worker, noticed in May 1914 a lump in the breast. It increased rapidly in size and was painful [case no. 3]. She came to the hospital in June, less than a month after the appearance of the symptoms. Clinical examination did not reveal any of the classical signs of advanced breast cancer such as attachment of the growth to the skin, retraction of the nipple or enlarged lymph nodes in the axilla. The surgeon decided to start with a simple amputation of the breast. The growth was classified as benign—fibroma or fibro-adenoma.—on the basis of gross anatomy. It was sent nevertheless for a frozen section which revealed malignancy. The patient underwent therefore a radical mastectomy. The pathology report states that several cross sections showed the typical appearance of fibro-adenoma, infiltrated in places by more or less numerous cancer cells, "a typical case of carcinoma that originated with an adenofibroma." The pathologist adds that, "this is an instance of a malignant growth of which the primary benign growth dominated the picture to such an extent that an error in gross diagnosis occurred. The case illustrates the danger of grounding a diagnosis on analysis of a resected portion of a tumor. If the first frozen section had been only a few millimeters shorter, the case would have passed as benign fibro-adenoma."[68]

Frozen section was also used during surgeries for other tumors, even in cases when the diagnosis seemed relatively straightforward:

A 44-year-old male, painter, was admitted May 11, 1920, with complaints, of constipation and pain [case no. 271]. 2 weeks ago his doctor found tumor in rectal examination. Considered operable. Roentgenological report [before the surgery] revealed irregularity in proximal sigmoid. Pathology report: frozen section presents the features of adenocarcinoma of the rectum. This diagnosis was confirmed by fixed specimen that show extensive invasion of the rectum wall.[69]

In the late 1920s, frozen section became the standard procedure in breast surgeries performed in the New York Hospital. Between 1914 and 1918, doctors usually felt obliged to justify the use of this technique. In the late 1920s they felt compelled to justify the—relatively rare—absence of frozen section, by referring to the obviously malignant or obviously benign gross aspect of the tumor. Nevertheless, the results of frozen section were not always reliable. Sometimes a paraffin section—seen as more trustworthy—provided a different verdict. For example, a 43-year-old woman came to the hospital in June 1928 complaining about a swollen and painful breast. A frozen section performed during the surgery was interpreted as showing atypical cells. Her surgeon proceeded with a radical mastectomy. The diagnosis was not confirmed by paraffin section: the pathologist's verdict was "mastitis" (inflammation of the breast).[70] In another case, the patient was luckier. A 46-year-old housewife was diagnosed during her surgery with suspicious proliferative changes of the breast. She was spared a radical operation and underwent a partial mastectomy. Her paraffin section did not reveal malignancy.[71]

The development of frozen section meant that the pathologist—in New York Hospital, Dr. Esler—was present in the operation room. If the tumor could be shelled out easily and the tissue around looked healthy, the sample submitted to frozen section was the lump only. If this was not the case, the surgeon either excised a portion of the breast, or, in many cases, the whole breast:

> A 52-year-old woman was admitted to New York Hospital in July 1931. She had noticed small lump in the breast, two weeks ago, while bathing [case no. 125]. Immediately consulted a physician, who advised her to see a surgeon. Clinical examination revealed an ill-defined small mass. Tentative diagnosis was carcinoma. Frozen section was made during the surgery. The pathology report states: "the first specimen received in the operating room consists of a rather small female breast, $11 \times 9 \times 2$ cm in size, there is one hard area in the upper quadrant of the breast about 1.5 cm in diameter. Immediate frozen section shows carcinoma in large amounts, chiefly of tubular and small accinar arrangements, There is marked fibrosis and round cell infiltration. Report made in operating room by Dr. Elser. Decision to proceed to radical mastectomy, that is, ablation of pectoral muscles and axillary nodes." Supplementary pathology record, written five days after surgery following the examination of a paraffin section, confirmed the diagnosis of carcinoma. No cancer was found in lymph nodes selected for their hardness in the axilla.[72]

In another typical case, a woman complained about a breast lump. During surgery this lump was found benign, but her doctor detected another smaller lump, diagnosed as malignant during the surgery. The patient then underwent a radical mastectomy:

> A 32-year-old woman was admitted to New York Hospital in September 1931 [case no. 128]. She had a lump in her left breast, present for one year and a half.

The lump increased in size 6 months ago. She had consulted three doctors and a quack who gave her "serum" injections, but the tumor continued to increase in size. Clinical examination, characteristic signs of carcinoma. Two masses felt, one large and one much smaller, freely mobile, especially the small mass. Pathology report from the frozen section: two excised tumors—large excision, with margins. One, a cyst 2.5 cm diameter, which has been cut open, contains a papillary, cauliflower like mass, easily broken. A smaller specimen, a chunk of tissue containing 1 × 1 × 1.5 cm nodule, came from region close to axilla. Frozen section of the papillary tissue contains closely packed epithelial cells. Invasion of the base is not certain in this preparation(s). The smaller node contains epithelial cells stretching to the stroma. It was estimated invasive. Diagnosis was, "intracystic papilloma and carcinoma of the breast." Paraffin section confirmed this diagnosis.[73]

Biopsy and Frozen Section at the Curie Foundation, Paris

Medical cultures vary as least as much as national cultures do. One can argue that it is easier to homogenize a medical subculture than the behavior of all the citizens of a given country. It is difficult to define what a typical "French" or "American" cultural behavior is, if such a thing exists at all. By contrast, it is easier to assume that a group of professionals who underwent a similar training will react in a comparable way. In France, the existence of standardized qualifying exams for all the doctors (*internat*) is a powerful element of homogenization of knowledge and practices. In the United States and in the United Kingdom, professional associations, board examinations, and rules of good clinical practice play a similar role.[74] Moreover, surgery, a practical skill acquired through master-apprentice relationship, may be particularly susceptible to be affected by local and national variables. French surgeons, unlike their U.S. colleagues, did not perceive a two-stage operation for breast cancer as a very dangerous procedure. Consequently, they often felt free to excise a suspicious lump, to send it to the pathology laboratory, and, if it was found malignant, to perform a more extensive operation a few days or a few weeks later.[75] They were therefore less interested in adopting the frozen section, a technique they perceived as a less reliable diagnostic tool than the paraffin section. One should add that in the interwar era, French surgeons were less submitted to pressure to adopt uniform rules of good surgical practice than their U.S. colleagues were expected to follow rules of good clinical practices issued by American College of Surgeons. The absence of regulatory bodies probably contributed to an important variability of local practices, reflected in articles published on this topic in French medical journals in the interwar era. At that time, some French doctors proposed more conservative treatment of small localized malignancies, while others advocated radical surgery. Advocates of the radical approach viewed the methods employed their more conservative colleagues as bordering on criminal neglect and accused them of favoring such approaches to attract patients unwilling to undergo a mutilating operation.[76]

The surgery books of the Curie Foundation for 1919–39, indicate that frozen section was rarely employed in this institution, even in the late 1930s. The Curie Foundation was a clinical service attached to the Radium Institute, headed by Marie Curie. Founded in 1919, it was among the first institutions in France to specialize in cancer therapy.[77] The Foundation's activity was focused on radium therapy, and the volume of surgeries performed at that institution was relatively low. It is possible that French surgeons who worked in specialized surgical wards had different practices. The Foundation's doctors, however, were keen to introduce innovative treatments of cancer and were also interested in cytological investigations. Claudius Regaud, the founder and the first director of the Curie Foundation, studied histological preparations of tumors, as did his assistant and successor Antoine Lacassagne, while the institute's chief pathologist, Georges Gricouroff, had surgical training and occasionally participated in surgical operations. Gricouroff also took an active part in the Foundation's research activities. The local conditions could have favored the integration of frozen section into surgical routines. The fact that this did not happen may reflect the experts' conviction that such emergency diagnosis was not very useful. When in doubt, they excised the suspected lesion and sent it to the pathology laboratory before undertaking further therapeutic decisions.

In the majority of cases, the Foundation's surgeons were confident in their ability to make decisions during the operation on the basis of gross anatomy findings alone. They conducted the surgery first and then sent the excised tissue to a pathology laboratory.[78]

Usually the Foundation's surgeons believed that observations made during a surgery could rectify misleading clinical impressions. A typical case follows:

A woman [surgery notebooks, case no. 861], was first seen in July 1932. She had a breast tumor that at first seemed benign. During the surgery it became clear that the small tumor for which the operation was done indeed looked benign, but the same breast contained another tumor, adherent to the skin. Her doctors decided therefore to proceed with a radical mastectomy with ablation of the pectoral muscles and axillary ganglions.[79]

Occasionally gross appearance of the tumor during a surgery did not dispel the surgeons' doubts, but in the 1920s they did not perform frozen section to clarify diagnosis:

A young woman [surgery notebooks, case no. 146] was operated on in June 1925 had a diffuse granulated breast tumor, looking like fibroadenoma, but with fuzzy boundaries and without lymph node involvement. Because of a difficult diagnosis and the patient's age, we decided to perform a mastectomy limited to the suspicious zone.[80]

In a different case, decisions were influenced (but not modified) by information provided by the evolution of the biopsy scar. Here a biopsy (surgical excision of the tumor alone) became a diagnostic tool not only because it made a cytological analysis (paraffin section) possible but also because it became a test for the patient's physiological reactions:

A 53[-year-]old woman [surgery notebooks, case no. 153] was first seen in March 1925, had an ulcerated and bleeding nipple and an enlarged lymph node in the axilla (probably a Paget's disease of the nipple). First biopsy revealed a benign tumor, but it was nevertheless decided to proceed with a mastectomy with ablation of axillary lymph nodes. Nevertheless, just before the surgery her doctors were stricken by the fact that the biopsy scar healed well, the nipple was less inflamed and the size of the lymph node diminished. After hesitation, they decided to proceed with the scheduled surgery, because of patient's age.[81]

Frozen section is not mentioned at all in the 1920s and is explicitly mentioned only in three descriptions of breast surgeries from the 1930s. Two of these surgeries were in women:

Case no. 743 of November 1930. A mobile tumor of the breast. The tumor was eliminated through a partial mastectomy that includes the nipple. The tumor looked benign, and a frozen section performed by Dr. Gricouroff confirmed diagnosis of fibro-adenoma.

Case no. 1074, of January 1936. A small breast tumor which nevertheless looked suspicious because it adhered to the skin. Frozen section, made during the surgery by Dr. Gricouroff confirmed malignancy. Lymph nodes, excised during radical mastectomy seemed suspicious too.[82]

The third was a surgery for a breast tumor in a man:

A male patient [no. 349 in the breast radiotherapy series] was first seen in May 1939 with suspicious tumor of the breast. His doctors confirmed the diagnosis during the surgery by a frozen section, then proceeded to a radical ablation of the breast, underlying muscles and axillary lymph nodes, and completed the treatment with radiotherapy.[83]

In the interwar era Curie Foundation doctors seemed to believe that in the case of breast cancer a cytological diagnosis was not an obligatory precondition for therapeutic decisions.[84] The diagnosis of cervical tumors differed. The Foundation was one of the main sites of development of radiumtherapy and radiotherapy for this malignancy. Radiation therapy of this type of tumor—locally called "Curie-therapy"—was directly linked with Pierre and Marie Curie's work and was seen as one of the main achievements of the new institution. Claudius Regaud and Antoine Lacassagne were proud of the high scientific standards of evaluation of therapy results of cervical tumors at the Foundation. A precise cytological diagnosis was seen as indispensable for maintaining such high standards. Among the 678 women treated for cervical cancer at the Curie Foundation between 1919 and 1935, only in fifteen cases (all between 1919 and 1922) did doctors initiate radiumtherapy without a previous cytological diagnosis, usually because the attempt to secure tissue for a biopsy failed.[85] Therapeutic success in such cases did not count as cures in the Foundation's statistics. By contrast, patients diagnosed with borderline or undetermined cervical lesion and whose clinical symptoms disappeared following a radiumtherapy usually were viewed as successfully cured because the Foundation's doctors classified these cases as an "early cancer."[86] In a typical case:

A 49-year-old woman, with symptoms of irregular bleeding for four months [case no. 366 in the cervical cancer notebooks] was seen at the Foundation's clinics in July 1923. Two biopsies did not yield positive results: one was negative, one presented "doubtful" cells, but no definitive signs of malignancy. A tentative classification was "stage I cervical tumor" She was treated with radiumtherapy, then with hysterectomy. No cancer was found in the uterus, but this result can be attributed either to absence of malignancy, or, alternatively, to the fact that all tumor cells were killed [i.e., "sterilized"] by radiation. She was alive and well thirteen years later.[87]

From 1925 on, all the cases described in the "cervical cancer" notebooks of the Curie Foundation were histologically confirmed malignancies.[88]

British doctors were more suspicious than their French colleagues were of two-stage breast surgeries. An official memorandum of the British Ministry of Health from September 1926 explained that such operations increased the danger of the dissemination of cancer. The same memorandum presented frozen section as insufficiently precise and therefore a potentially misleading technique. The safest diagnostic method, the memorandum's authors stated, is a careful examination of the tumor during the surgery. [89] However, some of the files of British hospitals of that period studied by statistician Janet Lane-Claypon mention results of a frozen section for breast tumors, indicating that this technique was occasionally employed to facilitate surgeons' decisions.[90]

In the 1930s, the pathologist's verdict became an obligatory condition of diagnosis of a breast malignancy. Such verdicts, especially in the United States, were increasingly provided by a frozen section performed during a breast surgery. Bloodgood revoked in the 1930s his earlier warnings about the two stage procedure. When the surgeon and the pathologist are in doubt, he proposed, the only reasonable solution is "to remove the tumor only, and to submit the sections to a number of pathologists of larger experience."[91] The danger of such a procedure, he explained, is much smaller than it was thought, especially when the biopsy is combined with an irradiation of the axilla and the wound: "Halsted's rule, 'when in doubt, perform the complete operation for cancer of the breast,' no longer holds true. In the case of doubtful tumors doctors should submit slides to a number of the best microscopic diagnosticians and wait for their verdict . . . this statement is absolutely the reverse of what I have advocated in previous publications, but it is forced upon me by facts, just as previous statements were."[92]

The clinical diagnosis of malignant tumors continued to be grounded in observation of numerous variables, but the "best microscopic diagnosticians"— surgical pathologists—became the only group of experts entitled to pronounce a definitive diagnosis of cancerous and precancerous lesions.

CHAPTER TWO

Classifications

Diffusion of Biopsies in Determining the Presence of Cancer

As discussed in the previous chapter, the first element that shaped the concept of precancer was the generalization of cytological diagnosis of malignancy in the early decades of the twentieth century. The second, and equally important element, was the collection of epidemiological data on malignancies, coupled with attempts to correlate diagnoses and outcomes. Data that were collected seemed to lend credence to the claim that treatment of early (that is small and localized) tumors was much more efficient than treatment of late tumors (larger and more extended ones). Extrapolating from this, these data favored the effort to detect and eliminate the "earlier than early" premalignant lesions. These two developments—the rise of cytological diagnoses of cancer and collection of data on outcomes of therapies—were connected through statistical investigations and the development of cancer registries. To compare results of treatment and produce statistical evidence, doctors needed not only to accumulate data but also to ascertain that they were comparing similar cases. They strived therefore to make cancer diagnoses more uniform.[1]

In the 1920s and 1930s, pathologists acquired a greater familiarity with a wide range of breast lesions and improved the classification and the codification of such lesions.[2] A homogenization of histological diagnoses, pathologists and surgeons hoped, would favor quantitative and comparative studies of the distant fate of premalignant or borderline breast lesions.[3] The goal to make the classifications of tumors more uniform was, however, hampered by the great morphological and clinical variability of these lesions. The classification of subsets of malignant transformations of the breast, French surgeon Pierre Masson maintained, is to some extent fictional, because it is grounded in a very partial knowledge. Pathologists can dedicate only a limited amount of time to the examination of excised tumors or amputated breasts. They study, therefore, a small number of sections from each sample. According to Masson, this technique may produce biased results: "Analysis of larger sections of the breast shows that breast malignancies are, as a rule, polymorphic. Fundamental, glandiform, atypical and metaplasic forms can be found in the same breast, together with numerous intermediate forms . . . The names that we give to these various forms may be useful for classification, but one should beware of perceiving them as truly distinct entities."[4]

Worse, experts had found that it was difficult to find stable correlations between cytological analysis of breast lesions and clinical data. As James Ewing put it: "The anatomical types of the disease [breast cancer] are so numerous, the variations in clinical course so wide, the paths of dissemination so diverse, the difficulty of determining the actual conditions so complex . . . as to render impossible in the majority of cases a reasonably accurate adjustment of means to ends."[5]

The complexity of differential diagnosis of breast lesions contrasted with the relative simplicity of clinical decisions: radical mastectomy, simple mastectomy (amputation of the breast alone, without underlying muscles), or the excision of the tumor alone, with more or less wide margins. The ultimate responsibility for therapeutic decisions increasingly belonged to the pathologist and often was the result of rapid examination of tissues excised during a surgery. However, occasionally, such an examination failed to provide a definitive answer. In such cases, some surgeons would perform a radical surgery to limit the danger of spread of malignancy, but others, including some of those who usually objected to two-stage operations, would elect to remove the tumor only and to wait for the results of a paraffin section. Results of such unplanned two-stage procedures indicated that fears about this procedure were exaggerated. Janet Lane-Claypon's 1928 study, discussed in detail below, of results of breast cancer surgeries had shown that people with small, localized tumors who underwent a two-stage surgery not only did not fare worse than those who underwent a one-stage operation, but they actually had a slightly better five-year survival rate. Lane-Claypon attributed this rather unexpected result to the supposition that patients who underwent a two-stage procedure often had a very early cancer, especially difficult to recognize in a frozen section.[6] Lane-Claypon's study illustrates a gradual integration of breast biopsy into surgical practice. It also indicates the growing importance of the collection of statistical and epidemiological data about outcomes of treatment of cancer and of the standardization of cytological diagnoses of malignant growths.

Cytological Classifications of Tumors: Tracing Origins

In the early twentieth century, surgeons who treated cancer became persuaded that it was easier to cure beginning tumors than more advanced ones. But how accurate was this supposition? And how does one separate beginning tumors from more advanced malignancies? To demonstrate that treatment of an early stage of a malignant tumor was more effective than the treatment of a later stage of an identical tumor, doctors needed to agree about the meaning of the terms "early stage" and "identical tumor." Similarly, if physicians wanted to compare two competing cancer treatments, it was important to ascertain that these treatments were administrated to people who were at an identical stage of the same malignancy. Accordingly, experts developed two classifications of tumors: cytological classifications that defined which kind of cancer the patient had, and clinical classifications that defined how advanced this cancer was. Cytological classifications, the domain of the surgical pathologist, were rooted in the supposition that malignant cells maintain many of the traits of tissues from which they originated. Clinical classifications of malignancies ("staging"), the domain of the clinician and the surgeon, were grounded in the assumption that cancer progresses gradually from a localized to a generalized disease.

A cytological classification of tumors was first proposed in the 1870s by German pathologist Julius Cohenheim.[7] All subsequent classifications of tumors paid attention to the type of tissue that gave rise to the tumor (epithelium, muscle or bone, glandular) and the organ in which the tumor was developing (skin, stomach, kidney, uterus). Tumors were usually divided into four major groups: epithelial tumors (carcinoma, epithelioma), mesenchymal tumors (sarcoma, endothelioma), germ cell tumors (seminona, teratoma), and tumors originating in highly differentiated tissues, such as nervous or glandular tissue. Cytological classification put benign and malignant tumors derived from the same tissue in a single classificatory group. Cytological classifications of cancer in the first (1911) version of the *Bellevue Hospital Nomenclature of Diseases and Conditions* divided tumors into four broad categories: "benign," "malignant," "mixed benign," and "mixed malignant."[8] Each group of tumors (bone, nervous tissue, connective tissue, skin) was included all the four categories.[9] The 1929 revision of the Bellevue classification maintained a similar principle. It attributed a single number (30) to all tumors and a second number according to the tumor's tissue of origin. Tumors in each group were then qualified verbally according to their level of malignancy.[10]

In the 1910s and 1920s, the majority of cancer experts believed that malignant tumors usually derived from benign growths. French cancer expert Goustave

Roussy was among the rare specialists who questioned this quasi-automatic supposition. His 1929 textbook of oncology adopted the general principle of classification of benign and malignant tumors according to tissues in which they
develop.[11] Roussy rejected, however, the idea, that such a classification is a statement on etiology of malignant growths. In the majority of the cases, the presence
of a benign tumor such as papilloma of the bladder or fibromyoma of the uterus
does not seem to increase the chances of development of a malignant growth.
Malignant tumors can occasionally develop in scar tissue, and a stimulus, such as
irritation, can sometimes transform a benign growth into a malignant one, but
such an evolution was exceptional. Usually malignant and benign tumors were
distinct, unrelated phenomena.[12] The opposite view, namely that malignant tumors always develop from benign ones, was frequently grounded in an observation of an invasive lesion in the immediate proximity of a noninvasive one. In
such cases, specialists assumed that the malignant tumor evolved from noninvasive proliferative changes. Such a conclusion, Roussy argued, was unproven and
may be erroneous. When one finds benign and malignant tumors in close vicinity, "we have no proof whatsoever that the benign neoplastic forms developed
earlier and not later than the malignant ones . . . One should also keep in mind,
that the so called pre-cancerous states do not always lead to cancer and that true
cancer can develop in a healthy tissue, sometimes very rapidly."[13]

To reduce the incidence of cancers, people should avoid conditions that favor
malignant transformation of normal tissues, such as mechanical, physical and
chemical irritation, in Roussy's view.[14] In parallel, Roussy stressed the importance of an early diagnosis of invasive cancers, because "cancer is curable if
treated in time" (le cancer est guérissable si traité à temps).[15] Terms employed by
Roussy had more than one meaning. "Curable" does not indicate whether all or
only some cancers can be cured, while "à temps" may be translated "while it is
time" or "at the right time," a circular claim, because only a cure can prove that
the time was indeed right. This ambiguity notwithstanding, Roussy's statement
reflected the shared conviction of cancer experts that a rapid detection of a malignancy greatly improved the patient's chance of recovery. Initially, this conviction was mainly based on anecdotal evidence. In 1929, when Roussy wrote his oncology textbook, it was also grounded in precise statistical data.

Janet Lane-Claypon on Correlations between the Tumor's Stage and Cure

The conviction that early detection of cancer promotes cures was contradicted by
a parallel observation that many cancer patients who underwent successful rad-

ical surgery for small, localized growths died from distant metastases.[16] James Ewing's pessimism about results of surgical treatment of cancer was grounded in his familiarity with such cases. So was the description of cancer, made in 1923 by Robert Le Bret, the general secretary of the main French cancer charity, Ligue Française Contre le Cancer, who called the disease "a frightening mystery that from remote times remained as dark as ever." [17] Demonstration of the efficacy of early treatment of malignancies was needed to dispel therapeutic pessimism. Such demonstration was provided by statistical studies conducted in the 1920s in the United Kingdom by Janet Lane-Claypon.

Lane-Claypon had a double training, in medicine and physiology. In the 1910s she became interested in epidemiology. During research on infant nutrition, she developed a new way to conduct epidemiological investigations: cohort studies.[18] In 1923, British Minister of Health Neville Chamberlain set up a committee to look into causation, prevalence, and treatment of cancer. The committee hired Lane-Claypon to gather information on this subject. Her surveys, conducted with great methodological care, were the first systematic investigation of their kind.[19] They became influential in the United Kingdom and elsewhere. Lane-Claypon was a prominent member of the statistical committee of the Cancer Commission of the League of Nations, and her findings were reproduced in the League's publications and in medical journals in numerous countries.

Lane-Claypon's first study of breast cancer was a systematic collection of data from medical literature (in several languages) about the length of survival of women who underwent radical mastectomy. She compiled data about the fate of more than seven thousand women who were diagnosed with breast cancer and whose diagnosis was confirmed by a cytological analysis. In absence of homogenous criteria of clinical evaluation of malignant tumors, comparison of data collected in medical journals was an arduous task. Lane-Claypon decided therefore to create such criteria, probably the first attempt at "staging" malignancies. She excluded from her study inoperable cases (women with distant metastases or a locally advanced tumor) and divided the operable ones into three categories: stage I growth (a small nonadherent tumor without palpable lymph node), stage II growth (an adherent tumor with palpable glands in the axilla), and stage III growth (a tumor adherent to skin and muscles, often with involvement of supraclavicle lymph nodes in addition to the axillary ones).[20]

Lane Claypon found that 43 percent of the patients in her sample survived three years after a radical mastectomy. The length of the survival varied however greatly according to the stage of disease. Sixty-five to 80 percent among women diagnosed with stage I cancer were still alive three years after the operation.

However, only 30 percent of those diagnosed with stage II cancer and 8 to 9 percent of those with more advanced tumors were still alive. Lane-Claypon was aware that her conclusions were based on analysis of highly heterogeneous data. Criteria used to diagnose breast cancer varied in different hospitals, as did surgical techniques. Nevertheless, she affirmed that the aggregated data pointed to a clear-cut trend. When the disease had already spread to lymph nodes (as was the case for the great majority of patients operated on at that time), radical mastectomy usually extended life by two or three years at most. By contrast, when the malignant tumor remained confined to the breast, mastectomy could lead to long-term survival.[21] Lane-Claypon's analysis faithfully mirrored descriptions in the analyzed medical texts. Accordingly she divided breast tumors into localized and extended, rather than early and late ones. Her results were, however, immediately translated into the "do not delay" axiom that shaped professional thinking about breast cancer from the early twentieth century on.[22] The chairman of the committee on cancer of the League of Nations, Sir George Newman, explained that "in all countries the proportion of women who present themselves at a sufficiently early stage of the disease to give a good prospect of cure is much too small. Without doubt many factors combine to produce this lamentable delay, but it is probable that popular ignorance is not the least important."[23]

In a subsequent study, Lane-Claypon analyzed hospital files to assess the results of radical surgery for breast cancer in general hospitals in England and Wales.[24] In this study she refined the definition of lymph node involvement, by adding the requirement that such involvement (and not only the presence of a cancerous lump in the breast) had to be confirmed by a cytological diagnosis. Stage I of breast cancer was accordingly defined as an absence of histologically detected lymph node involvement, stage II as the presence of histologically confirmed cancer in axillary lymph nodes, and stage III as histologically confirmed lymph node involvement coupled with an extensive local or locoregional spread of the tumor.[25] The analysis of hospital files confirmed the conclusions of her bibliographic study. When a woman was diagnosed with a breast tumor that had not spread to lymph nodes, a radical surgery often led to long-term survival: Nearly 80 percent of women diagnosed with stage I breast cancer were alive three years after their mastectomy, 71.3 percent were alive five years later, and 62.5 percent ten years following their operation. However, once cancer cells were found in lymph nodes, radical mastectomy was not a very efficient treatment: Thirty-eight percent of women diagnosed with stage II breast cancer survived for three years, 22.6 percent for five years, and 11.5 percent for ten years. In this series, women diagnosed with stage III cancer had similar survival rates to those diagnosed with stage II malignancy: A little more than 33 percent were alive three years after mastectomy, 20.5 percent after five years, and 11.4 percent after ten years. The decisive element seemed to be the presence or the absence of cancer cells in lymph nodes, not the size of the tumor.[26]

The study of hospital files also includes data on the fate of "untreated patients"—women who were diagnosed with breast cancer but did not undergo breast surgery. These women fared somewhat worse than those treated for stage II and III breast cancer, especially when one compares survival rate for ten years. Of untreated breast cancer patients, 34.4 percent were alive three years after their diagnosis, 16.1 percent five years later, and 4.9 percent ten years later. However, it is reasonable to assume that the group of untreated patients was composed mainly of women classified as inoperable, that is, those who suffered from more advanced tumors than women in the operable group (although the untreated group might have also included women who refused mastectomy). In an introduction to Lane-Claypon's new report, Sir George Newman reiterated his interpretation of localized cancer as an early one: "the all important factor in success is that the treatment should be applied in the earliest possible stage of the disease, before it has spread beyond the confinement of the breast."[27] The French Ligue Contre le Cancer similarly employed Lane-Claypon's data to stress the importance of an early diagnosis and to bring to the foreground the "do not delay" principle.[28]

Breast cancer rapidly became a model malignancy of the crucial role of early detection. The case of cervical cancer was more complicated. Lane-Claypon's survey of literature on cancer of the cervix failed to demonstrate clear-cut correlations between the disease's stage and therapeutic success. The main reason for this failure was probably technical. Cervical cancer was recognized by the presence of symptoms such as bleeding and pain. When such symptoms appeared the tumor had usually already spread, at least locally. In the interwar era, the principal difficulty in cervical cancer treatment was not how to make an accurate diagnosis (symptomatic women usually harbored a well-defined tumor, easily recognized in a cervical biopsy) but how to detect this malignancy at a stage at which a medical intervention was still possible. Accordingly, the main dividing line was not between localized and nonlocalized cervical tumors, but between treatable and untreatable ones. About half of the women diagnosed with cervical tumors were classified as inoperable cases (and as poor candidates for radiotherapy or radiumtherapy) and received palliative care only. People who were classified as operable, and who received their treatment in a specialized institution, had a 40 percent chance to be alive five years after the therapy.[29] Lane-Claypon's analysis of data from the files of the Samaritan Free Hospital, London, confirmed the trend observed through the compilation of medical literature. Only 52.8 percent women treated for cervical cancer in this institution were diagnosed at an operable stage.[30] Dealing with cervical cancer, doctors set up a relatively modest goal: to educate women to see a doctor before their tumor reached a stage in which the main medical intervention was a liberal supply of morphine.

Cancer Registries and the Rise of the TNM System

Lane-Claypon's effort to provide clinical classification of breast malignancies was tailored to the needs of her specific investigation. The first cooperative effort to homogenize clinical staging of cancer was international classification of cervical tumors developed by the Cancer Commission of the League of Nations in the 1920s and 1930s.[31] While all the experts agreed that the optimal treatment for breast cancer was radical surgery, opinions on the best way to treat cervical tumors varied. In the early 1920s, radiotherapy specialists complained that they were unable to convince their colleagues that their approach yielded better results than surgery did, because they were unable to prove that they treated the same types of cases: "There is no uniform classification of malignant tumors, or a universally recognized description of their properties, or even a way to compare different terminologies. As a result a research report may be fully understood only by its author."[32] Homogenization of clinical and pathological diagnoses was, however, a difficult task, because it relied on the tacit knowledge of the expert. It was easier to homogenize such diagnoses in a single institution than across sites, but even doctors who worked in the same place did not always agree. In 1936, when Claudius Regaud, Curie Foundation's director and one of the main promoters of the international classification of cervical tumors, reviewed notes on results of treatment of uterine cancers made by his close collaborator Antoine Lacassagne, he penciled several objections to the staging proposed by Lacassagne. In a typical case he had written:

> Case no. 3. Classified as stage II. It looks like a typical stage I cervical epithelioma. But there is also a small node, size of a coffee grain, in the conjunctive tissue near the ischeo-public branch of the pelvis, on the right hand side. This small node was treated by radium therapy at a distance. The nature of this small node was not defined with precision. This is an unusual location for a cancerous lymph node in cervical cancer. If this node should be nevertheless viewed as a cancerous lymph node, this a stage III and not stage I cancer. If we

do not take this node into consideration, this is indeed a stage I—this is my proposal. But there is no place in this case for a stage II.[33]

The desire to compare different therapeutic approaches and assess their effects increased the need for a standardized evaluation of the progress of cervical malignancies. The Cancer Commission of the League of Nations appointed a subcommission, composed of Professor J. Heyman of Radiumhemmet in Stockholm, Lacassagne of the Curie Foundation, and Professor F. Voltz of Munich, tasked with creating such a standardization. Its report became the basis of the Heyman's International System. This system defined four stages of progression of cervical tumors: In stage I the growth was strictly limited to the cervix; in stage II there was a limited local spread; stage III included extensive local spread and isolated metastases; and in stage IV a massive spread of the tumor to surrounding organs and distant metastases.[34] In the 1930s Heyman's International System was adopted by the majority of specialists. Until the 1950s, it remained however, an isolated attempt to homogenize a clinical classification of tumors. The generalization of staging of malignancies after the Second World War was linked to the development of cancer registries.

National death records, such as those established in England by William Farr, were employed in the nineteenth century to extract data on cancer mortality. However, until the 1920s, cancer was not separated from other causes of death. The establishment of a systematic registration of cancer deaths in the interwar era was a reaction to a growing awareness of an increase in such deaths. Cancer registries had multiple goals. Their main aim was to gather data on the prevalence of malignant tumors to portray an accurate picture of cancer morbidity and mortality, follow epidemiological trends, and plan the construction of centralized cancer services and supply of expensive radiotherapy equipment. Another goal was a search for geographic and familial clusters of malignancies and links between specific occupations and cancers. Finally, it was hoped that data collected in cancer registries would contribute to the perfection of diagnosis and classification of malignant tumors and to the improvement of evaluation of results of preventive and therapeutic interventions.[35] At first registries were seen mainly as tools for better targeting distribution of resources. With the growing importance of cancer epidemiology in post–World War II era (especially in the context of debates on links between cigarette smoking and lung cancer), registries became increasingly important elements in decisions about cancer prevention and cancer treatment.

A regional registry of cancer was created in Hamburg in 1926 and in Mecklenburg in 1937, but both these registries were discontinued during the Second World War. The first in North America, the Massachusetts Cancer Registry, was established in 1936. It was followed in 1941 by the Connecticut Cancer Registry, which was active until the late twentieth century. The development of cancer registries in the United Kingdom was promoted by the main British cancer charity, British Empire Cancer Campaign (BECC). In 1934, the clinical research subcommittee of BECC proposed to gather data collected by some hospitals: records, statistics, and methods of follow-up of cancer cases.[36] This idea was transformed in 1935 into a project "to pool out all the statistics in London and centralize them by a 'Central Committee'"—that is, a coordinating BECC committee for London, which would be dedicated to the collection of statistics and standardization of classificatory criteria.[37] The project was adopted by BECC's direction, and in 1937, BECC decided to hire a medical registrar to supervise the collection of data and a statistician to help him in this task. Before starting his job, the newly appointed registrar, Lt. Col. W. L. Harnett, visited the United States to study North American experience of keeping patient's records and cancer registries.[38] The U.K. registry became operational in 1938. Its activity was slowed down, but not stopped, during the war, and it resumed immediately after the end of hostilities. One of the main achievements of the U.K. registry was the unification of inscriptions and the homogenization of classification of tumors. At first some clinicians resisted such homogenization, fearing that the introduction of new classificatory categories would destroy locally accumulated knowledge about relationships between the morphology of tumors and clinical outcomes.[39] Later, however, all the hospitals adopted BECC's rules, a trend that reflected a general tendency to standardize patients' records, accelerated by the development of the National Health Service in the late 1940s.[40]

Other Western countries also developed their own national cancer registries.[41] The majority of these registries included, like that of BECC, only the initial diagnosis (stomach cancer, breast cancer, bone tumor) and then the final outcome (cure or death). The French registry included, however, an additional element: the clinical stage of the tumor. From 1943 on, the recording of cancers in France was centralized by the Permanent Cancer Survey (L'Enquête Permanente Cancer). A typical product of the Vichy bureaucracy committed to modernization and rationalization of the French state (and partly inspired by the reorganization of the German state apparatus by the Nazi regime), the Enquête was affiliated with the Institut National d'Hygiène (INH). INH was initially created by Petain's government to stop the "demographic decline" of France. Later it was also made responsible for the control of major public health problems.[42] Cancer was classified, together with tuberculosis, as a "social disease," and a young Parisian surgeon, Pierre Denoix, was hired to collect data about this pathology. Denoix realized that the existing hospital records were too heterogeneous and could not be used to construct an efficient database. He decided therefore to develop an entirely new approach. In 1944, after the liberation of France, Denoix and his collaborators introduced a single classification for all malignant growths, an approach they perfected in 1948.[43]

The system proposed by the Permanent Cancer Survey in 1948 was partly inspired by Heyman's International System of classification of cervical tumors, energetically promoted by leading French cancer experts. The main classificatory elements were the anatomical location of a tumor, its size, and its degree of invasiveness (superficial, infiltrating, aggressive). Each cancer was designated by an arabic numeral that defined an organ (digestive system, respiratory system, skin), a capital letter that described an anatomic site (stomach, mouth, breast), a Roman numeral that characterized the level of local spread, and a lowercase letter (a, b, c) that denoted the presence and the degree of lymph node involvement. Thus 46.D.II.b was a digestive tumor, localized in the stomach, adherent to stomach lining, and with a partial lymph node involvement and 53.A.II.a was a skin tumor on the face that had invaded the hypodermis and had had no lymph node involvement.[44]

In 1952, the classification of tumors proposed by the Permanent Cancer Survey was modified to include information about the presence of distant metastases (the 1948 classification recorded local spread, but it did not distinguish invasion of nearby organs from distant metastases). The final version of the French classification became the basis of the International Classification of Malignant Tumors, the TNM classification (for Tumor, Nodes, Metastases). TNM classification was elaborated in 1953 by the International Union Against Cancer (IUAC), in close collaboration with the American Joint Committee on Cancer (AJCC).[45] Denoix, IUAC's director in the 1950s, played a central role in the promotion of this classification. The TNM system took into consideration clinical findings only. Thus T1N1M0 was a small tumor with some lymph node involvement and no distant metastases, T2N2M0 was a bigger tumor with more lymph node involvement and no metastases, and T4N3M1 was a large tumor with important lymph node involvement and a few distant metastases. According to this nomenclature, N and M could have 5 levels, from 0 to 4, while T could have four levels, from 1 to 4. Below T1, the disease was not a clinical cancer and was, therefore, outside the scope of TNM.

The Inclusion of Precancerous Lesions in Classifications of Cancers

International standardization of clinical classifications of cancers after World War II was paralleled by a standardization of cytological classifications of malignancies. The latter classification kept the principle of proximity between malignant and nonmalignant tumors that originated from the same tissue. Each group of tumors of similar histological origin included benign and malignant growths and also an "indefinite" subgroup, composed of tumors that cannot be clearly defined as either benign or malignant. "Classification by anatomical location, malignancy and histology," proposed by the World Health Organization Expert Committee on Health Statistics in 1956, ascribed a three-digit number to an anatomical site (ovary, esophagus, brain), a two-digit number to histological origins (epithelial, hemopoietic, nerve tissue), and one-digit code (from 1 to 6) to the estimated level of malignancy.[46] The *Manual of Tumor Nomenclature,* published by American Cancer Society in 1951, proposed a similar system. It gave each tumor a double classification. The first two numbers indicated the tissue of origin, while the last number, separated by a period, described the degree of malignancy. Tumors were graded from 1 to 9: those with grades 1 and 2 were benign, 3 and 4 indefinite, and 5 and higher, malignant. According to this classification, ductal carcinoma in situ (a noninvasive breast lesion) was 00.5 and an infiltrating ductal carcinoma (a malignant breast tumor) was 00.6. This classification, like that of the World Health Organization, indirectly hinted that an infiltrating carcinoma is just one additional step on a linear trajectory that leads from fully normal to fully malignant tissue.[47]

The first versions of the TNM classification included only confirmed malignancies, and the less advanced tumors were described as T1N0M0. The exclusion of precancerous lesions from TNM classification was challenged, however, by the widespread adoption of Pap smear, a method that detects the presence of abnormal cells in a vaginal smear. Suspicious findings on the Pap test—a frequent event—were usually checked by a cervical biopsy. Consequently, many women underwent such biopsies and were diagnosed with noninvasive proliferative lesions of the cervix.[48] These lesions, some experts proposed, have very similar structure to the invasive lesions of the cervix and should therefore be named "stage 0." The term *stage 0* had two distinct meanings. For some specialists, the main reason for the establishment of this classificatory category was the exclusion of results of the treatment of noninvasive lesions from statistics of cancer cures. People diagnosed with noninvasive lesions were occasionally classified as being treated for a beginning cancer. In fact, however, they were treated for a lesion with an unclear future and unknown potential to become malignant. They, therefore, received a preventive, and not a curative, therapy. The inclusion of these patients in statistics of cancer therapies artificially increased the number of cures and provided an inaccurate picture of the efficacy of treatments.[49] According to this interpretation, the meaning of "stage 0" was "not a true cancer," and the main accent was on "0," not on "stage." However, other experts viewed noninvasive cervical lesions as preinvasive ones and assumed that given sufficient time all such lesions would become malignant.[50] For these specialists, the meaning of "stage 0" was "a very early cancer," and the main accent was on "stage," not on "0."

Noninvasive cancerlike lesions were occasionally found in other organs as well. In the late 1950s, the TNM classification incorporated the term "stage 0." This stage was renamed "pre-invasive carcinoma" or "the so-called carcinoma in situ." Later versions of TNM changed the name of this lesion. People diagnosed with in situ tumors were classified T1S (there was no need to provide information on nodes or metastases, by definition absent when the lesion is not invasive). The category T0 was attributed to cases in which the someone had obvious signs of the presence of a malignant growth such as tumor-positive lymph nodes or distant metastases, but doctors were unable to find the primary tumor. Such a person (classified, e.g., T0N3M1) has an advanced, disseminated cancer with a poor prognosis.

The inclusion of the T1S stage in the clinically based TNM classification had a somewhat different meaning than the inclusion of tumors of unknown or intermediary malignancy in cytological classifications of tumors. The recognition of the fact that some tumors cannot be defined as malignant or benign on the basis of their microscopic appearance alone attests to the existence of a gray zone between the normal and the pathological. It indicates that malignant transformation, like other complex biological phenomena, cannot be adequately described in simple binary terms. The inclusion of T1S stage among the categories of TNM, a classification which, by definition, deals exclusively with the clinical disease of cancer, is a statement about the nature of in situ (noninvasive) tumors. T1S is defined implicitly as being the stage that precedes the development of an invasive tumor, T1N0M0. The inclusion of in situ tumors in an official classification of malignancies has practical consequences as well. For example in France categories produced by the national health insurance (Sécurité Sociale) directly follow the TNM classification. People diagnosed with in situ tumors are treated by the health system in the same way as those diagnosed with invasive tumors. They have the same rights and an identical access to health services. Experts continue to discuss whether the term *carcinoma in situ* is accurate, and some have proposed replacing it by a more neutral expression that does not evoke the dreaded "carcinoma."[51] In the meantime, health administrators are not bothered by such subtle distinctions. For them people diagnosed with in situ lesions are bone fide cancer patients.

Coda: Classifications of Malignant Tumors and Life Insurance

Doctors and their patients were not the only people interested in the distinction between benign, premalignant and malignant lesions. Insurance companies were also directly concerned by this distinction. They had a strong financial motivation in the evaluation of epidemiological data to assess the long-term effects of physiological conditions. To use the language of risk, first introduced by insurance companies, insurers aspired to identify elements that transform a potential client into a "poor risk."[52] A 1943 textbook destined for doctors who worked for insurance companies, *Medical Insurance Examination: Modern Methods and Rating of Lives,* evaluated data on numerous tumors to differentiate lesions that have a high probability of becoming cancerous from those that will remain benign and do not disqualify a future customer.[53] The author's tendency was to treat the majority of proliferative lesions as potentially cancerous. Chronic mastitis—a condition associated with cystic and lumpy breasts, which will be discussed in length in the following chapter—was classified as precancerous, as were polyps of the rectum, papillomatous tumors of the bladder, and benign tumors of the uterus. Only rodent ulcers (skin cancers) were seen as an acceptable risk for the insurer, because this category of tumors had a good prognosis if properly excised. It was, therefore, possible to offer insurance to people who had been diagnosed with rodent ulcers in the past and were free from recurrence for five years.

Medical examiners were advised by the textbook's author to be especially suspicious of the history of operations for cysts or growths in premenopausal or menopausal women. In such cases, the medical examiner should talk with the surgeon and the pathologist connected with the case to exclude the possibility of malignancy. If the medical examiner observed a doubtful cyst or tumor in a candidate for insurance, even a young and healthy person, insurance should be delayed until the clarification of the nature of the suspicious growth. In such cases, a family physician or a surgeon should be asked to obtain some scrapings of tissue, and the medical examiner—or, alternatively, the family doctor—should examine them under the microscope and assess the nature of the growth. If an operation was contemplated for such a condition, the textbook advised rejecting the application for an insurance policy or at least postponing the question of insurance until after the surgery. The manual stressed that a medical examiner should systematically reject applications of people who had a malignant tumor in the past, whatever its nature, cytological grade, stage, and treatment. When the risk was a financial one and the bottom line was the company's profit, the textbook concluded that "there is little ground for intelligent insurance."[54]

The insurers' approach may be seen as parallel to an approach promoted by advocates of a preventive elimination of precancerous lesions. Clinicians, like insurance companies, aspired to reduce risks. They wanted to limit the risk of cancer death for their patients and of professional failure for themselves. While their frame of reference was different from the one of the insurers, clinicians often arrived to similar conclusions: one should aggressively deal with all the malignant tumors, however minimal, and attempt to eliminate all the premalignant lesions. In the interwar era these principles were adopted by the majority of cancer experts. Specialists held nevertheless divergent definitions of premalignant lesions, divergent views about the desirable threshold of intervention, and divergent opinions about the best way to limit the danger of malignancy.

CHAPTER THREE

Borderline Lesions

Radical Solutions: Surgery for Female Cancers

Until the last two decades of the twentieth century, the principle of early detection and surgical elimination of precancerous lesions was applied mainly to the detection and preventive treatment of female malignancies. Biopsies continued to be employed to diagnose other tumors (head and neck, lower digestive tract), and, in selected cases, surgeons asked for frozen sections of suspicious tissue during a surgery for variety of conditions, malignant or not. Nevertheless only the management of female cancers (those of the breast and uterus) included systematic efforts to diagnose and to eliminate premalignant lesions.[1] In the interwar period, such efforts were hampered by the difficulty of defining what a premalignant lesion of breast or cervix was and how it should be treated.

In the nineteenth century, cancer was seen mainly as a women's disease, a perception linked to the ease of diagnosing women's malignancies.[2] In absence of modern diagnostic methods such as medical imagery, cancers of internal organs—such as the lung, the liver, the stomach, the colon, and the pancreas—were seldom recognized as malignant growths. People with these tumors became very sick and died from an organic failure: shortness of breath, jaundice, bleeding, blocked intestine, or general weakness. Many cancer deaths were accordingly seen as age-related demise. By contrast, female cancers were frequently diagnosed before the patient reached a terminal stage, and they produced visible and highly distressing symptoms: wounds that failed to heal, discharge of blood or pus, ulcers, necrosis, and a foul smell. Cancer, represented as it was by these pathologies but also by head and neck tumors, was indeed a "dread disease": frightening, degrading, repulsive, and associated with a loss of control. In the early nineteenth century the word "ancome," which described earlier a swelling or a tumor, was occasionally confused with the word "income," a curious comment on one of cancer's main characteristics, reckless growth.[3] Social scientists and literary critics put forward the role of cancer as a metaphor of individual failings and societal ills. However, an excessive accentuation of metaphorical meaning of cancer may be misleading. This disease did not unfold in an abstract discursive space but within a living body of a patient, and physicians attempted to cure it with all the concrete means at their disposal. The history of cancer therapies is more closely related to the development of specific medical practices than to broader cultural trends.

Doctors who attempted to deal with the harsh manifestations of cancer often felt that they need to be matched by similarly harsh therapeutic means (chasing evil with evil). Halsted's radical mastectomy became a model of other surgical interventions such as the Wertheim hysterectomy for uterine malignancies. This operation, improved by the Austrian surgeon Ernest Wertheim in the early twentieth century, was seen as a gynecological equivalent of radical mastectomy. Wertheim affirmed that to achieve a cure of a locally extended cervical cancer the surgeon should resect the uterus, the ligaments (parametria), and the nearby lymph nodes. In advanced cases the surgeon also eliminated the surrounding fused organs. The surgery had a high rate of mortality. In Wertheim's early attempts, nearly 40 percent of the people undergoing the surgery died as a direct consequence of the operation. Later the mortality due to surgery stabilized at around 10 percent. This result was seen as acceptable when the alternative was a painful and lingering death, less so when it became possible to treat cervical cancer through less deadly methods, such as radiotherapy and radiumtherapy.[4]

In the 1920s and 1930s, the great majority of French and Swedish women diagnosed with cervical cancer were treated with x-rays or radium, as were some (but not all) British patients.[5] In these countries, the coexistence of radiotherapy and surgery lessened the pressure for heroic operations. By contrast German and Austrian doctors believed that surgery was the only efficient way of dealing with cervical cancer. Radiotherapy was employed only to treat patients diagnosed with extensive tumors that could not be removed by surgery (e.g., growths that were fixed to the pelvic wall). Important differences in therapies of cervical cancer prompted international comparisons of curative techniques. Such comparisons indicated, however, that radiotherapy and surgery had a similar efficacy. In the hands of the best specialists, 40 percent of women diagnosed with a cervical cancer before it had spread beyond the cervix were alive five years after the initial diagnosis.[6] Consequently, cancer experts maintained their respective national traditions. The majority of French women diagnosed with cervical cancer under-

went radiotherapy, while, until the 1960s physicians in German-speaking countries proposed a radical surgery to all the women diagnosed with cervical carcinoma. They continued to be persuaded that a large excision increased the probability of cure: "Surgical radicalism focused on excision of the parametrial tissue
and the largest possible vaginal cuff. Surgeons prided themselves in photographs
of their surgical specimens, with the parametrial tissues spread out, and the vaginal cuff opened. In those days the histological diagnosis of a biopsy specimen
needed only to contain the word 'carcinoma' to justify radical surgery. At many
places, pre-invasive intraepithelial carcinomas were treated as aggressively as the
most locally advanced but still operable cases."[7]

In the interwar era many French, British, and American experts contested the
efficacy of radical or ultraradical surgery for cervical cancer. By contrast, radical
mastectomy for breast cancer continued to be perceived in all the three countries
as the gold standard of treatment of breast malignancies.[8] This operation was
nevertheless questioned by a small number of specialists, among them one of the
leading U.S. oncologists, James Ewing. The results of radical surgery for breast
cancer, Ewing stated, are often disappointing: "the experience of patients accomplishing a cure of an early cancer is generally a severe one, while the fate of fail-
ures is passed over in silence."[9] Other experts also noted that radical mastectomy
for small, localized breast tumors frequently failed to save the patient's life.[10]
Hence came the wish to intervene at an earlier stage and to excise precancerous
lesions of the breast. An even better solution was to prevent the development of
such lesions by eliminating the underlying cause of proliferative changes in the
breast—chronic irritation.

Irritation Theory and Precancerous Changes in the Breast

The irritation theory of carcinogenesis continued to dominate the understanding of cancer in the interwar era. It explained the origins of abnormal proliferation of cells, the variability of the produced lesions, and their prognostic instability. In parallel, it made preventive interventions possible. Cancer experts and
cancer charities argued that the most efficient way to reduce the incidence of cancer was to prevent chronic irritation. James Ewing explained thus that tumors of
genital organs, both male and female, were the result of poor hygiene, repeated
infection, and, in women, the laceration of the cervix by repeated childbirth,
while tumors of the mouth resulted from a neglect of teeth and of the oral cavity.[11] Sampson Headley similarly believed that cancer could be prevented through
the elimination of all the sources of chronic irritation. He called to pay a special

attention to the lack of appropriate dental hygiene, for him the main cause of mouth and throat tumors. In 1935 he argued that "until dental hygiene is universally secured we cannot count ourselves a really civilized race. In spite of the work of Sir William Hunter, the laity has not realized the host of evils that spring from decaying teeth and infected gums. The slums of the body must be abolished as well as those of the city."[12]

Claudius Regaud shared this view. Benign tumors, he proposed, morph into malignant ones only if they are submitted to a constant irritation. The most efficient way to prevent cancer is to avert the development of chronic lesions, and, if they do arise, to eliminate them surgically.[13] Education materials disseminated by the British Empire Cancer Campaign (BECC) stressed the threat of chronic inflammation produced by bacterial irritants, mechanical injury, or corrosive chemicals.[14] Women's magazines propagated similar message and warned their readers against the dangers of poor personal hygiene and of excessively tight clothes.[15]

The observation that radiation can induce malignant tumors did not challenge the irritation theory. X-rays and radium were known to produce burns and, therefore, trauma and irritation. Sampson Handley explained in 1936 that doctors who observed that exposure to x-rays or radium led to the development of rodent ulcers (skin cancer) were at first puzzled by this supposed deviation from the dominant theory of chemical carcinogenesis. Later, however, "the radiation cancers were brought under the fold of the irritation theory of cancer by a simple expedient. It was admitted that the irritation might be chemical or physical."[16] Similarly, the observation that tobacco users more often have tumors of the bucco-pharyngeal region was interpreted as an indication that tobacco contains irritants for mouth and throat mucous tissues. The tumor-inducing action of tobacco, the specialists proposed, was amplified by poor oral hygiene. The latter effect was believed to be a contributing factor of the high incidence of mouth cancer among working-class men. Or, as Joseph Colt Bloodgood put it in 1932: "the modern woman who keeps her teeth clean and in good shape teaches men how one should smoke with a minimal risk of cancer."[17]

A chronic irritation could have an internal, physiological cause as well. In such cases, preventive action was more difficult. It was, however, still possible to prevent malignancies through a surgical elimination of partly transformed tissues. Such tissues had already developed abnormal pattern of proliferation but had not yet acquired the capacity to invade surrounding tissues. Their surgical excision may be thus less extensive than the one of fully malignant tissues, an additional argument in favor of prophylactic surgery.

Chronic Cystic Mastitis: A Malignant Inflammation?

Chronic cystic mastitis, a disease characterized by multiple cysts and often by breast pain, was seen as a perfect illustration of carcinogenic effects of a persisting inflammatory state. According to Ewing, "mammary cancer practically never arises in a previously normal breast, but always in an organ altered by involution and inflammation."[18] Breast cysts were seen as one of the consequences of such involution (that is, degeneration of tissue), frequent in an organ that expands during pregnancy and lactation and then shrinks with age. Cystic mastitis was known to surgeons in the nineteenth century. An 1831 text of Sir Astley Cooper described the characteristic blue tint of mastitis cysts. Alfred Louis Velpeau defined in 1856 "a serous cyst of the breast" and proposed the treatment of smaller cysts by extirpation and larger cysts by iodine.[19] Pierre Reclus, another known expert on breast diseases, provided in 1878 a detailed description of the "cystic disease of the breast"; in France this condition later was called "la maladie de Reclus" (Reclus's disease).[20] The name *chronic cystic mastitis* was coined in the late nineteenth century. At that time this lesion was already linked with cancer or rather with the danger of developing cancer. Curt Schimmelbusch, a German surgeon who investigated breast cysts, stated in 1892: "it is indeed possible that cystadenoma may be placed in the category with certain epithelial conditions of irritation . . . which are in a sense benign, but have a tendency to become malignant." Accordingly he proposed that, in some cases at least, a chronic inflammation of the breast should be treated with a bilateral mastectomy.[21]

In 1906, Joseph Colt Bloodgood described a "senile parenchymateus hypertrophy of the female breast," a condition that, he explained, approximately parallels "la maladie de Reclus" or Schimmelbusch's disease. According to Bloodgood, the "diffuse parenhymatous hypertrophy of the senile breast" is seen most frequently in women between the ages of 40 and 50, the usual age of menopause.[22] Pathologists disagree about the exact definition of this condition: inflammation, benign tumor, or hypertrophy, but these debates are not very important from a practical point of view. One should merely keep in mind that this lesion has a benign and a malignant stage. The malignant stage is not different from other cancers of the breast. The benign stage has two distinct forms. One is characterized by a few big, smooth-walled cysts. This form seldom degenerates into malignancy and can be safely treated with an excision of the cyst alone. By contrast, in the second form, called by Bloodgood "adenocystic type," the breast is filled with hypertrophic tissue and multiple, small cysts: "in this form carcinoma is so frequent that I believe that in every instance the entire breast should be removed, and in some cases the two breasts . . . an early recognition followed by a proper operative intervention will undoubtedly increase the number of permanently cured cases."[23]

For James Ewing, cystic mastitis was a perfect illustration of precancerous changes of the breast that develop from inflammatory conditions.[24] Careful analysis of breasts amputated for cancer, especially small and atrophic ones, often revealed simultaneous presence of cystic mastitis, transitory forms between mastitis and adenomas or carcinomas, and distinct miniature carcinomas: "the gradual passage by many transitional stages of the nutritional and inflammatory changes of chronic mastitis into cancer has been traced by many observers and in such detail as to leave no reasonable doubt that these authors have been describing stages of the same process."[25]

Half of the breasts excised for cystic mastitis, Ewing claimed, showed such pronounced precancerous changes, a finding that fully legitimated a surgical removal of mastitis-containing breasts: "while some unnecessary surgery may thus be done, I think that the study of precancerous lesions in this organ fully justifies the radical procedure."[26]

Other experts agreed. M. C. Tod and E. K. Dawson from Edinburgh Royal College of Physicians noted that French surgeons often pronounced chronic mastitis a benign disease, and advocated, at most, the resection of the diseased part of the breast. Such a view, Tod and Dawson argued, is misguided. Breasts with mastitis often contain foci of malignancy, and a biopsy of excised tissue does not provide the necessary security: "partial extirpation for chronic mastitis must be regarded as only partial insurance of the life of the patient."[27] By contrast it was believed that a simple mastectomy, a technique that eliminates all the breast tissue, but not breast muscles or lymph nodes, and leaves intact the skin and nipple, does provide adequate safety margins.[28] British surgeon Sir Lenthal Cheatle, proposed in 1922 the surgical removal of inflamed and cystic breasts. Cheatle believed that the term "proemial" (prior, ahead of, antecedent, anterior, anticipatory) was more accurate than "precancerous" and "precursory." He stated: "I look upon it [the proemial breast] and treat it precisely in the same way and for the same reasons that compel surgeons to remove an appendix that has been inflamed. The proemial breast bears exactly the same relationship to cancer and papillomate of the breast as the proemial appendix does to general peritonitis."[29] In an influential textbook, *Tumours of the Breast*, of 1931 (written with U.S. surgeon Max Cutter), Cheatle and his coauthor proposed that when a breast contains a single "blue dome cyst" it is usually safe to remove only the cyst. By contrast, when a woman suffered from a generalized cystic disease, it was wiser to remove the whole gland. His own clinical experience, Cheatle added, supported this view. Several times, he found unsuspected carcinoma in a breast amputated for multiple cystic disease.[30]

Cheatle and Cutler probably represented the surgeons' point of view. Columbia University pathologist Arthur Purdy Stout advocated a more nuanced approach to treatment of cystic mastitis. This condition, he explained, is often found in young women, a population with a low occurrence of breast cancer. When planning a surgery, one should take into account the woman's age, the psychological effects of the loss of a breast, and the overall condition of breast tissue. If the person only has cystic mastitis, Stout believed, the chances of cancer are remote, and an excision of the cysts should be sufficient. By contrast, when cystic mastitis is accompanied with other changes in breast tissue, it may be safer to perform either a simple or, in advanced cases, a radical mastectomy. Frozen section during surgery can help therapeutic decisions, but one should also bear in mind that it is not a foolproof diagnostic technique. Stout mentioned two cases of people who underwent partial mastectomy for lesions diagnosed as benign during the surgery and who later developed metastases in axillary lymph nodes. Finally, when the woman harbors an excessive fear of malignancy, it was thought that a simple mastectomy might be an efficient cure for cancerophobia.[31]

Stout advocated a wide range of therapies for cystic mastitis. Patients' records from the 1920s and 1930s display a great variability of treatments for this condition. Such variability might have reflected the diversity of clinical situations, but it also might have reflected dissimilar beliefs held by surgeons and divergent interpretations provided by pathologists. The latter faced a challenging task: to provide a firm diagnosis of a morphological entity with an unclear definition and fuzzy boundaries.

Lumpy Breasts and Ambivalent Images

During their training, pathologists learn how to recognize forms and patterns and to classify shapes. Such skill is grounded in individual expertise and is not transferable. As U.S. pathologist William Sternberg put it: "A cancer is a cancer, histologically, not because it fulfils certain a priori criteria, but because of its resemblance to other lesions that have proved to be clinically malignant. The criteria of malignancy vary in different sites of the body and must be modified from organ to organ. The technique is essentially that of natural historian, or of you will, of the sophisticated bird watcher."[32]

Some surgeons contested the privileged status of cytological diagnosis of cancer. An excessive reliance on pathologist's judgment, William White argued in

1930, may be misleading: "I question very much any histological diagnosis of cancer that is not supported by some gross evidence such as gritty feeling to the knife, yellow dots in the cut section, and absence of capsule." White's proposal can be seen as an attempt to turn the clock backward and to give the surgeons the control over cancer diagnosis they had around 1900. He advanced, however, a new argument to legitimate a macroscopic diagnosis of malignancy. Exclusive reliance on cytological evidence may lead to a mistaken diagnosis of benign tumors as malignant: "I believe that many so called cancers seen in chronic cystic mastitis were not malignant growths, but merely a chronic inflammatory reaction."[33]

Surgical pathologists are aware of the difficulty of providing an unambivalent distinction between normal and pathological tissues, especially when they examine borderline lesions. The history of diagnosis of such lesions is that of visual ambiguity. "Magnification," art historian Barbara Stafford explained, "drives to the center of the major aesthetic problem faced by all natural history descriptions. What do you do with beings that are neither one thing nor the other?"[34] The chapter on cancer in a recent textbook of general pathology reproduces M. C. Escher's print *Angels and Devils*, with the caption "interwoven angels and devils, the nightmare of the pathologist examining a tumor that appears neither benign, nor malignant."[35] Such a use of Escher's image may, however, be misleading. The ambivalence of Escher's white-and-black drawings is grounded in the principle of a gestalt shift of the "duck or rabbit" kind. Looking at the angels and devils picture one can see either the angels or the devils but not both simultaneously. By contrast, pathologists are confronted with ambiguous, indeterminate forms, dominated by shades of gray.

Fundamental scientists who study microscopic preparations, Stafford argued, grapple with the "ethics of esthetics": they look for ways to produce order and legibility in visual representations of highly variable manifestations of life, without robbing them of their uniqueness and without undue simplifications. Practitioners face a different dilemma. For them the main problem is not the heterogeneity and ambiguity of images seen through the microscope, but the need to produce an unambivalent knowledge. Medicine, unlike biology, is a normative discipline, and the distinction between the normal and the pathological has far-reaching practical consequences. The pathologists' main concern is not the "ethics of esthetics" but the ethics of medical intervention. They often observe ambivalent images, but their duty is to interpret these images within a coherent analytic framework and to provide a verdict that will guide the clinicians' actions. Pathologists' language—or rather their multiple languages—mirrors the double need to accurately describe observed phenomena and to translate representation

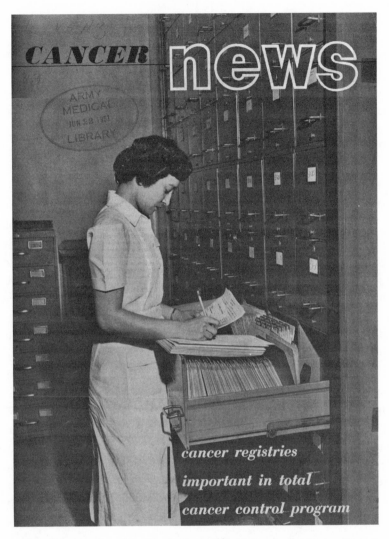

The cover of *Cancer News,* showing the importance of cancer registries. *Cancer News* 5, no. 3 (1951): cover. Reprinted by permission of the American Cancer Society, Inc. All rights reserved.

into intervention. This task was especially arduous when dealing with the highly variable and poorly defined breast lesions.[36] Descriptions of proliferative lesions of the breast, produced in three pathology laboratories—London Hospital, Addenbrooke's Hospital, Cambridge, England, and the Curie Foundation, Paris (after Second World War, the Curie Institute)—illustrate different styles of depicting ambiguity through words.[37]

Pathology Styles

The surgical pathology laboratory of the London Hospital was founded by Hubert Maitland Turnbull, professor of Morbid Anatomy at London University and head of the pathology laboratory at London Hospital from 1906 to 1946. Turnbull studied pathology in Germany and then transposed German methods, and probably also German-style linguistic constructions, to the United Kingdom.[38]

The "so called chronic mastitis," Turnbull explained in his teaching notes, is not a chronic inflammation but an abnormal evolution and involution of the breast. Turnbull linked a tendency to develop breast hyperplasia not only to the absence of changes in the breast induced by pregnancy but also to a lack of sexual stimulation: "That such morbid deviation occurs more frequently in older virgins, has been attributed to the omission of the evolution associated with pregnancy—an evolution which should under normal conditions occur during the life of every woman. It may be added that there is evidence that such evolutionary changes are instigated by the sexual act unaccompanied by pregnancy."[39]

Turnbull stressed the fluidity of boundaries between normal and pathological proliferative conditions of the breast. Hyperplasia, he explained can be divided into two main types, benign and adenomatous. Both types are almost always clinically diagnosed as chronic mastitis. On the one hand, the benign type should be considered a normal consequence of sexual activity: "Lenthal Cheatle calls the simple tubular hyperplasia with slight epithelial cathartic 'mazoplasia': it is of no significance: for him, 'every girl who does a little masturbation has it.' "[40] On the other hand, some adenomatous lesions are very close to true malignancies. For example, an intracystic papillary adenoma is classified as a cancer when found outside milk ducts and as premalignant lesion if it is diagnosed as a duct papilloma or a cystic duct adenoma. In some cases, multiple cysts of chronic mastitis are defined as benign polycystoma, but when the proliferation is more intense, the usual diagnosis is of a true carcinoma.[41] Terms employed in pathological practice at London Hospital in the early twentieth century mirrored Turnbull's views on close relationships between proliferative conditions of the breast and cancer. The most frequent borderline diagnosis of a breast lesion was "carcinomatous hyperplasia," a broad category that included numerous lesions, among them chronic cystic mastitis. The juxtaposition of "carcinomatous" and "hyperplasia" probably sent an appropriate message to surgeons.[42] Approximately half of the women with these conditions treated at London Hospital in 1909 and in 1919 underwent an amputation of the breast.[43]

The pathology laboratory of London Hospital provided as a rule detailed descriptions of macroscopic aspects of each sample: the consistency of the tissue, its surface, its resistance to cutting, and equally detailed descriptions of forms seen under the microscope.[44] Early descriptions of breast specimens were rich and complex. They attempt, one may propose, to mimic the complexity of the studied biological material. Here is a typical example from 1909:

> Macroscopic: the nipple is flattened, but not retracted. The breast tissue is un-even, some nodules can be felt. On section, one can see hard breast tissue with a few cysts. The surface of the cut bulges. The cysts contain a clear, glare-like liquid. No signs of cancerous growth. There are no enlarged lymphatic glands. Microscopic: cystic disease of the breast and acinar papilloma. There are bunches of abnormal accini and ducts in the fibrous breast tissue. One of these bunches show a number of dilated ducts with a lining of flattened cubical cells and lumen full of blue-stained debris. Others are traversed by fine branching showing tree like processes covered by tall columnar cells; this appears defini-tively like papilloma. The cells show a great affinity for eosin. In the prepara-tion, one can find an intermediate stage between cysts, and papilloma like structures.[45]

In 1919, pathology reports often introduce composite terms: "lobular adeno-matous hyperplasia," "intracanalicular fibroadenoma," "lobular and cystic ade-nomatous hyperplasia," "lobular, adenomatous and carcinomatous hyperplasia." The descriptions of borderline lesions are usually shorter than in 1909 and skip detailed descriptions of macroscopic aspect of the studied tissue. However, the introduction of the practice of analyzing several samples (usually three to five) from a single amputated breast favored the display of the coexistence of several kinds of proliferative lesions, adding a new layer of complexity. For example, one 1919 report describes: "lobular, tubular and solid tubercular, cubical and polygo-nal celled, adenomatous and carcinomatous hyperplasia and infiltrating carci-noma of the breast, near the nipple. Lobular and cystic adenomatous hyperpla-sia of the peripheral breast."[46] In 1929, one may observe somewhat greater standardization of descriptions of borderline lesions. The language is still very rich, but the expressions are more codified. Typical example is: "Intracanalicular myco-fibroadenoma of the breast. Slight adenomatous hyperplasia in the neigh-boring mammary tissue."[47] Finally, in 1939, London Hospital pathologists in-creasingly employed the term *precancerous* to describe proliferative lesions of the breast, for example, "extensive precancerous hyperplasia in ducts of breast, but no definite infiltrating carcinoma."[48]

The Curie Foundation's pathologist, George Gricouroff, also elected to provide detailed cytological descriptions of breast lesions, although he seldom employed composite terms ("peri- and intra- canalicular adeno-fibroma") and had chosen more straightforward definitions ("epithelioma of a canalicular origin, stratified and muciparous").[49] For example: "a beginning cancer. Epidermic epithelium was replaced by simple prismatic epithelium. Malignant transformation of pavimanteux stratified epithelium. Invasion by budding of cervical stroma by the transformed epithelium. It is certain that the presence, in the same site, of regressing and degenerating muciparous elements and proliferating malignant epidermic elements produces a mixture of secretion products and of cells, and of the two kinds of cells."[50]

Pathological diagnoses of cancer in the archives of Addenbrooke's Hospital in Cambridge, England, display yet another style of description of borderline lesions, less exuberant and more concise. Addenbrooke's pathology books start in the late 1930s, and the entries were provided by the hospital's pathologist Dr. C. H. Whittle.

Typical descriptions of borderline breast lesions from 1937 are "hyperplasia within cystic spaces of somewhat flattened epithelium" or "dense fibroma with irregular masses of material staining almost black, and with massive glandular hyperplasia. The cells are columnar and arranged in duct-like form." Descriptions from 1942 are also relatively short and tend to rely mainly on the existing classificatory categories. Examples include "fairly regular massive hyperplasia of the cubical epithelium" or "hyperplasia in fold of columnar epithelium. Chronic inflammatory changes inside cystic spaces."[51]

Pathologists' publications similarly reflect differences of individual style. Legends of photographs in a 1905 article on proliferative lesions of the breast by J. Collins Warren provide relatively detailed descriptions of such lesions: "papillary cyst adenoma: microscopic appearances. Note the exuberant growth of epithelium over papillary outgrowth of connective tissue from the wall of cyst cavity"; "fibro-cyst-adenoma. Note the cyst cavities and exuberant growth of epithelial ducts in lobular arrangement in a stroma of a periductal tissue"; "papillary cyst-adenoma."[52] Legends to photographs in Bloodgood's 1906 article on hyperthrophic lesions of the breast are less detailed: "intaracanalicular myxoma"; "adenoma," "diffuse virginal hypertrophy," "single cyst in early stage of parenchymatous hypertrophy," "senile paranchymatous hypertrophy."[53] Usually legends of photographs of cytological preparations provide only a description of the depicted material. Legends of photographs in Bloodgood's 1932 paper on borderline breast tumors offer, in addition, information on the person's ultimate fate:

Case I. Section of wall of chronic lactation mastitis abscess. Diagnosed cancer in 1894. The patient is well, no recurrence today.

Case III, section from a wall of a blue domed cyst, large solid duct adenoma. Diagnosed by Bloodgood at St. Agnes Hospital. Cyst removed. No recurrence in 1930.

Case VII. Thick walled cyst. Excised from breast seven years ago. No recurrence since. Pathologists differ as to malignancy.[54]

At that same time Bloodgood had started to doubt the wisdom of systematic ablation of breasts with chronic mastitis. The inclusion of data about clinical outcomes in legends of photographs depicting cytological preparations probably aimed at strengthening the main argument of his paper: images seen under the microscope do not always "speak for themselves."

Diagnostic Mastectomies

Advocates of mastectomy for proliferative conditions of the breast, above all cystic mastitis, legitimated their position by the danger of cancer. An additional, more practical reason to favor an amputation of a mastitis-containing breast was the difficulty of diagnosing an already existing malignant tumor, hidden among cysts and lumps. Partial diagnostic procedures, such as the excision of a lump or breast lesion, Ewing argued, may be too dangerous for the patient, because the examination of the excised nodes and nodules may still miss areas of malignancy: "it is usually safer to excise the whole breast, to make the diagnosis *complete*, and to remove the source of anxiety or actual danger."[55] Robert Greenough from Massachusetts General Hospital agreed. In some supposedly benign lesions, such as cystic disease, an adequate gross and microscopic examination cannot be conducted without the removal of the whole breast.[56]

British cancer experts Tod and Dawson held a similar opinion. Precancerous conditions of the breast, they explained, are often associated with the presence of small foci of carcinoma. Only the removal of the breast and the subsequent careful analysis of the entire tissue of a breast tissue by competent pathologists can confirm that premalignant lesions are not intermingled with a true cancer and that there is no need to perform a radical surgery.[57] They called this approach "diagnostic mastectomy" and argued that it a much safer approach than the resection of the suspicious area alone. It was thought that doctors who were too anxious to avoid mastectomies might put the lives of their patients at risk: "that the psychological effect of such removal might be injurious can hardly be denied, but in our view this possibility has been allowed to weigh too heavily, and it is noteworthy that the women surgeons with whom we have discussed the matter, lay little stress on this factor."[58]

The term *diagnostic mastectomy* highlights the interdependence between therapeutic choices and diagnostic and surgical techniques. Many experts believed that a frozen section, however useful, did not provide sufficient information about presence of microfoci of malignancy in a cystic or otherwise modified breast. In such cases, surgeons often elected to remove the whole breast to allow a thorough examination of this organ in the pathology laboratory. Moreover, when biopsy was conducted as a part of the surgery, the standard procedure was to pack the wound with gauze soaked with formaldehyde while waiting for pathologist's verdict. If a malignancy was found, the patient was redraped, and the surgeon changed his instruments and proceeded with radical mastectomy. If the tumor was declared benign, the surgeon was still obliged to eliminate the formaldehyde-soaked (and thus dead) tissue, that is, to make a very extensive excision. When the lesion was large or the breast small, the only cosmetically acceptable solution was to perform a simple mastectomy.[59] The choice to carry out an increased number of exploratory surgeries for suspicious breast conditions, coupled with a reluctance to conduct two-stage procedures, might have led to an increase in frequency of simple mastectomies.[60] A complex interplay between material constraints, technical variables, theoretical presuppositions, surgical cultures, and the perception of the female breast as a useless organ may account for a high number of mastectomies for benign growths of the breast in the 1920s and 1930s.

The records of Huntington Hospital, Cambridge, Massachusetts, illustrate the trend of amputating breasts with benign proliferative changes. The hospital, which was founded in 1913 and affiliated with Harvard University, specialized in the treatment of cancer. Between 1920 and 1940, the number of patients diagnosed with invasive breast cancer at this hospital remained stable: between eighty and one hundred cases per year. By contrast the number of diagnoses of benign conditions of the breast increased steadily, from ten to twenty cases per year between 1920 and 1926, forty to sixty per year between 1927 and 1936, more than eighty between 1937 and 1940.

The hospital records reveal in tandem a sharp increase of amputations for benign conditions of the breast, a trend that started in 1931. Before that date there were very few breast amputations for this indication (four for the whole period

1920–30). In 1930–31 there were ten amputations (22 percent of women diagnosed with nonmalignant breast disease); in 1931–32, fourteen (27 percent); in 1933–34, eighteen (27 percent); in 1934–35, seven (17 percent); in 1935–36, thirteen (19 percent); in 1936–37 twenty-two (27 percent); in 1937–38, thirteen (15 percent); in 1938–39, ten (12 percent); and 1939–40, seven (10 percent). The main indication for breast ablation was cystic breast disease; other less frequent indications were diagnoses of fibroma and fibroadenoma.[61] It is reasonable to assume that the increase in mastectomies for benign breast conditions in the 1930s may reflect contingent variables such as the opinion of the surgeons and the pathologists active at that time at Huntington Hospital. It is, however, equally reasonable to suppose that the rise in number of simple mastectomies mirrored the increase in the number of women who consulted physicians for suspicious changes in their breast and a parallel augmentation of the number of exploratory surgical procedures that occasionally led to an ablation of the breast for diagnostic or cosmetic reasons.

Proliferative Lesions of the Breast in New York

Breast lesions such as cystic mastitis and akin proliferative conditions were unstable diagnostic categories, with multiple and sometimes incommensurable definitions. It is not surprising that doctors' choices to treat these lesions varied in different settings. Such choices were probably influenced by shifts in perception of a given pathology, national and local traditions, and idiosyncratic differences between practices of surgeons and pathologists. Files of the New York Hospital and Presbyterian Hospital, both in New York, the Addenbrooke's Hospital, Cambridge, England, and the Curie Foundation, Paris, display a heterogeneity of medical practices. These hospitals were selected because they were leading cancer treating centers in their respective countries, but also because they conserved their patients' files, an important consideration for a historian.

Let's look first at a selection of cases, among those found in the New York Hospital files. In a 1914 case, a tumor diagnosed during breast surgery as malignant on the basis of its gross appearance was reclassified in the pathology laboratory as containing elements of true carcinoma and of cystic mastitis, a possible indication of pathologists' conviction that the two lesions are closely related:

N.H., a 48-year-old woman, working as a house maid, was first seen at the New York Hospital in June 1914 [case no. 2]. She had a lump in her breast for 5 or six years: it was asymptomatic, but a month ago, started to cause slight pain. Clinical examination revealed a hard, elastic mass in the upper quadrant of the left breast, attached to skin, another mass in the same breast and several palpable axilla lymph nodes. Because of the movable character of the tumor it was deemed wise first to remove the breast in masse and to make a gross examination of this tumor. On dissection, the tumor was found to be undoubtedly carcinomatous, and her surgeons proceeded to radical mastectomy and a dissection of the axilla. The pathology report [paraffin section] confirmed the presence of malignancy. The main nodule, in lower portion of the breast was classified as scirrous carcinoma. The resected breast also contained a diffuse mass, classified as an area of cystic mastitis with no evidence of cancerous growth. No cancer was found in lymph nodes.[62]

In a 1918 case, a frozen section during a surgery led to diagnosis of cystic mastitis, and surgeon decided to perform a simple mastectomy:

A 32-year-old female clerk was admitted to New York Hospital in March 1918 [case no. 29]. She had accidentally found a tumor in her breast five days ago, has no other symptoms. Her physician advised her to go to the hospital. A frozen section was made during breast surgery and the pathologist reported that the tumor was non malignant. Nevertheless her breast was removed, because it contained one large cyst and several smaller cysts. Pathological diagnosis [paraffin section] was chronic interstitial mastitis with fibroadenoma of the breast.[63]

In a case treated in 1924, New York Hospital doctors performed simple mastectomy for a recurrence of cystic mastitis and presented this surgery as a treatment of premalignant changes in the breast:

A 42-year-old housewife was admitted to New York Hospital in April, 1924 with a tumor in her breast [case no. 214]. She had a duct papilloma excised in June 1922, and the tentative diagnosis was the recurrence of papilloma in the nipple region. Her doctors decided that this time the right treatment would be a simple mastectomy: "in view of the recurrence after resection of the mammary gland for duct papilloma, it seems wise to remove the nipple and the segment of the breast containing the papilloma. If the nipple was removed, it seemed wise to remove the whole mammary gland to avoid leaving a useless area of epithelial tissue which may become the site of a malignant growth or, in the event of pregnancy, give rise to a galactocele." Analysis of pathology slides revealed multiple papillary cysts, adenoma of the breast of the benign type and mastitis with atypical proliferation of glandular epithelium. The pathologists also noted that some of the glandular areas showed marked atypical "borderline" proliferation of the lining epithelium. Such proliferation can be viewed as a recurrence of a disease of the breast, but not the recurrence of the tumor previously removed. Her discharge notice states: "chronic mastitis or the so-called precancerous lesions."[64]

In a 1928 case, the patient's clinical examination led to a presumption of malignancy, and a frozen section indeed detected suspicious proliferative changes. The surgeon performed a radical mastectomy; paraffin section did not reveal malignancy.

A 43-year-old cook was admitted to the hospital in July 1928 with a swollen, painful left breast. Her symptoms had started 10 days before hospitalization. Doctors who examined her suspected malignancy, also noted the enlargement of axillary lymph nodes. The pathologist who performed frozen section had found papillary proliferation in the ducts and atypical cells elsewhere, together with an evidence of a widespread chronic mastitis. The surgeon accordingly performed a radial mastectomy. Paraffin section did not confirm these findings. It displayed adenoma with papillary proliferation and mastitis in the whole organ, but no malignant cells. Microscopic examination of axillary lymph nodes shows an inflammatory hyperplasia. Final diagnosis, "papillary cytadenomata of the breast, with chronic mastitis." Final summing up of the case: "removal of breast for chronic mastitis."[65]

In a similar case, also from 1928, a frozen section during breast surgery had shown cystic mastitis and other proliferative changes. The pathologist believed that these elements did not justify a radical mastectomy and recommended a simple ablation of the breast. He was, however, aware of the fact that a pathologist's judgment of borderline cases vary.

A 46-year-old housewife was admitted in June 1928 with a lump in the right breast. She has serous discharge from the breast for 20 years, and was aware of the presence of a tumor for the last five years. Recently she suffered from mild pain in the breast. A frozen section revealed a chronic cystic mastitis and the presence of intracystic papilloma but no true malignancy. Upon the pathologist's advice, the surgeon decided to refrain from radical mastectomy. Paraffin section revealed the presence of some suspicious areas in which cells had undergone fibrous changes. The pathologist, Dr. Elser, concluded that the experience of this department had been that such changes should not be seen as true malignant tumors, though in some laboratories they are classified as such.[66]

In many cases an amputated breast contained zones of cystic mastitis together with invasive carcinoma. In a case from 1930, the patient was diagnosed as suffering from a true malignancy; the invasive lesions were intermingled with cystic mastitis lesions:

> A 38-year-old woman was admitted to New York Hospital in October 1930. She had a mass in the right breast, noticed last February. Clinical examination did not provide a definitive evidence of malignancy. Frozen section made during the surgery section revealed malignant changes, and surgeons proceeded with a radical mastectomy. Pathology reports explained that the "first specimen is a mass of breast tissue representing the near-totality of the breast, with mass 5 × 4 × 3 cm, not encapsulated. Microscopic analysis found lesions of carcinoma and cystic mastitis of the breast. Three nodules removed from the contra-lateral breast during the surgery were diagnosed as benign adenofibroma.[67]

The boundary between cancerous and precancerous changes was sometimes fluid. In another case, from 1930, a frozen section revealed very similar lesions in both breasts, with somewhat clearer evidence of invasion in the right breast. The pathologist's verdict was "left breast—chronic cystic mastitis with marked hyperplasia, probably pre-cancerous but not definitively malignant; right breast—chronic cystic mastitis with probable malignant changes." Accordingly the surgeon decided to perform a radical ablation of the right breast and simple ablation of the left one. The patient died a few days after the operation from postsurgical complications.[68]

Case studies in the files of Maurice Lenz, a radiotherapy expert of the Presbyterian Hospital (affiliated with Columbia University), display dilemmas of accurate diagnosis of breast tumors. One solution for diagnostic uncertainty was a close medical surveillance of women diagnosed with proliferative changes in the breast. The head of the surgery department at the Presbyterian hospital, Dr. Cushman Haagensen, often recommended long-term surveillance. In one such case, doctors suspected malignancy, reclassified the breast lesion as mastitis, then decided, on the basis of clinical evolution of the disease, that after all this was probably a carcinoma:

A 47-year-old nurse was seen March 1923 at Columbia's Presbyterian Hospital, New York. She was diagnosed during her surgery with a cystic disease of the breast with epithelial hyperplasia of the so-called "dangerous" sort. Her doctors decided to proceed with a radical mastectomy. Pathological diagnosis of the paraffin section revealed an extreme grade of active cellular proliferation, considered probably non-malignant. She was followed in the clinics until 1932, then her follow up was discontinued on the grounds that she had a cystic disease. In December 1935, she came back to the clinics contra lateral breast with 8.5 cm mass, slightly hot and red, retracted, fixed nipple, reduced mobility of the breast and "pig skin" lymphoedema. Two axillary nodes showed metastases. Pathological report was similar to the findings 13 years ago. A review of her 1923 slides made in light of the new clinical findings, resulted in a change of opinion. Her old tumor was reclassified as carcinoma of the so-called comedo type. She underwent radiotherapy in 1936.[69]

Facing unclear or contradictory findings experts frequently elected to err on the side of prudence and to perform a radical surgery:

A 31-year-old woman came to the Presbyterian Hospital in September 1923, because of bleeding from a nipple that started three weeks ago. She was diagnosed wit an intraductal papillary growth, and her doctors advised observation rather than surgery. The patient failed to appear to control visits, returned finally to Presbyterian hospital only in 1930 with a mass in the breast. She was then examined by Dr Arthur Purdy Stout, concluded that she suffered from cancer, and recommended an exploratory dissection of axillary lymph nodes. The dissection did not find any sign of malignancy. Nevertheless, Lenz recommended a radical mastectomy on the basis of the clinical findings. Tumors formed by papillary intraductal growths, Lenz explained, should always be looked at with an extreme suspicion; mastectomy is therefore highly indicated. And, he added, "the only question that arises is whether there should be radical operation or simple mastectomy. In this instance I think it is wise to do a radical mastectomy, because of the lack of faith I have in my ability to be sure, even after the breast has been removed, how to classify such cases as regard malignancy. It is by all odds best to give the patient the benefit of doubt."

Analysis of the amputated breast did not resolve the doubt about the status of breast lesions. No cancer was found. The pathologist explained that this was an interesting case of a papillary cysto-adenoma of the breast with clinical signs of malignancy but which, on gross and microscopic examination, showed no evidence of cancer. He added nevertheless, "I feel that this type of cystic disease with epithelial hyperplasia is the nearest thing to cancer that there is in the breast."

In April 1937 Lenz reviewed the patient's slides with two colleagues, and they decided to revise their original judgment:

> On re-examination of these sections Dr. Stout, Dr. Haagensen and I now feel that this is a carcinoma. The process of intraductal papillary growth is not confined to the large cyst, but is extensive throughout the duct system of the breast. In some areas that are remote from the larger tumor mass, there is what now seems to us to be a definitive evidence of invasion. Diagnosis: Carcinoma of female mammary gland.[70]

In this case, at first pathological data contradicted the clinical ones. A retrospective reexamination of the original slides set the record straight, and aligned the treatment—a radical mastectomy, with the cytological diagnosis—a carcinoma. One may assume that the woman herself was not aware of the complexities of her case and, after her first radical mastectomy (a treatment systematically presented as indispensable and life saving), she was simply informed that she was successfully treated for breast cancer.

Proliferative Lesions of the Breast in the United Kingdom

Janet Lane-Claypon's 1926 survey of files of women operated for breast cancer in nine hospitals in London and Glasgow provides insight into treatments proposed to women diagnosed with suspicious changes in the breast.[71] Lane-Claypon lumped together cytological analyses of problematic cases provided by nine pathology laboratories. One group was composed of women with confirmed or suspected nonmalignant lesions. Seventeen women were diagnosed with chronic cystic mastitis confirmed by a biopsy. Lane-Claypon did not provide information on treatment of three of these women. Five patients underwent lumpectomy (the removal of the cyst alone), two a partial mastectomy (an ablation of part of the breast), four a simple mastectomy (ablation of all the breast tissue), and three a radical mastectomy (ablation of the breast, axillary lymph nodes, and pectoral muscles). Eight additional women were diagnosed with unspecified borderline breast lesions. Five women of this group underwent radical mastectomy, while the treatment of the remaining three others was not mentioned.[72]

The second group included women initially diagnosed with benign lesions but later reclassified as having a malignancy. Five women were originally diagnosed with a benign growth, but a frozen section performed during surgery led to a diagnosis of malignancy and an immediate radical mastectomy. In seventeen women who underwent lumpectomy and in three who underwent a simple mastectomy (probably without a frozen section), a paraffin section of the excised tissue revealed malignancy.[73] In all these cases but one, their surgeon performed a radical mastectomy shortly after the original operation. The sole exception was a woman who, on learning that her tumor was reclassified as malignant, refused the radical operation.[74]

The third group is composed of women diagnosed with benign growths who later developed a cancer of the breast. Twelve women diagnosed with a benign tumor (often cystic mastitis) developed an invasive tumor shortly after their initial diagnosis. These cases, Lane-Claypon proposed, point to the difficulty of differential diagnosis of proliferative lesions of the breast. Five women, initially diagnosed with cystic mastitis and treated by removal of the affected part of the breast only, many years later developed (in one case, twenty-seven years later) a malignant tumor in the same breast. In these cases, Lane-Claypon explained, cystic mastitis was in all probability a precursor of an invasive cancer of the breast. She had recorded also thirty-five cases in which pathologists had found in the amputated breast zones of well-defined malignancy surrounded by areas of cystic mastitis.[75] The implicit message conveyed by her data is that breast cancer may be confused with cystic mastitis, breast cancer may be intermingled with this lesion, or cystic mastitis may evolve into cancer, all observations that could have been interpreted as a justification of surgical radicalism.

Files from Addenbrooke's Hospital confirm that women diagnosed with proliferative lesions often underwent a surgical ablation of the breast, usually a simple mastectomy. Here is a description of a typical case:

A 43-year-old woman, seen August 1937. Six months ago she noticed discharge from nipple. No lump felt. Operation [by Mr. Butler, the surgeon in many breast cases], simple mastectomy. Pathology report: "this breast shows fibroadenomatous changes only. No signs of malignancy."[76]

Sometimes the pathologists' report recognized the difficulty of providing a precise diagnosis:

A 54-year-old woman was seen in Addenbrooke's Hospital in October 1937. She noticed a lump in her breast one year ago. No enlarged lymph nodes in the axilla. The patient underwent a radical mastectomy [modified Halsted]. The surgeon observed that her breast tissue was very fibrotic with many involved cysts. Pathology report stated: "rather irregular hyperplasia of squamous epithelium with some down growths into the sub-cutaneous tissue and with much fibrous tissue formation. This is suggestive of the type of change occurring in Paget's disease, but not absolutely diagnostic."[77]

In other cases the surgeon decided to remove the breast, while the pathologist found out that the breast tissue was not malignant. The hospital records seldom mention frozen section during surgery. One may assume thus that Addenbrooke's Hospital's surgeons often made their decisions on the basis of clinical data and gross anatomy of the breast:

A 45-year-old woman came to Addenbrooke's Hospital in January 1937, complaining of pain in the breast & lumps. The breast was removed surgically. Pathology report states: "this breast shows fairly regular hyperplasia of columnar epithelium several layers deep, with duct like channels lined by these cells. I think that it is innocent and adenomatous only.[78]

In some cases, cystic mastitis was treated by radical mastectomy, especially when the patient had enlarged axillary lymph nodes, a symptom that is not infrequent in a chronic inflammation. Occasionally the pathologist seemed to be displeased by an unnecessary radical surgery:

A 56-year-old woman came to Addenbrooke's Hospital in January 1942, with a small lump in right breast, discovered 7 weeks ago. She underwent a radical mastectomy [made by Mr. Ghey]. Pathology report states: "The breast tissue appears to consist of fat only. The gland appears to show no carcinoma. *Will Mr. Ghey please see me about this section?*"[79]

In other cases the opposite was true: a surgeon decided, on the basis of gross anatomy of the lesion, to perform a conservative surgery, while the pathologist contested the wisdom of this decision in spite of the fact that the lesion was not invasive:

A 60-year-old woman came to Addenbrooke's hospital in July 1942 with lump in the left breast, present for 10 months. Clinical examination displayed a small hard lump, attached to the skin, not attached to deep fascia, and a dimpling of the breast [usual clinical signs of malignancy]. Surgery: local excision of the lump. On a naked eye account it was cystic, with an area of mastitis around. Sent lump for pathological report. Pathology: "this section shows duct like spaces filled with papilliforous gland-cell proliferation. The hyperplasia is regular, and there is no evidence of transgression of the basement membrane, but the cells are deeply stained and rather atypical and suggest potential malignancy." The patient was discharged five days after hospitalization.[80]

In the late 1940s, surgeons of the Addenbrooke's Hospital continued to view chronic mastitis as a lesion that increased the possibility of developing breast malignancy:

A 47-year-old woman came to Addenbrooke's Hospital in September 1947 with a lump in the left breast. A segment of the breast was removed. Pathology report states: "mammary dysplasia, adenosis type [i.e., "chronic cystic mastitis"]. This is the type of mastitis which is associated with an increased liability to carcinoma, but I have not seen evidence of malignancy in these sections."[81]

The decision to surgically remove a mastitis-harboring breast was sometimes presented as self-evident:

A 51-year-old woman came to Addenbrooke's hospital in July, 1947. She noticed a lump in the breast 3 weeks ago, and also had palpable glands. During the surgery, the breast was removed as well as suspicious glands. Frozen section found no malignancy, only chronic mastitis. Letter from her surgeon, Mr. Ghey to her physician: "the microscopic report following simple mastectomy for this patient who had a vague mass in the breast associated with hard axillary glands shows chronic mastitis only. There was no sign of any malignant disease in the breast, nor in axillary nodes."[82]

In another case, a simple mastectomy for cystic mastitis was justified by cosmetic considerations:

A 46-year-old woman came to Addenbrooke's Hospital in July 1947 with a lump in the breast. The surgeon first performed a lumpectomy; the lump was examined macroscopically and microscopically and was found benign. The surgeon then proceeded with a simple mastectomy. Pathology report states: "mammary dysplasia [mastodynia type], with some features of adenosis. Some of the lobules are larger than normal, but on the whole there is relatively little evidence of epithelial hyperplasia. Some of the small cysts are lined by cubical epithelium, others by epithelium of the sweat gland type. No evidence of malignancy." In a letter to the patient's physician, her surgeon explains: "you will remember that we were a little unhappy about the lump in her left breast. A frozen section was done to this, and I'm happy to say that this proved to be chronic mastitis and nothing worse. In view of the fact that she had such a small breast we felt that a simple mastectomy would be advisable, and this was done."[83]

After the Second World War, Addenbrooke's doctors stressed the importance of surveillance of women with potentially dangerous changes in their breast:

A 66-year-old woman came to Addenbrooke's hospital in November 1947 complaining about a discharge from the breast. A lump removed from her breast was found benign on frozen section. Letter from the surgeon Mr. Ghey to her physician, states: "I explored this patient's right breast from which the blood stained discharge has been coming and found that there were many dilated ducts containing old blood, but there was no any sign of neoplasm. In view of this, the affected sector of the breast has been excised, and on microscopic examination the pathologist is unable to find any definite evidence of malignant disease. *In view of her age and the nature of her condition, I think that it would be as well that she should see me again in the outpatient department from time to time, as I think that the condition may be a premalignant one.*[84]

Mr. Ghey gave very similar advice to a much younger woman:

A 31-year-old woman was seen at Addenbrooke's Hospital in April, 1947, with a lump in her breast. The lump was excised by Mr. Ghey and examined by frozen section. Pathologist's report affirms: "mammary dysplasia, adenosis type, with much epithelial hyperplasia and multiple intra cystic papillomata. I see no definite evidence of malignancy, but this type of lesion is regarded by many as precancerous; and the degree of hyperplasia is rather disquieting." Letter from Ghey to the patient's doctors explains: "I removed the nodule from the lower margins of this patient's left breast. The pathologist's report states that this is a condition of chronic mastitis with considerable capillary hyperplasia. *This is certainly an innocent condition at present, but is one which the pathologist con-*

siders might become malignant, so that she should be followed up from time to time in the outpatient department."[85]

In the late 1940s surgeons at Addenbrooke's Hospital incorporated the surveillance of suspicious proliferative conditions of the breast into strategies of dealing with these conditions. In the1930s, a benign breast lesion was treated as a unique event and the physician's task was to react to this event. The approach developed in the hospital in the 1940s was focused on the dynamics of growth of proliferative breast lesions, on the long-term danger represented by such lesions, and on the management of danger-harboring bodies.

Proliferative Lesions of the Breast in Paris

Curie Foundation surgeons Jean-Louis Roux-Berger and André Tailhefer were strongly committed to radical—and sometimes ultraradical—mastectomy for a confirmed cancer of the breast. They were, however less keen to amputate breasts with nonmalignant lesions. Roux-Berger and Tailhefer did not view simple mastectomy as a desirable option. If the patient suffered from cancer, for them the only acceptable solution was a "complete operation," and any lesser surgery was equal to a criminal neglect. If the growth was benign, a mutilating operation was useless. For Roux-Berger and Tailhefer borderline lesions presented the main difficulty. In one such case, the therapeutic decision was grounded in observation of the tumor's physiology, rather than its morphology:

A 33-year-old woman suffered for two years from intermittent secretion of liquid from the nipple, then noted the presence of a hard lump in her breast. Her physician reassured her that this was a benign cyst. The tumor increased rapidly in volume, and became painful; she also suffered from pain in the arm. Dr. Tailhefer, diagnosed (tentatively) a potentially malignant intracanalicular tumor, and proposed an x-ray treatment followed by a radical breast surgery. The patient's doctor was informed that her prognosis was reserved, mainly because of her young age. The x-ray therapy induced an extended radiodermitis, but the size of the tumor remained stable. This was seen as a good sign: malignant tumors are radiosensitive, while benign cysts are not. Dr. Tailhefer decided then to excise the tumor alone. The histological diagnosis confirmed that the tumor—fibro adenoma with intracanalicular proliferation—was not malignant, and her doctor was reassured that the outlook was in fact very good.

The patient did not come for follow up visits, but one of her nurses met her accidentally two years later; she was in excellent health.[86]

In a different case, the woman diagnosed with a borderline tumor underwent a conservative surgery. She developed then several other tumors of the breast (presumably benign or borderline) and was treated with surgery and radiotherapy. The treatment was a success but she suffered from permanent side effects of radiation.

A 52-year-old woman, Mrs. B came for the first time to Curie Institute in May 1947. She was diagnosed with a small benign and well encapsulated tumor of the left breast [fibroadenoma]. Treated by lumpectomy, she failed to appear for control tests. In November 1948, she came back to the Curie Foundation with two tumors in the emplacement of the previous one and a suspicious lymph node. X-ray examination does not reveal metastasis. Clinically the tumors seem benign, but the rapidity of their growth is suspicious of malignancy. They were excised with large margins, and the pathologist decided that this was not a recurrence of a previously eliminated tumor but a different growth, a moderately malignant papillary epithelioma. It was treated by X-ray radiation. Two years later, the patient developed another small tumor in her right breast. The tumor was excised and found to be benign. In 1954, six years after her original radiotherapy, she developed severe signs of late post-radiation reaction: necrosis of the skin in irradiated zones of the breast, edema of left arm and a chronic pain. Questioned about her health in August 1968, she reported: "my present health status: monoplegia of the left arm, a consequence of radiotherapy of the left breast. This monoplegia is a source of constant suffering." The patient died in 1979 at the age of 84.[87]

This was not an isolated case. The routine treatment of benign breast conditions at the Curie Foundation in the 1930s was a local excision of the tumor, and, if the lesion was a diffused one, x-ray radiation. The latter therapy induced occasionally iatrogenic complications such as chronic pain or purulent ulceration of the breast.[88]

Another woman was initially diagnosed with a benign tumor of the breast, then her tumor was reclassified as probably malignant following a new development:

A woman was diagnosed in May 1939 with a breast tumor seen as benign. The tumor was excised, analyzed in pathology laboratory and diagnosed as cystic adenofibroma. She then developed an enlarged lymph node. A cytological analysis of this node revealed suspicious epitheloid cells. Her doctors then decided to perform radical mastectomy.[89]

It is reasonable to assume that in the latter case the choice to perform a radical mastectomy stemmed from the supposition that the quasi-simultaneous presence of a breast tumor and suspicious cells in the axillary lymph node was probably not a coincidence and was too evocative of the possibility of malignancy to be ignored. While the final decision was grounded in a cytological analysis, its ultimate logic was a clinical one: the reading of signs displayed by the body. By the late 1930s, French doctors usually reacted to an already existing disease rather than to a danger of such a disease.

Management of Cystic Mastitis: Alternative Solutions

The therapeutic options following a diagnosis of chronic cystic mastitis were prophylactic mastectomy or the excision of the cyst only. In the interwar era, many experts favored the first solution, especially when dealing with "lumpy" breasts. Faced with the reluctance of women to lose a breast following a diagnosis of cystic mastitis, some doctors attempted to develop alternative therapeutic solutions. Two such solutions were proposed in the interwar era: hormonal manipulation and irradiation of the cyst-containing breast. Dr. Howard Taylor, from Memorial Hospital in New York, pointed out similarities between the endometrium (the lining of the uterus) and the breast. It is well known that the proliferation of endometrium is stimulated by female sex hormones secreted by the ovary, and he argued that the same was probably true for breast tissue. Taylor proposed therefore in 1930 to treat cystic mastitis by irradiation of ovaries, a treatment that would put an end to the secretion of hormones by these glands. Such approach "was considered to be rational because of certain apparent similarities in the nature of endometrial hyperplasia and the diffuse hyperplastic processes in the breast, and because of the beneficial effect of ovarian irradiation on the endometrial condition." He described a case of a "colored female of 37 years" who underwent an incomplete hysterectomy: her uterus was removed but her ovaries remained in place. The patient developed cystic mastitis three years later, cured by an irradiation of her ovaries.[90]

British surgeon and cancer expert Sampson Handley proposed in 1936 an x-ray treatment of cystic mastitis. Handley was persuaded that a chronic cystic mastitis is a precancerous lesion, but he was also aware of women's reluctance to undergo mastectomy for this condition. The irradiation of the affected breast provided a less drastic therapeutic alternative. He started to apply this therapy as early as 1910 and claimed that he treated several hundreds of women. Alas, the results of these early attempts were problematic. Several women developed breast cancer, possibly as a side effect of radiation. Handley returned to his attempts to cure mastitis with radiation in the 1930s, this time employing better controlled radiation sources. He claimed that he obtained excellent results: the mastitis disappeared, while none of the treated women developed breast malignancy. Handley was persuaded that, when given in low doses and under well-controlled conditions, radiation of the breast is harmless and can even be used to prevent cancer in the general population. He was aware of the fact that his colleagues did not share his enthusiasm for a prophylactic x-ray treatment and were reluctant to irradiate breasts of healthy women. It is quite reasonable, however, he argued, to propose such preventive treatment to women who have higher than average chances of developing breast cancer: "a preventive course of X-rays to both breasts is in any rate harmless, and should certainly be given when the breast has done its work to all the women with a strong family history of cancer, or suffering from chronic mastitis."[91]

Doctors who discussed treatment of chronic cystic mastitis assumed that this condition increased the chances of developing breast cancer. But how accurate was this supposition? The evolution of Joseph Colt Bloodgood's opinion on cystic mastitis illustrates the changing perception of its danger. In 1906 Bloodgood uncritically adopted Schimmelbusch's definition of the "small cyst variant" of chronic mastitis as a precancerous condition.[92] He changed his mind in 1921, when he noted that untreated patients with this condition did not develop breast malignancies. Nevertheless at that time he still affirmed that, facing a borderline proliferative condition of the breast, the surgeon should avoid above all "a mistake that should not be made," that is, the classification of a malignant growth as a benign cyst. It is preferable to make the opposite mistake and to classify a benign growth as malignant, since such a mistake, "produces no harm but mutilation."[93]

In the 1930s, Bloodgood further radicalized his opposition to mastectomy for cystic mastitis. This move paralleled his growing support for a systematic use of frozen sections during breast operations to prevent unnecessary mastectomies.[94] In his 1934 comments on the history of chronic cystic mastitis, Bloodgood explained that initially radical surgery for cystic mastitis was motivated by the fear of missing a true malignancy and the belief that cystic mastitis is somehow linked with breast cancer. Such opinion guided Halsted's, Schimmelbusch's, and his own clinical decisions. In retrospect, Bloodgood concluded that this fear was grounded in mistaken premises and faulty observations: "we failed to confirm our diagnosis of malignancy by a follow up of the ultimate results."[95] Radical mastectomy for invasive tumors, even small, was an imperfect treatment. In spite of the most careful dissection, many patients had had a recurrence of their tumor. Whereas women operated on for chronic cystic mastitis practically never experienced regional recurrence or distant metastases. This observation might have led to a belief that surgical removal of a presumed precancerous lesion was an especially efficient therapeutic approach. Bloodgood arrived at the opposite conclusion. A condition that never spread to lymph nodes or produced metastases cannot be a true cancer. The women operated on did not develop complications because they were never sick in the first place. Bloodgood decided thus that an extensive surgery to confirm cystic mastitis was unnecessary. Sadly, he added, other experts are still at the point where he was nearly thirty years ago: they fail to notice that women with this condition do not have an increased tendency to develop breast malignancies.[96]

Writing his comments on cystic mastitis in 1934, Bloodgood was aware of the fact that many specialists disagreed with his views and favored radical surgical options.[97] His view was vindicated later. The diagnosis of chronic cystic mastitis became less frequent in the 1940s and became rare from the 1950s on, as were mastectomies for this pathology. In the post–World War II era, chronic cystic mastitis quietly disappeared from the list of precancerous lesions of the breast. It was primarily replaced by in situ ductal and lobular carcinoma but also by ductal hyperplasia and atypia. The shifting definition of what a dangerous lesion of the breast was did not eliminate, however, the core problem identified by Bloodgood: the need to ground therapeutic decisions about premalignant lesions in solid epidemiological data. Specialists agreed that, in principle, this should be the case, but their practices continued to be guided by the wish to excise dangerous body parts. The switch to diagnosis of in situ cancer increased the distance between a lived and a "biomedical" disease. Women diagnosed with cystic mastitis usually consulted a doctor because they had painful, swollen, "lumpy" breasts, and, some at least, because they feared that these symptoms revealed the presence of a malignant tumor. Women diagnosed with an in situ carcinoma of the breast usually did not have any distressing symptoms and developed such symptoms only as a result of a preventive treatment. The unproblematic acceptance of painful and sometimes mutilating treatment by asymptomatic women attests to the success of the principle of prophylactic elimination of precancerous lesions.

CHAPTER FOUR

In Situ Cancers

Proliferative Lesions of the Cervix before the Era of Mass Screening

In the second half of the twentieth century, "carcinoma in situ" became the most visible and most often debated precancerous lesion. The term *carcinoma in situ* describes a cluster of cells that, when examined under the microscope, look exactly like cancer cells but do not invade surrounding tissues. In situ cancerlike lesions were first observed in cervical malignancies. Gynecologists who detected such lesions viewed them at first as a rare phenomenon. From the 1940s on, the efforts to screen healthy women for the presence of cervical malignancies led, however, to frequent diagnoses of such lesions and to dilemmas linked with these diagnoses. Observations made on cervical tumors were then transposed to the breast. Again, initially the diagnosis of in situ proliferative lesions of the breast was a rare event, but the introduction of mass screening for breast malignancies led to rapid increase of diagnoses of carcinoma in situ of the breast and to a need to deal with these problematic diagnoses.

The first instrument that allowed physicians to look directly on the cervix—the speculum—was developed in the early nineteenth century. Gynecologists equipped with a speculum were able to perform cervical biopsies. Pathologists who studied such biopsies occasionally uncovered superficial (that is, noninvasive) proliferative lesions of the cervix. Probably the first description of such a lesion was made by British professor of midwifery John Williams in 1886. In his Harveian Lectures on uterine cancer, Williams described a superficial lesion of the cervix: "This is the earliest condition of undoubted cancer of the portio vaginalis which I have met with, and it is the earliest condition which is recognizable as cancer. It presented no distinctive symptoms, and was discovered accidentally; its nature was not recognized with certainty, but it was held in suspicion."[1] In early twentieth century, several authors (W. Schausenstein, K. Pronai, I. C. Rubin) defined these lesions as "surface carcinoma" and as the earliest stage of squamous carcinoma of the cervix.[2] Surgeons encountered such lesions in a routine clinical practice:

A 52-year-old cook was admitted to New York Hospital in September, 1920. Her main complaint was back pain and occasional abdominal pain. She did not have abnormal vaginal bleeding, only a heavier period, seen by her as related to a "change of life." An exploratory surgery revealed a diffuse growth in the uterus. Frozen section of the cervix had indicated that the macroscopically opaque area was covered with atypical epithelium that is sharply marked off from normal epithelium. The growth was, however, confined to the surface only and did not invade deep structures of the cervix. The pathologist concluded that further sections were necessary to decide whether this was an early carcinoma or a precancer. The patient underwent a complete hysterectomy. Paraffin sections of the cervix displayed the same condition as the frozen sections, but one or two places showed the beginning invasion, strongly suggesting a very early carcinoma.[3]

Curie Foundation files of cervical tumors from the 1920s, which contain data about more than a thousand people, describe two such cases, an indirect indication of the rarity of these observations:

Patient no. 629, first seen in May 1926, histological diagnosis was "a probable epithelioma of the cervix, a very early stage." Ulterior classification of the case, made in 1936, when results of radium therapy were prepared for a publication, was "stage I." She was treated successfully with radiumtherapy and hysterectomy, and remained healthy (last report from 1939).

Patient no. 766, first seen in November 1927, diagnosed with ulcerations of the cervix. Histological diagnosis was "hyperplasia of the cervical epithelium." The ulterior 1936 classification of the case, was "stage I"—after hesitation. The notes in the cervical cancer notebook first state "stage 0" with a question mark, then "stage 0" was crossed over, replaced by stage I. The patient was treated with radium and did well. She died in 1950 at the age of 78.[4]

In the 1930s, Viennese gynecologist Walter Schiller became interested in the superficial proliferative lesions of the cervix. He was the first to follow the devel-

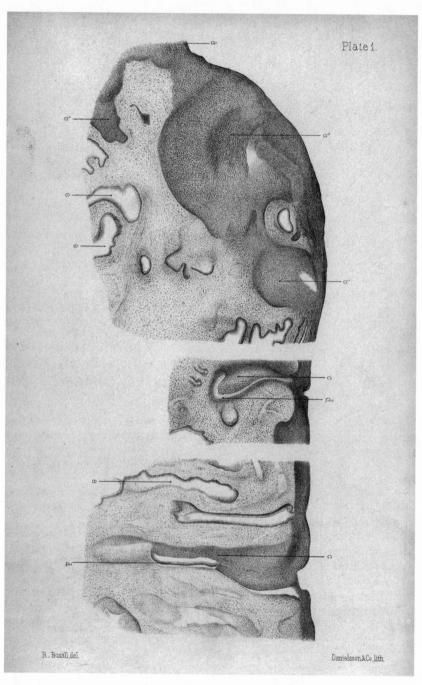

The first image of in situ cancer of the cervix, which was drawn in the late 1880s.
John Williams, *On Cancer of the Uterus* (London: HK Lewis, 1888), plate I.

opment of such lesions over time. Serial biopsies from the same person displayed several stages of transition from a normal epithelium to a malignant one. Observation of such intermediary stages, Schiller argued, proves that pre-invasive lesions of the cervix were true precursors of malignant tumors. Carcinogenesis (the development of a malignant tumor) is analogous to embryogenesis (the development of an embryo). A few-day-old embryo of an animal looks very different from a newborn animal. Scientists are nevertheless fully confident that the embryo is an early stage of development of the newborn, because they possess complete series of intermediary stages of the embryo's intrauterine development. An identical comparative method can be applied to the study of natural history of malignant growths.[5] Schiller was persuaded that his series of slides demonstrated without any possible doubt that superficial lesions of the cervix are very early stages of cervical cancer. He proposed therefore to call these changes "young carcinoma" and strongly rejected the argument that the word "carcinoma" should be reserved for invasive lesions only: "The objection that the carcinomatous layer is not carcinoma because it does not penetrate deeply is equivalent to saying that the embryo of a mouse has not the characteristics of a mouse because the embryo does not breathe through his lungs as a grownup mouse does. . . . We do not speak about 'prehuman' embryo but a 'human' embryo, and I believe that the same thing applies to cancer: there is a 'carcinomatous' layer, but not a 'precancerous' layer."[6]

The dynamic vocabulary employed by Schiller in his descriptions of superficial lesions of the cervix accentuated the presumed capacity of these lesions to become invasive: "early carcinoma of the cervix consisting of a larger superficial layer and two small projections that *dip deeply* into regions of the external bone with strong inflammatory infiltration of the surrounding tissue"; "a beginning carcinoma consisting of an extended superficial layer which *has penetrated deeply* in one place only"; "a carcinomatous layer of tissue which was found *penetrating* into the long side of a gland"; "a carcinomatous layer with large, plump plugs *rowing towards* the cervical glands."[7]

Faithful to radical surgical solutions advocated by Austrian and German surgeons, Schiller affirmed that the only acceptable treatment for a "young carcinoma" was a radical hysterectomy by Wertheim's method, followed by radiotherapy. Using this approach, he achieved a complete cure in 90 to 95 percent of the cases.[8] Not all the gynecologists adopted Schiller's point of view. Some were not persuaded that superficial proliferative lesions of the cervix were indeed early stages of a carcinoma. They proposed a more conservative treatment of such lesions: either a local removal of zones of proliferation or the amputation of the cervix alone, without hysterectomy.[9] The observation that some of the women who underwent conservative surgery developed invasive cervical tumors, however, led to a change of policy and to a wider adoption of an aggressive treatment of superficial lesions of the cervix. In the 1940s the majority of the specialists believed that such lesions should be treated by hysterectomy, with or without radiation.[10]

Pap Smear and Carcinoma In Situ of the Cervix

A cancer is, by definition, an invasive lesion. Carcinoma is a tumor derived from epithelial cells (like those of the skin or lining of the body's cavities) that has acquired the capacity to cross the basal membrane that separates the epithelium from other tissues. In the absence of such capacity, a lesion theoretically should not be called carcinoma. From a strictly logical point of view, the term *carcinoma in situ* can be viewed as an oxymoron. Nevertheless, this term was coined in the 1930s to stress the close relationship between invasive and noninvasive lesions. Experts believed at first that in situ cancers were an unusual and presumably rare phenomenon, a pathological curiosity rather than a clinical problem.[11] The development of new diagnostic approaches—the Pap test for the detection of cervical cancer and then mammographic screening for the detection of breast malignancies—greatly increased the frequency of the observation of cancerlike noninvasive lesions. At the same time, the desire to promote an early diagnosis of cancer probably favored the choice of the emotionally charged term "carcinoma" to describe these lesions. The adoption of this term had in turn a practical consequence: a growing identification of noninvasive cancerlike lesions with carcinoma per se.[12]

Carcinoma in situ was first coined to describe proliferative changes in the breast. In the interwar era debates on precancerous lesions were focused on borderline breast lesions. However, in the 1940s and 1950s, the focus of such debates shifted to cervical cancer. Summing up in 1952 controversies on the treatment of carcinoma of the cervix, New York cancer expert Howard Taylor nostalgically remembered the not-so-distant past when this issue brought much more agreement. Thanks to the activity of the League of Nations Commission of Cancer in Europe and parallel efforts of the Cancer Campaign Committee (the precursor of the Committee on Cancer, or COC) in the United States, "the principles of treatment were widely agreed upon, and the chief effort seemed to be towards the raising of general therapeutic performance rather than towards the discovery or the testing of new methods." Sadly, this harmonious edifice was shattered in the

1940s "as a result this formerly most standardized area in cancer therapy is now perhaps the most controversial."[13]

The unraveling of the solid consensus around cervical cancer, Taylor proposed, started with the contestation of criteria of histological diagnosis of this disease, a development directly related to the diffusion of a new diagnostic test for cervical cancer, the Pap smear. Named after the physician who developed it, New York pathologist Dr. George Nicholas Papanicolaou (1883–1962), this test initially aimed at improving the diagnosis of confirmed cancers. Papanicolaou had a double training, in medicine and in zoology. He first developed vaginal smears to study cyclic changes in female laboratory animals, an approach rapidly adopted by numerous researchers in reproductive biology and endocrinology.[14] Papanicolaou then extended his method to study changes induced by the sexual cycle in women (in his words, the "human female") and called it "exfoliate cytology."[15]

Papanicolaou's first report on the possible correlation between the presence of abnormal cells in a vaginal smear and the presence of cervical malignancy was made in a 1928, at the Third Race Betterment Conference in Battle Creek, Michigan.[16] In this paper he explained that when he tried to extend the method of detecting hormonal changes from animals to women he had found that "unfortunately, the organ in the woman is a little more complex than it is in most other mammals, especially in rodents." To study changes induced by the hormonal cycle in women's vaginas Papanicolaou was obliged to familiarize himself with gynecological diseases. During this process he noticed that vaginal smears from women with cervical malignancies contained abnormal cells and numerous leucocytes and that such abnormal cells were found only in women with cervical malignancies: "in a case of a benign tumor, everything you find in a vaginal smear is more or less normal." Papanicolaou's 1928 report, "New Cancer Diagnosis" was not well received, partly because it was based on the observation of a small number of cases. He improved his method in the 1930s, and in 1941 he published, together with gynecologist Herbert Frederick Traut, another description of his diagnostic approach, this time grounded in a study of a greater number of women.[17] Papanicolaou attempted to extend the use of exfoliate cytology to the diagnosis of other malignant tumors, such as cancers of the respiratory, urinary, and gastrointestinal systems.[18]

The Pap smear was rapidly adopted by gynecologists. The Boston City Hospital opened in 1947 a clinic for an early detection of cervical cancer: "all the departments of the hospital have been requested to refer as many women over thirty five years of age as possible to the Gynecological Clinics for 'screening.'" This was probably the first use of the term *screening* in this context. Women with suspicious vaginal smears were subjected to a biopsy by curettage, a cervical biopsy, or both. In many cases this method led to a diagnosis of previously unsuspected malignancies. At first, the sole aim of exfoliate cytology was the detection of invasive carcinoma.[19] With the generalization of this method, many women who underwent biopsy following an abnormal Pap smear were diagnosed with either well-defined pre-invasive cervical lesions (carcinoma in situ) or less pronounced proliferative changes (dysplasia). Both diagnoses were problematic, because experts were not sure what the status of such lesions was.[20] Some viewed them as irreversible developments that always led to malignancy; others believed that some lesions might stabilize, or even disappear.[21]

In spite of these differences, in the 1940s the majority of the gynecologists favored radical therapies of noninvasive cervical lesions. They assumed that even if some of these lesions grew so slowly that they would never produce invasive cancers in the woman's lifetime, it was safer to view them as true malignancies and treat them accordingly.[22] In 1950, Randolph Hoge from the Medical College of Virginia mailed a questionnaire about the treatment of carcinoma in situ of the cervix to seventy-nine approved medical schools in the United States and in Canada. Seventy-seven schools answered this questionnaire. In two medical schools, gynecologists treated this pathology exclusively by excision of suspected lesions by cone biopsy (conization) and in one by the amputation of the cervix. Gynecologists in twelve additional medical schools occasionally provided a conservative surgery, especially if the person to be operated on was young. The overwhelming majority of the experts were, however, favorable to hysterectomy. Hoge concluded that "the present consensus is that total hysterectomy with a conservation of the ovarian function in the younger woman is the treatment of choice."[23]

A year later Carl Henry Davis from Miami mailed a more detailed questionnaire on the same subject to 160 American gynecologists and pathologists and collected seventy answers. The results of this survey were similar. The great majority of the surveyed experts viewed "cancer in situ" as a pre-invasive stage of a genuine cancer, and a slightly smaller but still considerable majority believed that this lesion was unable to regress spontaneously. Accordingly, only four gynecologists saw a local treatment—electroconization and coagulation or cervical amputation—as adequate. All the other specialists were persuaded that the only safe therapy was a simple or radical hysterectomy (for a small minority, followed by radiotherapy). When the cervical lesion was found in very young women, and especially in pregnant ones, some gynecologists were willing to consider a more

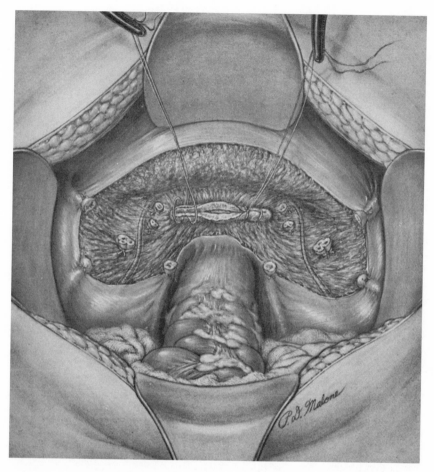

A drawing showing the method of performing a hysterectomy for in situ cancer of the cervix. Joe V. Meigs, ed., *Surgical Treatment of Cancer of the Cervix* (New York: Grune & Stratton, 1954), 135.

conservative treatment, but this option was seen as a pragmatic compromise, not as an optimal solution. During a discussion that followed the presentation of these data at the annual meeting of the American Gynecological Society in 1952, only one specialist, Dr. T. C. Peightal from New York, was explicitly opposed to a routine treatment of pre-invasive cervical cancer by hysterectomy. Conization biopsy, Peightal argued, is at the same time a diagnostic and a curative tool. In the absence of malignancy, such biopsy is usually sufficient to definitively eliminate a cervical lesion. All the other specialists viewed hysterectomy as the only safe therapeutic solution.[24]

Dilemmas of Treatment of In Situ Cervical Lesions

Clinical results strengthened the U.S. experts' conviction that radical elimination of a premalignant lesion is the best way to produce a cure. Practically all the women diagnosed with "stage 0" carcinoma of the cervix in the early 1950s and treated by hysterectomy remained cancer free. Some specialists contested nevertheless the principle of a similar treatment for noninvasive and invasive cancers. French gynecologists were more often disinclined to perform hysterectomies for premalignant lesions of the cervix than were their Central European or North American colleagues, an attitude that was probably related to a more general reluctance to excise female reproductive organs. One possible reason might have been French gynecologists' support of pronatalist policy and unwillingness to sterilize fertile women. Another might have been the conviction that a skilled gynecologist is able to propose specific cure, not merely remove diseased body parts.[25] It is not at all certain, Georges Gricouroff argued, that all or even the majority of such lesions will became malignant in the future.[26] His colleague at the Curie Foundation, Antoine Lacassagne, was even more categorical. He refused to recognize the notion of "carcinoma in situ": "It is not possible to affirm, when confronted with epithelial hyperplasia or dysplasia, that this epithelium did or did not became cancerous, in the absence of an invasion of neighboring tissues . . . in the absence of invasion of the chorion, it is impossible to make a definitive statement on the nature of this epithelium."[27] For Lacassagne, either one deals with a cancer or with something else, and the decisive criterion that defines a lesion as a cancer is its ability to transgress the basal membrane and invade other tissues.

The director of the Radium Centre, Copenhagen, Jens Nielsen, shared this opinion. In 1943, he explained that: "in clinical practice, precancerosis is a disagreeable concept. It involves only two possibilities, either (1) to be treated as cancer or (2) to be followed without treatment. So long as we lack well-founded and comprehensive data as to how often, with how long a latent period and in what manner the so called precanceroses became frank cancer, we must be reserved in our therapeutic efforts, restricting them mainly to a conservative follow up."[28]

In order to provide such "well founded and comprehensive data," Nielsen initiated a prospective clinical study of the development of precancerous lesions of the cervix.[29] The study was conducted by Dr. Olaf Petersen and was financed by the Danish Anti-Cancer League. Petersen identified 212 women diagnosed with an epithelial hyperplasia with nuclear abnormalities. Nearly all these women came to the Radium Centre clinics with gynecological complaints, and 71 percent bled outside menstrual periods (metrorrhagia). All underwent cervical biopsies and were diagnosed with precancerous conditions. Eighty-five of these women— mainly those diagnosed with borderline malignancies—underwent a treatment, usually a radical one—radiumtherapy (sixty-six) or hysterectomy (eight); eleven women underwent a conservative therapy, either deep conical electroexcision or the amputation of the cervix. One hundred twenty-seven women were left untreated, but underwent an annual gynecological and clinical examination and a cervical biopsy. People were not randomly distributed between the untreated and the treated group. Petersen's publication does not explain on which basis women were allocated to each group and does not mention consent for participation in this trial. The majority of the women were recruited circa 1943 and observed for ten years. A few women who belonged to an earlier group were diagnosed in the mid-1930s and were studied for more than fifteen years. A few additional participants were recruited later and observed for at least five years. Petersen's study ended in 1953.

Thirty-four of the 127 untreated individuals selected for this study developed invasive cancer of the cervix (33 percent). The frequency of malignancies increased with time.[30] Most of the diagnosed tumors were stage I or II, but some women developed stage III and IV tumors in spite of annual checks. The latter finding indicated that a stagnation or a slow development of pre-invasive lesions does not determine an equally slow development of a malignancy. The lesions of many other women in this group remained stable or regressed. After three years, thirteen women in the untreated group developed cancers, while all those in the treated group remained cancer free. The clinical experiment continued however. After five years there were twenty-two cancers among the untreated women and one case among the treated ones. In spite of the great number of malignancies, the observation of the untreated group continued for an additional four years, in which twelve more women in the untreated group (and none in the treated group) developed cervical cancer.[31]

The single case of carcinoma among the eighty-five treated women was retrospectively attributed to a probable presence of invasive cancer at the moment of diagnosis, because this woman had clinical signs of carcinoma that were not confirmed cytologically. Treated by radiotherapy, she was healthy for five years. She then developed localized cervical malignancy and was again treated successfully with radiation.[32] There were no other cases of malignancy in the treated group. However, radical treatment of noninvasive cervical lesions was far from innocuous. Two of the eight women who underwent radical hysterectomy died from complications of this operation, and six among the sixty-six women treated with radium experienced severe side effects of this therapy; one remained permanently incapacitated. Among the thirty-four individuals who developed cancer in the untreated group, five died of the disease, and one was alive in 1953 with a metastatic tumor; others went into a remission after treatment.[33] The average latency period between the diagnosis of symptomatic noninvasive cervical lesions and the development of an invasive tumor was 3.4 years for stage I cancer and five years for more advanced cancers. Peterson's main conclusion was that the treatment of such lesions was not an emergency. When a woman who complains about irregular bleeding or other gynecological problems is diagnosed with a noninvasive cervical lesion, there is no need to make hasty decisions. She can be safely observed for a year at least. During this period she should be examined at short intervals to see if her lesions regress or progress before deciding which treatment will suit her best.[34]

In the 1950s, oncologists grappled with the clinical meaning of carcinoma in situ in different anatomical sites. Preparing in 1959 his teachings at the University of California Medical Center, San Francisco, a young radiologist, Frantz Bushke, became concerned about the status of carcinoma in situ of the larynx. He wrote to known experts in his area—Lederman, Lampe, Winyarder, Stout, Altman, and Baclesse—asking for their opinion; he concluded that the consensus seemed to be that for practical purposes carcinoma in situ of the larynx should be viewed as a very early stage of a true carcinoma. He added that this does not seem to be the case for in situ carcinoma of the cervix: "the latter appears in average in patients ten years younger than carcinoma patients, while the age of patients with in situ carcinoma of the larynx is the same as the age of patients with infiltrating carcinoma."[35] Experts generally agreed that the in situ proliferative changes of the cervix were true precursors of a malignant transformation, but they were not sure in what percentage of cases such transformation took place. A 1962 volume summarized the available data on these lesions:

1. It is actually a cancer, even though it may lack one of the conventional hallmarks of the disease, i.e., invasiveness.
2. Some—but by no means all—carcinoma in situ lesions may progress to become invasive cancer. Estimates vary widely.
3. Most, if not all, invasive cancers go through an early phase of carcinoma in situ.
4. Contrary to expectation, the time that it takes for the average lesions to progress from carcinoma in situ to invasive cancer is quite long.
5. Although in situ lesions may progress to invasion, they may remain stationary, regress or disappear spontaneously.

6. There is no precise way of separating the indolent from the potentially aggressive lesion.[36]

The last of these statements—the most important from a practical point of view—was grounded in long-term prospective follow-up of women with cervical lesions and in retrospective examination of cervical biopsies of women who later developed cancer.

Leopold Koss and his colleagues at Albert Einstein College of Medicine, New York, followed the evolution of cervical lesions in untreated women. They attempted in parallel to correlate cytological diagnoses—mild, intermediary, or severe dysplasia—and outcomes—that is, aggravation and progression to cancer versus stagnation or regression. Such attempts failed: they were unable to uncover stable correlations between a morphology of a lesion and its fate. Petersen's study had already indicated that the behavior of cervical lesions was erratic and unpredictable and that lesions that looked remarkably similar could have very different long-term outcomes. Observations made by Koss and his colleagues confirmed that some mild-looking lesions suddenly changed their pattern of growth and became more aggressive, while some aggressive-looking lesions became less aggressive with time. In one especially telling case, a cervical lesion showed a distinct pattern of decrease of abnormalities for four years, then half a year later, the patient developed an invasive carcinoma in the same site: "the last case is of utmost importance in demonstrating that the level of epithelial abnormality may be of no prognostic significance."[37] The authors concluded that "the belief that there is a correlation between the aggressiveness of carcinoma in situ and the degree of surface differentiation has not been borne by our study. Comparing the histological patterns of persisting lesions with those of disappearing lesions failed to reveal any histological difference of prognostic value."[38]

Other researchers made similar observations. Ralph Richard from Columbia University left people with mild cervical dysplasia untreated and discovered that several of these women developed an invasive cancer. Richard concluded that each case of cervical dysplasia, however mild, was an indication for a therapeutic intervention.[39] C. Gad, from the department of gynecology and obstetrics at the Fredrikberg Hospital in Copenhagen, studied the evolution of cervical lesions in thirty women with severe dysplasia or in situ carcinoma of the cervix who did not receive any treatment (his publication does not explain why they were not treated) between 1951 and 1972. Nine of these women developed invasive carcinoma and two died. He similarly concluded that gynecologists should treat all cervical lesions, however superficial.[40]

Studies grounded in reexamination of old pathology slides led to a similar conclusion. Researchers from the department of gynecology at the Johns Hopkins Medical School identified thirteen women with cervical cancer who had undergone a cervical biopsy several years before the diagnosis of malignancy (usually because they complained of abnormal bleeding). Their biopsies were originally classified as normal. When the same biopsies were reexamined after a diagnosis of cancer, pathologists had found carcinoma in situ or dysplasia. In some individuals, cellular changes were observed many years (up to sixteen) before the diagnosis of malignancy. A few women in this sample underwent several consecutive biopsies. These biopsies documented a gradual progression from noninvasive changes to full malignancy. The authors of this study concluded that, if a cervical lesion is treated at the pre-invasive state, a person's chances of being cured are almost 100 percent. They added, however, that a retrospective investigation conducted on women who did develop a cancer does not provide data on the percentage of pre-invasive lesions that do progress to malignancy or a definitive proof that invasive lesions evolve directly from pre-invasive ones.[41]

The growing consensus about the need to intervene in each case of proliferative cervical lesions did not lead to an agreement about the nature of such an intervention. French gynecologists, faithful to a local tradition that did not favor indiscriminate removal of the uterus and the ovaries, often advocated conservative therapy for noninvasive proliferative changes in the cervix, while their North American colleagues often recommended a hysterectomy.[42] U.S. gynecologists (at that time, nearly exclusively men) had a general tendency to recommend hysterectomy with oophorectomy (the removal of the ovaries) for "female complaints" to all women who no longer considered pregnancy. This trend was legitimated, among other things, by the argument that the removal of organs they considered "useless," the uterus and the ovaries, eliminated the danger of deadly gynecological cancers.[43] When faced with a precancerous lesion—that is, an already existing and not a hypothetical danger—American experts usually recommended hysterectomy. This operation, a 1962 U.S. text explained, is the "definitive treatment" for an abnormal cytology of the cervix. A young woman who wishes to have children can be offered a more conservative therapy, but only if she is willing to accept frequent clinical examinations and repeated cervical biopsies.[44] A tradition of radicalism in gynecological surgery in German-speaking countries produced similar practices. Austrian gynecologist Erich Burghart recalled that in the 1950s "histological specimen needed only to contain the word 'carcinoma' to justify radical surgery. At many places, pre-invasive epithelia carcinomas were treated as aggressively as the most locally advanced but still operable cases"—that is, with extensive elimination not only of the uterus, but also surrounding tissues and lymph nodes.[45]

Nevertheless, in the late 1960s and 1970s, gynecologists, including those in the United States, started to advocate more conservative therapies of cervical lesions. This gradual and uneven change in practice—many gynecologists continued to advocate hysterectomies to all women with abnormal Pap smears even in the 1980s—originated in the finding that cervical lesions were very fragile. It was not possible to conduct long-term observation of the same lesion, Leopold Koss and his colleagues proposed, because a biopsy nearly always led to its definitive disappearance.[46] Or, to put it otherwise, it was not possible to find out what the fate of an individual lesion would be if left in place, but it was possible to ascertain what its fate would not be if removed—it would not became an invasive tumor. Koss and other gynecologists who made similar observations developed quasi-accidentally a conservative treatment of proliferative changes of the cervix. Around 1980, in the United States, too, conservative therapies of cervical lesions—conical biopsy, thermocoagulation, and laser therapy—became the clinical norm.[47] The growing popularity of these therapies was probably also related to the growing hostility of women to radical gynecological surgeries.[48] In the 1970s, a gradual retreat from aggressive surgical treatment of in situ cervical lesions was paralleled by the rise of a more conservative surgical treatment for breast cancer—but paradoxically not always by a conservative treatment of in situ carcinoma of the breast.

Pathologists and Breast Lesions in the 1940s and 1950s

The practice of removing cystic breasts, already criticized by some experts in the 1930s, was on the wane in the 1940s. A 1945 U.S. textbook, *Diseases of the Breast,* explains that "the incidence of mammary cancer in patients with chronic cystic mastitis is too low to warrant a mastectomy." Surgical ablation of the breast, the textbook explained, may nevertheless be considered in advanced or recurrent or proliferative changes, especially when the microscopic examination of the breast tissue is inconclusive and is unable to rule out the presence of malignancy. In such cases, doctors frequently chose the safe solution of mastectomy.[49]

In the postwar era, "chronic cystic mastitis" gradually disappeared from oncology textbooks and specialized journals.[50] In the late 1950s, precancerous lesions of the breast were still gathered under the heading "cystic hyperplasia," but pathologists did not view that condition as a distinct cytological entity, but as a composite aggregate of tissue changes, some probably linked with a transition to malignancy with others devoid of such links.[51] The main indication for a preventive ablation of suspicious breast tissue shifted to in situ breast carcinoma. This shift was slow and incremental. Many of the interwar classificatory categories of proliferative lesions of the breast remained in place after the war, and inscriptions in pathology laboratory notebooks from the 1940s and 1950s reveal more continuities than ruptures.

Descriptions of "intermediary" breast conditions in reports produced by the Pathological Institute of London Hospital for 1949 are similar to those from 1939, although they tended to be slightly shorter and to provide a definitive statement: "no malignancy" more frequently.[52] Pathologists continued to employ complex terms such as "solid trabercular and acinar, rarely tubular polygonal cells" or "lobular epithelial hyperplasia with cyst formation" and provided detailed descriptions such as "lobular and intraduct epithelial hyperplasia of the breast with considerable focal luxuriance of epithelium confined within basement membranes"; "diffuse fibrosis of breast: dilated ducts, slightly epithelial hyperplasia and perilobular chronic inflammation"; or "lobular and intraduct epithelial hyperplasia of the breast with considerable focal luxuriance of epithelium, but this confined within basement membranes." Pathology records of Addenbrooke's Hospital display similar continuities.[53] Thus in 1947 the list of borderline breast conditions diagnosed at that hospital included such items as "small cysts lined by the 'sweat gland' type of epithelium with periductal mastitis"; "hyperthrophic epithelium in which the normal two layers of the cells are often unusually conspicuous"; and "irregular and abnormal epithelium of the ducts with some giant cells."

Addenbrooke's breast pathology series ends in the late 1940s. Reports from the pathology laboratory of London Hospital from the 1950s and 1960s indicate a growing tendency to simplification and a striving for more definitive diagnosis. The concise aspect of the notes may be reinforced by the fact that from the 1950s on, records were typed by a secretary who transcribed pathologists' notes, an arrangement that probably facilitated a posteriori corrections. Descriptions of proliferative lesions of the breast became more straightforward and less often conveyed an impression of complexity and ambiguity. Typical diagnoses from 1959 include "fibrocystic hyperplasia without evidence of malignancy," "lobular and cystic hyperplasia of breast with some chronic inflammatory infiltrate around the larger cyst," "well marked fibrocystic hyperplasia with some intraduct hyperplasia," or "fibroepithelial hyperplasia with large and small cysts and some intraduct hyperplasia." Those from 1969, even more concise, contain descriptions such as "lobular and cystic hyperplasia of right breast," "fibroadenosis of right breast," "lobular and cystic hyperplasia of the breast," or "pericanular fibroadenoma and fiboradenomatosis." The shift from the vague diagnosis of cystic mastitis to the more precise one of "in situ carcinoma" probably reflected a similar trend.

In the post–World War II era, cancer experts gradually abandoned the irritation theory of carcinogenesis. They increasingly adopted the view that malignancies are induced by permanent changes in the hereditary material of the cell.[54] Such changes were attributed either to external elements, such as radiation, or to a physiological disturbance, especially a hormonal one. In the 1930s, 1940s, and 1950s, "hormones" occupied the place taken today by "genes." Scientists had hoped that hormonal manipulation of the body would open the way to the enhancement of human potential and victory over disease. Hormones were also seen as holding the key to the "mystery of cancer." The new focus on hormones favored a smooth transition between "irritation" and "mutation" theories of carcinogenesis. In the 1930s, such researchers as Alexander Haddow in Britain and Antoine Lacassagne in France induced experimental cancer of reproductive organs in laboratory animals treated with high doses of sex hormones. They pointed to structural similarities between sex hormones and known chemical carcinogens. Sex hormones, they proposed, can act as "internal irritants," and cancer may arise from a deregulation of the internal milieu and its potential carcinogenic effects.[55] In previous periods, scientists believed that mechanical blocking of the milk duct led to irritation, inflammation, and then to the development of malignancies. According to the new view, substances retained in milk ducts contained hormone-like carcinogenic agents. Their accumulation could therefore lead to malignant transformation of cells.[56] Henceforth, the key event was a malignant transformation and not chronic inflammation of the breast (mastitis), and the important observation was the presence of transformed cells.

In Situ Carcinoma of the Breast: From Pathological Curiosity to Clinical Problem

In the 1950s, debates on the links between noninvasive lesions of the cervix and cervical cancer were paralleled by those on noninvasive lesions of the breast and breast malignancies. Cervical cancer became progressively established as a model of a gradual transition from precancerous conditions to cancer and a proof of validity of cancer schemata. A 1962 textbook on early diagnosis of cancer stated that "in the earliest phase the disease consists of microscopic lesions confined to the tissue of origin. This in situ cancer may persist for a long period of time before either local invasion or distant metastasis can take place. In the case of cervix uteri, where intraepithelial carcinoma has been most extensively studied, it has been demonstrated that the pre-invasive stage may persist for many years. . . . It is possible that all cancers originating in a single tissue or organ pass through such a primary focal stage.[57]

Noninvasive breast lesions were first described by pathologists who analyzed tissues removed during a mastectomy. They occasionally found areas that contained modified, but not fully malignant, cells. With the rise in the number of breast biopsies, proliferative changes such as breast hyperplasia, atypia, lobular carcinoma in situ (LCIS), and ductal carcinoma in situ (DCIS) were also observed in intact breasts. Before the development of mammographic screening, an observation of these conditions was nearly always accidental. Typically, a woman underwent a biopsy for a suspicious lump. The lump was found to be benign, but a detailed histological analysis of the biopsy sample revealed proliferative changes in the surrounding tissue.

The first description of DCIS of the breast was made in 1932 by U.S. pathologist Albert Borders, who described "a condition in which malignant cells and their progeny are found in or near positions occupied by their ancestors before the ancestors underwent a malignant transformation." Borders described in situ lesions of the cervix and of the breast. The latter were mainly lesions of the milk duct, a condition later named ductal carcinoma in situ. Borders argued that morphological features of cells were much more important than their ability to invade adjacent tissues. Carcinoma in situ, he explained, should be carefully distinguished from invasive penetrating epithelium, a benign breast pathology associated with inflammation. His description of carcinoma in situ accentuated the fact that those were malignant cells and downplayed the lack of invasion of surrounding tissues, presented merely as a particular spatial arrangement. Borders was persuaded that morphological traits of these lesions, combined with the fact that in some slides they were observed in the immediate vicinity of foci of invasive cancer, were sufficient to classify carcinoma in situ of the breast as a true cancer and thus as an entity that represented a grave danger to the individual: "if it goes unrecognized, carcinoma is allowed to masquerade as benign or no more than a pre-carcinomatous process, with the possibility of its becoming too advanced to be amenable to treatment." The difference between a malignant and nonmalignant lesion, Borders concluded, is grounded in the nature of the cells, not in their spatial arrangement: "it is therefore imperative that the microsocopist takes into consideration the character of the epithelial cells above everything else in order to arrive at a correct diagnosis."[58]

The description of LCIS, made by Frank Foote and Fred Waldorf Stewart in

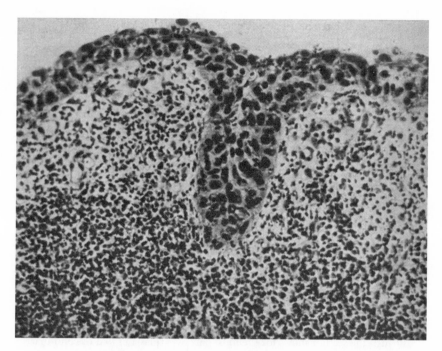

A photograph of carcinoma in situ and penetrating epithelium taken in the 1930s. Albert C. Borders, "Carcinoma in situ contrasted with benign penetrating epithelium," *Journal of the American Medical Association*, November 12, 1932, 1672. Copyright 1932 American Medical Association. All rights reserved.

1941, was similarly grounded in a careful observation of cells' morphology.[59] The condition, named "a rare form of mammary carcinoma," was, like DCIS, classified as a true malignancy on the basis of similarity between LCIS cells and those of invasive lobular carcinoma.[60] Some specialists supported the redefinition of cancer as a disease of the transformed cell. Surgeons Lenthal Cheatle and Max Cutter, authors of an important textbook on breast cancer, explained in 1931 that "cell transformation is the most important event, not the ability to invade tissues."[61] Other experts contested, however, an unproblematic identification of the disease cancer with the presence of abnormal cells. Robert Greenough (from Massachusetts General Hospital, Boston) argued in 1934 that one should maintain the definition of carcinoma as an infiltration of epithelial cells beyond the basal membrane for the ducts: "it is wise to regard anaplastic morphology of a single cell or cells within their normal structural confines as evidences of hyperplasia, precancerous if you will, but not as justification for the diagnosis of cancer."[62]

Records from Addenbrooke's Hospital from the 1940s indicate that local pathologists viewed noninvasive breast lesions as true cancers:

A 38-year-old woman came to Addenbrooke's Hospital in July 1942, with a lump in her breast, present for 5 weeks. She underwent a radical mastectomy. The pathology report states: "this breast on section shows duct-like spaces filled with spheroid cells many layers deep, large and atypical. *There are no signs of infiltration,* and with the breast removed, I think that the prognosis is good, but the condition is, I believe, a duct carcinoma. The gland shows no secondary deposits.[63]

In a related case, the pathologist believed that he had detected a very early beginning of an invasion, that is, the point of passage from an in situ to invasive ductal cancer:

A 45-year-old woman came to Addenbrooke's Hospital in June 1942, with a lump in her breast. She underwent radical mastectomy. Pathology report affirms:" the section shows for the most part hyperplasia in fold of columnar epithelium inside cystic spaces, suggesting duct carcinoma, *but on one spot the growth has escaped,* shows typical invasion of tissue spaces and is carcinomatous. The gland shows no secondary deposit.[64]

Pathologists who wished to persuade their peers that in situ carcinoma was a true early stage of invasive malignancies employed a language that stressed this point. In his first description of carcinoma in situ, Albert Borders systematically attributed agency to transformed cells. This stylistic device conveyed the impression that the observation of stained and fixed (and thus dead) cells provided information on the dynamics of behavior of these cells within the body: "squamous cells carcinoma in situ of the uterine cervix in which the carcinomatous cells have replaced the normal cells and are appearing to function in a protective manner."[65] Borders added that it was a true cancer, in spite of the fact that the abnormal cells did not cross the basal membrane. Frank Foote and Fred Stewart employed the same approach when they described LCIS for the first time. Preparations of LCIS, Foote and Stewart insisted, directly display this lesion's capacity to evolve and became a full-fledged invasive tumor, with the *"invasive phase developing from lobular carcinoma in situ.* A terminal duct with 'pagetoid' cell is shown, with surrounding infiltrative cancer cells."[66] In another study of proliferative conditions of the breast, Foote and Stewart similarly deduced the direction of development of a precancerous lesion from its microscopic appearance: "*further progression* in formation of aporine epithelium. Shows focal areas of change."[67]

Surgical pathologists were usually confident in their ability to decide whether a given lesion was malignant, premalignant, or benign. Occasionally, however, a pathologist questioned the very basis of these classifications. Curie Foundation pathologist Georges Gricouroff held this skeptical view. Gricouroff stressed the intrinsic difficulty of defining benign or malignant tumors on the basis of histology alone or of tracing a boundary between normal and malignant tissue. Some tumors, like those in the salivary glands, are typically a mixture of benign and malignant cells. Benign tissue can occasionally invade neighboring tissues and in some rare cases nonmalignant tissues—such as the proliferating endometrium— and can even colonize lymph nodes through the blood. Gricouroff illustrated this permanent blurring of limits between the normal and the pathological with photographs of benign growths that bore a troubling resemblance to malignant tissues. He used the same rhetoric technique as Borders, Foote, and Stewart did but with an opposite goal: to point out the difficulty of relying exclusively on selected visual elements.

The captions of photographs that illustrate Gricouroff's article describe the depicted elements, but at the same time mimic faithfully descriptions of malignant growth: "benign *infiltrating* proliferation of cutaneous epidermis induced by an underlying fibroma of the dermis. Histological aspect of *baso-cellulary epithelioma*," "anaplastic cells produced by *budding ramifications of invasive epithelium* irritated by the presence of a fibroma," "benign *infiltrating* tongue mucosa on the level of granoulous cells," and "rhabodmyoma with a histological aspect of a *spinocellulary epithelioma*." Images and descriptions in Gricouroff's publications reinforce each other to trouble his readers and to convince them that there is no such a thing as a single, decisive cytological element that leads to a diagnosis of cancer. They lead the reader to the conclusion that "it is totally impossible to trace an absolute limit between benign and malignant structures."[68] Not only precancer, but cancer itself, Gricouroff proposed, is a conventional classificatory category, not a natural entity.

Treatment of In Situ Carcinomas and Proliferative Lesions of the Breast

From the 1950s to the 1980s, the recommended treatment for both LCIS and DCIS in the United States was a surgical ablation of the breast, either a radical mastectomy, or, more often, a simple one. Surgery was justified by a morpholog-

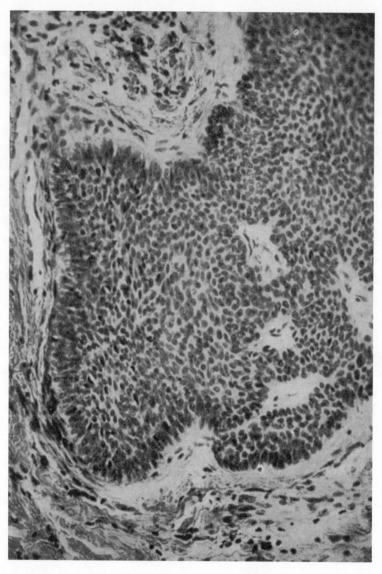

A photograph of cancer-like benign tissues. Georges Gricouroff, "Essai de définition de la prolifération cellulaire maligne," *Bulletin du Cancer*, 1955n 42(1), 100–101. Used by permission.

ical heterogeneity of breast lesions. Pathologists who studied amputated breasts often observed several types of proliferative changes in the same breast. This phenomenon, some specialists proposed, probably reflected the capacity of the neoplasm of the breast epithelium to differentiate simultaneously in several directions and to produce multifocal, morphologically diversified proliferative lesions. A diagnosis of one kind of lesion thus increased the probability that the same breast harbored additional, perhaps more dangerous, lesions.[69] In 1950, Fred Stewart, one of the leading U.S. breast cancer experts, explained that "the female breast is a pre-cancerous organ."[70] Robert Hutter reiterated this proposition in 1975: "In the broadest context, we must regard the female breast as a premalignant target organ when exposed to the physiological milieu of the female organism."[71] Stewart argued that the right treatment for both LCIS and DCIS was mastectomy, and this recommendation was adopted by nearly all the U.S. surgeons for more than thirty years.[72] A systematic simple mastectomy for LCIS—a lesion seen as less aggressive than DCIS—was justified not only by the danger of future tumor but also by the possible presence of microfoci of invasive cancer in LCIS-carrying breast and the difficulty of uncovering such microfoci through random sampling biopsies. Mastectomy was seen as a "safer and more thorough biopsy technique."[73]

A 1964 report by Edward Lewinson, from the Breast Clinics of the Johns Hopkins Hospital, reviewed the dilemmas of LCIS treatment under the revealing title, "Lobular Carcinoma In Situ of the Breast: The Feminine Mystique."[74] The more doctors look for LCIS, Lewinson explained, the more often they find it. The frequency of diagnosis of this condition is directly proportional to the number of sections done and the care in which they are examined. It is not clear, however, what these findings mean: "Is LCIS a cold war precursor of a malign and monstrously destructive disease . . . or is there a possibility of peaceful coexistence?" It is probable, Lewinson argued, that only a minority of women with LCIS will progress to cancer, but in the absence of more reliable knowledge, "most surgeons consider that the boldest counsels are the safest." Simple mastectomy with or without axillary dissection became therefore the treatment of choice for LCIS despite the obvious disadvantages of mutilation. Doctors hoped to reach a more reliable understanding of the natural history of breast cancer soon and to quickly develop ways of controlling precancerous conditions of the breast through hormonal management, but in the meantime felt that "it is advisable, even if precautionary, to treat the many for the benefit of the few."[75]

Aggressive treatment of LCIS was grounded in long-term observations of women diagnosed with this condition, such as a twenty-three-year-long follow-up of a cohort of individuals diagnosed with in situ lobular carcinoma at the Memorial Hospital in New York. The results of this study, published in 1967 and cosigned by Foote and Stewart, were very persuasive. More than half of the women diagnosed with this condition and left without treatment developed an invasive cancer of the breast. The authors concluded that "this data supports our contention that the histological lesion designated in situ lobular carcinoma is a pre-invasive form of breast cancer. Patients who have such a lesion and are not treated by mastectomy incur a considerable risk of a later invasive carcinoma." The cure rate for an invasive carcinoma at the Memorial Hospital, they added, was 42 percent at ten years and 34 percent at twenty years. By contrast, the cure rate for LCIS treated by mastectomy is very near 100 percent: "in view of these findings, it seems most reasonable to accept in situ carcinoma as a real threat, but one that can be eliminated by appropriate therapy at the time of diagnosis."[76]

Pathologists noted that LCIS was occasionally discovered together with an invasive carcinoma. This observation suggested a possible causal link. Members of the "Arthur Purdy Stout Society of Surgical Pathologists," a New York–based group whose members gathered to discuss diagnostic puzzles, analyzed a typical case:

> 34-year-old woman. Mass in breast discovered at routine gynecological exam, and an area of indurations in the other breast. Biopsies revealed fibroadenoma in one breast, LCIS in other. Simple bilateral mastectomy. Pathological analysis uncovered a small infiltrating carcinoma in the same breast as the fibroma, and, in addition, bilateral foci of lobular neoplasia and diffuse hyperplasic lesions. Patient is symptom-free year after mastectomy. The participants discussed the association of atypia with risk of carcinoma.[77]

Another case analyzed in a meeting of the Arthur Purdy Stout Society illustrates the difficulty of tracing a firm boundary between proliferative changes in the breast and an invasive tumor:

> A woman first seen at the age of 36, when she noted a diffuse lumpiness of the left breast. Biopsy revealed an extensive papillary proliferation of the ductal epithelium; it was interpreted by several pathologists as a worrisome hyperplasia, "potentially pre-cancerous." The patient underwent a prophylactic simple mastectomy. Pathology examination of the amputated breast revealed the presence of the same histological lesions throughout the whole breast. Twelve years later, the patient noticed a deep seated nodule in the lower left maxillary region. The

nodule, measuring 1 cm in diameter, was removed and proven to be an infiltrating ductal carcinoma with a few foci of intraductal growth. She was then
diagnosed with bilateral pulmonary metastases. The subsequent course of her
disease was characterized by alternating periods of regression and reactivation
of the pulmonary and intracranial metastases that were treated by oophorectomy, hormonotherapy, hypophysectomy and radiotherapy. At present, 18
months after the removal of the axillary carcinoma, the patient is alive with a
questionable persistence of cerebral metastases.[78]

In the late 1960s and 1970s breast cancer experts were confronted with the
dilemma faced by gynecologists ten years earlier. Here too, a large-scale testing
of symptom-free women led to great increase in diagnoses of in situ cancers
and other proliferative lesions. With the development of mammographic screening, doctors felt compelled to do biopsies of all the suspected lumps seen on a
mammogram. Occasionally such a lump was found to be benign, but a biopsy accidentally revealed the presence of carcinoma in situ. Biopsies made for microcalcifications, entities that are visible on a mammogram only, also occasionally
revealed in situ transformations. Screening mammograms—like Pap smears—
led to an increase in the number of biopsies and to a parallel increase in the number diagnoses of in situ cancers.[79] Lewinson explained that while in former years
a diagnosis of LCIS was a clinical curiosity and pathological rarity, during the
past few years he saw personally more than twenty individuals with this pathology.[80] Doctors became increasingly aware of the difficulty of tracing a firm
boundary between cancerous and noncancerous transformations of the breast.[81]
Moreover, the majority of diagnoses of LCIS were made in relatively young
women, a finding that further complicated clinical decisions. The rise of the
movement for breast-conserving treatment of invasive breast tumors also contributed to the view that mastectomy was a problematic treatment of noninvasive lesions.[82]

A 1975 debate on management of precancerous lesions displayed the extent of
disagreement among experts.[83] Dr. Taylor set the tone by defining a borderline lesion as one that "somebody else calls cancer and I call benign. Or we could say
that borderline lesions are those about which a panel of experts could not agree."
The debates were focused on the best way to treat these lesions. The recommendation varied form radical mastectomy to surgical removal of the suspected
areas, with an additional debate on the desirability of removal of the second
breast, especially if a biopsy revealed some cellular abnormalities in that breast.
In the 1970s, decisions concerning treatment of premalignant lesions of the

breast increasingly included a calculus of individual's individual risk as well. Family history, the number of children, age of first period and of first pregnancy, and the use of hormones were related to the chances of developing breast cancer.[84] Specialists attempted accordingly to evaluate the relative contribution of these elements to the probability of transformation of a precancerous lesion into a malignant growth.[85] The 1975 debate was focused, however on a very different risk: the one taken by the physician who is treating a borderline lesion of the breast. Experts discussed their risk of making a medical mistake and facing the consequences of this mistake. As one of the participants, Dr. Powers, put it: "the upsurge of interest in breast cancer is going to make life a lot more difficult for pathologists and surgeons in making decisions on earlier and earlier cases. The fact is that with these diagnoses of probable cancer, *we have to take some risk.*"[86]

One possible way of diffusing such risk, Dr. Shingleton proposed, is to share it with women diagnosed with such borderline conditions: "I think that the patient should be taken into the radiologist's confidence, and the surgeons should not have to bear the brunt of the decision."[87] In the 1970s women diagnosed with breast cancer increasingly insisted on their right to participate in decisions about their treatment. The proposal to burden women with the responsibility of making a wrong decision when facing medical uncertainty might have been an unanticipated consequence of this demand.

In the 1970s and 1980s some specialists continued to advocate mastectomy—either unilateral or bilateral—as the only safe treatment of LCIS.[88] Other specialists increasingly recommended careful follow-up of individuals rather than a radical surgical intervention. Surgical removal of precancerous lesions such as LCIS, J. P. Sloane argued is not efficient, because the most dangerous lesions usually do not produce any clinical signs, while those detected more easily tend to be less aggressive.[89] In the 1970s, Cushman Haagensen from Columbia Presbyterian Medical Center also questioned the wisdom of treating LCIS by mastectomy.[90] Haagensen proposed distinguishing between benign forms of LCIS, without any perceptible infiltration, and malignant forms, with a beginning of an infiltration. The latter condition should be treated as cancer. The right therapy for all the invasive forms of breast carcinoma, however early, is a radical mastectomy, and this treatment should be proposed to women with "aggressive LCIS" (or rather a very early carcinoma), too. By contrast, the right treatment for a true LCIS is close surveillance. Women diagnosed with this condition should undergo a clinical examination of the breast every four months for the duration of their lives. Individuals who underwent mastectomy for an aggressive form of LCIS and who did not agree to a prophylactic removal of the second breast were expected also to be subjected to a rigorous surveillance: "mammography is performed at 6 to 12 month intervals, and physical examination of the remaining breast at six month intervals, for the duration of the patient's life. Repeated biopsy or a simple mastectomy is performed if the examination of mammograms became even minimally suspicious."[91]

Women with suspect breast lesions, Haagensen and other experts proposed from the 1970s on, could escape mutilation—or at least to keep one of their breasts—but the price was a permanent submission to the clinicians' gaze.[92] The intensity of this gaze was directly proportional to the extent of uncertainty about links between LCIS and invasive cancer of the breast. In 1994, the range of estimates of the chances of a woman diagnosed with LCIS of developing an invasive cancer varied between 6 and 67 percent.[93] One of the reasons for the gradual abandonment of definition of LCIS as a true precancerous lesion was the observation that women diagnosed with this condition had indeed greater than average probability of developing cancer of the breast, but often the cancer appeared in a different area of the breast than the zones of LCIS. This condition was therefore increasingly described as a sign of greater susceptibility to breast cancer rather than a direct precursor of a malignant growth.[94]

In the early 1980s, pathologists and surgeons redefined "morphological risk factors" for breast cancer. Some experts proposed dismantling the broad entity "fibrocystic breast disease" and replacing it with more precise descriptions of specific proliferative lesions.[95] Cushman Haagensen and his colleagues at Columbia University's hospital argued that only gross cysts with proliferation, multiple intraductal papilloma, and LCIS increased the risk of breast cancer. All other proliferative breast lesions—microcysts, gross cysts with some proliferation, fibrous tumors of the breast or intraductal papilloma—were totally innocuous.[96] Other experts resisted the claim that some proliferative lesions of the breast were totally harmless and divided such lesions into two groups: one included lesions, such as adenosis, fibrosis, fibroadenoma, cysts, and typical hyperplasia, which increase slightly (1.2- to 1.6-fold) the probability of developing a breast cancer; the second includes lesions, such as LCIS, atypia, and lobular hyperplasia, associated with a higher (four- to tenfold) increase of cancer risk.[97] Even the long-neglected chronic cystic mastitis found an unexpected new niche among potential risk markers. A 1976 study stated that women diagnosed with this condition and followed for thirty years had 2.5 times higher probability of developing breast cancer.[98]

In the 1980s, LCIS became mainly a marker of breast cancer risk. DCIS followed a very different path. The follow-up of women diagnosed with this condition who developed later an invasive cancer indicated that these two lesions developed in the same area of the breast. This spatial coincidence, together with a persuasive series of slides that showed intermediary forms between DCIS and malignancy, convinced the specialists that DCIS was a true premalignant lesion and a precursor of breast cancer and that it had to be eliminated surgically.[99] Women diagnosed with DCIS in the 1980s often underwent mastectomy. The choice of a radical surgery was justified by the observation that DCIS was often a multifocal condition, difficult to excise with "clean margins" (absence of atypical cells in the external part of excised area). In addition the observation that DCIS has a very good prognosis made it an especially appropriate target for a surgical radicalism, because doctors could argue that a surgery would surely bring a cure—and a peace of mind—to the patient.[100] Because the treatment for invasive and noninvasive cancers is very similar, women diagnosed with DCIS frequently view themselves as cancer patients and believe that their risk of dying from their disease is the same as the risk of women treated for an invasive malignancy.[101]

Some European surgeons shared the radicalism of their U.S. colleagues. A textbook of oncology written in 1983 by a Belgian specialist advocated radical mastectomies for women with "minimal mammary cancers, such as DCIS and LCIS." It defined DCIS and LCIS as "true cancers, although not infiltrating yet" and affirmed that a radical mastectomy is the best guarantee of a long-term survival of women diagnosed with such "minimal cancers."[102] Other European surgeons elected partial mastectomy with radiotherapy, an approach increasingly adopted by U.S. specialists, too. The rate of mastectomies for DCIS in the United States decreased from 43 percent in 1992 to 28 percent in 1999. However, according to a large-scale U.S. database "Surveillance, Epidemiology and End Results" (SEER), the frequency of this pathology in the United States had risen 7.2-fold between 1980 and 2001, with a very sharp increase in the 1980s (attributed to the generalization of mammography) and a more moderate increase (1.8 fold) in the 1990s. Consequently in the 1980s and 1990s, the absolute number of American women who underwent ablation of their breast following a DCIS diagnosis remained constant.[103] Treatments for DCIS varied from local excision to mastectomy with radiation and in some cases the ablation of lymph nodes.[104] According to 2006 SEER data, 33.9 percent of American women with DCIS were treated with total mastectomy, 63.9 percent with partial mastectomy (6.4 percent with axillary node dissection), and 35.5 percent of those received in addition radiation therapy.[105] SEER data also reveal that women treated for DCIS and who later developed an invasive breast cancer were diagnosed more frequently with advanced breast tumors (stages II and III) than were women in the general population.

This is a rather unexpected observation, because one may assume that these women undergo more frequent mammographic and clinical tests than women who were never treated for breast lesions. It may indicate that mammographic and clinical surveillance does not always lead to the detection of less advanced malignancies.[106]

Calling a lesion "in situ cancer," some pathologists proposed, may increase the tendency to treat it aggressively. The term *carcinoma in situ,* Chandler Smith argued, is deeply ambivalent. It does not reveal whether the lesion is already a cancer but has not yet became invasive or whether it is not a cancer but may became one at a later stage. The pathologist may think "cancer later," while the clinician may interpret the changes as "cancer now," a message conveyed to the person who lives with the burden of cancer diagnosis. A different name, such as "epithelial atypia" may alleviate such burden.[107] His colleague, Bernard Ackerman, disagreed. Ambiguity, polysemy, and ambivalence in pathology, he proposed, are not limited to in situ cancers. Expressions such as " 'cancer,' 'invasion' and 'atypia' " are no less ambiguous, subjective, and unclear than is "carcinoma in situ."[108] David Page similarly affirmed that the ambivalence of the terms LCIS and DCIS mirrors the ambiguity of biological situations. To adequately account for such ambiguity, the absolute language of a pathological diagnosis should be translated into the relative langue of risk, and words such as "precancer" should be replaced by an evaluation of probability of development of a cancer.[109] Finally, Arkady Rivlin argued that in spite of its ambivalence the term *carcinoma in situ* has a heuristic utility. Naming a lesion "carcinoma" is a call for an intervention and, "as pragmatic practitioners, we should convey through our terminology a proper course of action to our clinical colleagues." [110]

A surgical and radiological treatment of DCIS was often compared to the systematic surgical treatment of cervical dysplasia. This comparison may be inaccurate. Experts agree that the great majority of cervical tumors pass through a detectable dysplasia phase (the opposite is not true; the majority of cervical dysplasias do not became cancers). The causal relationship between DCIS and invasive breast cancer is more controversial. Moreover, population-based data indicate that, while the elimination of cervical lesions led to important reduction in incidence of cervical tumors, the treatment of DCIS has at best a marginal effect on the incidence of invasive breast cancer.[111] Doubts about the contribution of the elimination of DCIS to reduction of breast cancer mortality did not affect the principle of a systematic therapy of this condition. DCIS was presented as a "gold standard," the lesion against which all other breast lesions need to be compared.[112] Treatment of DCIS, however, is highly variable, and therapeutic choices are complicated by the lack of reliable estimates of the percentage of DCIS lesions that progress to malignancy. Recent evaluation varied between 14 percent and 60 percent progression ten years after the initial diagnosis.[113] The status of knowledge on this topic was summed up by an editorial in a January 2008 issue of *Annals of Surgical Oncology*: "Ductal Carcinoma In Situ: Through a Glass, Darkly."[114]

The consensus, established in the 1970s on the basis of epidemiological data, that LCIS is an indicator of an increased risk of cancer, not a true precursor of breast cancer, led to a less aggressive treatment of this condition. In 2006, 11.5 percent of American women diagnosed with LCIS underwent mastectomy (as compared with 33.9 percent of women diagnosed with DCIS). Mastectomy for LCIS was usually bilateral, because its goal was not to cure an already existing lesion but to prevent a future tumor. When filmmaker Yvonne Rainer was diagnosed with LCIS, her surgeon "wanted to take 'em both off. No breasts, no breast cancer."[115] The perception of LCIS as a risk factor was, however, partly destabilized in 2006 by analysis of SEER data. The conviction that LCIS is not a direct precursor of breast malignancies was grounded in observations that indicated that usually LCIS and breast cancers develop in different parts of the breast, whereas an analysis of more than 40,000 cases of in situ cancer in the SEER database failed to find major differences between DCIS and LCIS. In both cases invasive lesions developed often, but not always, in the same part of the breast as noninvasive ones. The authors of this study concluded that DCIS and LCIS seem to be more alike than was previously assumed and recommended a similar treatment for both.[116] Other studies also indicate an absence of qualitative differences between LCIS and DCIS and hint at difficulties of predicting the future of this lesion.[117] Such an understanding of LCIS may lead to radicalization of its treatment and the return of more aggressive therapeutic approaches, such as those promoted in the 1950s and 1960s.[118] There will be one important difference: before the generalization of mammographic screening, the number of women diagnosed with in situ lobular carcinoma of the breast was incomparably smaller.

Prophylactic Ablation of a Healthy Breast: Balancing Risks

The ablation of an LCIS- or DCIS-containing breast, one may argue, is not a true prophylactic mastectomy, since the amputated breast has already undergone pathological changes. The preventive ablation of the second, healthy breast, in a woman diagnosed with breast cancer is probably closer to the definition of a "true" preventive surgery. Women diagnosed with cancer in one breast have a higher than average chance of developing a malignant tumor in the other breast. In the 1950s and 1960s some cancer experts advised these women to undergo a bilateral mastectomy. Such surgery was especially recommended to women with a family history of breast cancer, those diagnosed with benign proliferative changes in the contralateral breast, and those with "good prognosis" cancers, such as lobular, comedo, colloid, and medullary breast tumors. The last, at first a somewhat surprising recommendation (a diagnosis of a "good" malignancy leads to a more extensive mutilation) was justified by the observation that cancers that developed in the contralateral breast were not detected in an earlier stage than the first tumor and were frequently of a different—and potentially less favorable—histological type.[119] A woman diagnosed with a "good" cancer who underwent a bilateral mastectomy had a near certainty of a long-term cure. If she conserved the healthy breast, she had a nonnegligible chance of developing a second—and perhaps more aggressive—breast tumor.[120] Moreover, cytological analyses of preventively removed contralateral breasts frequently displayed the presence of proliferative lesions. Such observations strengthened in turn the rationale for preventive surgery.[121]

Some experts actively promoted the preventive ablation of the other breast. Robert Pollack explained in 1958 that since all the women diagnosed with breast cancer had a higher than average probability of developing a malignancy in the second breast, ideally one should propose to them a preventive ablation of the unaffected breast, either at the same time as their radical mastectomy or a year or two after the first operation. Despite its obvious advantages, Pollack observed, preventive mastectomy is viewed with abhorrence by many women and, consequently, it was not performed as frequently as it should be.[122] George Pack—a surgeon known for his enthusiasm for aggressive surgery that earned him the nickname "Pack the Knife"—argued in 1952 that it is surprising that preventive mastectomy is resisted more strongly than preventive oophorectomy:

> The surgeon who knowingly removes a malignant tumor of one ovary and conserved the opposite ovary and the uterus is vulnerable to authoritative criticism, yet the sexual mutilation by bilateral oophorectomy is greater and more fundamental than by double mastectomy. By a strange paradox, women tolerate the loss of both ovaries better than the removal of both breasts . . . there is no valid excuse for retention of the opposite breast if one becomes cancerous . . . the sacrifice of an useless organ such as the remaining breast does not make the patient a functional cripple, as would the complete removal of other paired organs such as the testes. [123]

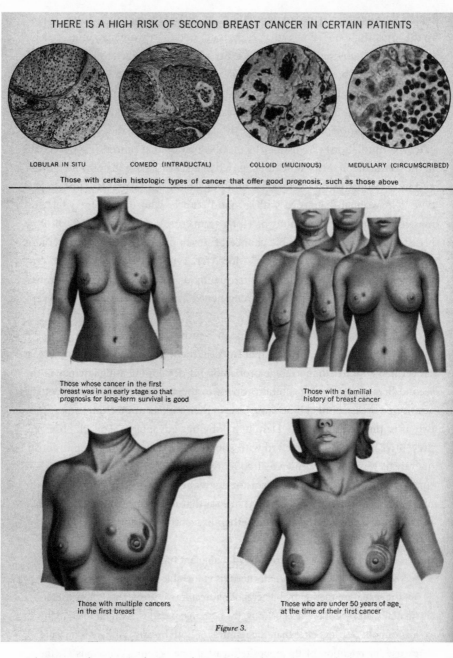

THERE IS A HIGH RISK OF SECOND BREAST CANCER IN CERTAIN PATIENTS

LOBULAR IN SITU   COMEDO (INTRADUCTAL)   COLLOID (MUCINOUS)   MEDULLARY (CIRCUMSCRIBED)

Those with certain histologic types of cancer that offer good prognosis, such as those above

Those whose cancer in the first breast was in an early stage so that prognosis for long-term survival is good

Those with a familial history of breast cancer

Those with multiple cancers in the first breast

Those who are under 50 years of age at the time of their first cancer

Figure 3.

A late-1960s drawing in the journal *Hospital Medicine* showing the best candidates for prophylactic removal of the contralateral, cancer-free, breast. Henry Patrick Leis, "Prophylactic removal of the second breast," *Hospital Medicine*, January 1968, 48. Used by permission.

Dr. Leis, from the New York Medical College, also viewed the reluctance of women diagnosed with breast cancer to undergo a bilateral mastectomy as an irrational reaction. The remaining breast remains as a useless and largely nonfunctional organ and a questionable psychosexual symbol: "few women are willing to show it as a questionable badge of sexual enhancement alongside their opposite mastectomy scar, and equally few women allow it to be used during the act of lovemaking."[124] It is difficult, Leis admitted, to persuade a woman who is on the verge of giving her consent to a radical mastectomy should the lump in her breast be found malignant, to give her immediate agreement for the loss of the second breast as well. But a few months later, many women spontaneously express concerns about their second breast. They are worried about pain, nodularities, and irregularities and express a deep concern about the possibility of developing a second cancer. This is the right psychological moment to talk with individuals about a radical way of eliminating such a danger and the possibility of freeing themselves of all their worries.[125]

Prophylactic mastectomy was also recommended to women especially prone to developing breast cancer in the future. Surgeons proposed to women a rough evaluation of their chances of developing a breast cancer, taking into account age, presence of breast cancer in relatives, and reproductive history. Doctors also recommended a preventive ablation of the breasts to women with "lumpy breasts" (fibrocystic disease of the breast) who underwent frequent biopsies, especially when such repeated biopsies led to an accumulation of scar tissue and breast deformity. Finally such surgery was seen as a cure for severe neurotic or psychotic fear of breast cancer.[126] Before the demise of Halsted's operation, one of the main arguments in favor of prophylactic removal of the breasts (especially in the United States) was that a preventive surgery is much less mutilating than a radical mastectomy. Women with high risk of developing breast cancer have the choice between certain, but not very traumatic, surgery now and high probability of a much more drastic surgery in the future. Another argument was the possibility of a good quality reconstruction of the breast. Women who underwent a prophylactic removal of their breasts in the 1970s and 1980s usually had a subcutaneous mastectomy, a surgery that conserved the skin and the nipple and made possible a more natural-looking reconstruction. As a *New England Journal of Medicine* editorial put it: "many patients who refuse more 'radical' operations may accept subcutaneous mastectomy as a compromise with which they can live."[127]

Some surgeons advocated immediate reconstruction of the ablated breast to save the stress of additional surgery and also because the cosmetic results were often better. An immediate reconstruction had a higher rate of complications, however, and was sometimes less well accepted by the individual: "For the reconstructive surgeons, there is an advantage in delaying the breast rebuilding. The patient who has to live with her deformity will be more understanding of the shortcomings of the reconstruction."[128] Articles on breast reconstruction usually brought to the foreground the quality of aesthetic results and rarely mentioned postsurgery complications, pain, or loss of sensitivity in the new breast.[129] There were exceptions, however. A 1982 article on prophylactic mastectomy for women with a family history of breast cancer discussed the advent of serious complications in up to a quarter of those who underwent breast reconstruction. It added that the most often employed procedure, the implantation of silicone prosthesis, occasionally induced intense fibrotic reaction that produced a ball-shaped, firm breast. This reaction can be relieved by compression and rotation of the prosthesis (capsuloctomy), but the latter procedure may provoke rupture of the silicon transplant and the formation of granuloma (an inflammatory reaction).[130] The article described a 29-year-old woman with a fibrocystic disease of the breast and a family history of breast malignancy who underwent a prophylactic bilateral mastectomy: "on the follow up, 7 months later, the patient was satisfied with the operation; however one breast was so painfully firm due to fibrous contraction that she had to cut a hole in her mattress in order to sleep prone. She finally found a surgeon familiar with this complication which he relieved by a closed capsuloctomy."[131]

Experts usually presented preventive mastectomy as the individual's choice. Some people with cancer who underwent mastectomy with reconstruction had chosen a bilateral surgery for esthetic reasons, especially when the surgeon was unable to produce a reasonably symmetrical result. Others feared a second cancer. Women concerned about a second breast tumor explained that they did not want to face the prospect of another mastectomy with an axillary dissection (an extensive surgery which frequently induces lymphedema, a painful swelling of the arm) and another course of chemotherapy.[132]

Doctors who dismissed such fears as excessive might have been reluctant to admit that one of the main causes of apprehension is not the disease itself, but the medical interventions that aim to control it.[133] Some might have also be unwilling to acknowledge their active role in promotion of preventive surgeries. A U.S. survey of women who underwent prophylactic mastectomy of the second breast indicated that the most frequently cited reason for such surgery was their physician's advice (30 percent). Their own fear of developing cancer in the second breast was a distant second (14 percent), cosmetic consideration was third (10 percent), and family history fourth (7 percent).[134]

U.S. breast cancer activist Rose Kushner was strongly opposed to prophylactic mastectomy. She learned that, according to one evaluation, the number of such surgeries had increased recently, and 10,000 U.S. women had undergone prophylactic ablation of the breast in 1983. The growing popularity of this operation was ascribed to a combination of increased detection of minimal cancer and precancerous lesions, the improvement of techniques of plastic surgery, and a greater acceptance of reimbursement of breast reconstruction by U.S. insurance companies.[135] Kushner was appalled by these data: she saw prophylactic mastectomy as "a pretty aggressive self-mutilation."[136] An article published in *Mother Jones* in 1985 with the suggestive title, "Indecent Proposal," similarly argued that preventive mastectomies were an unnecessary and risky procedure and strongly warned against high rates of surgical complications of breast reconstruction.[137] The practice of preventive mastectomy remained nevertheless popular in the 1980s, especially among women diagnosed with a "morphological risk" of cancer.[138]

Hoffman's and Pressman's 1982 discussion of advantages of prophylactic mastectomy starts with the statement: "A famous surgeon once said: 'if all women were to have their breasts removed at puberty, breast cancer could be eliminated.' While this approach is rather drastic and unacceptable in our breast-oriented society, there are indications for prophylactic mastectomy. Since it is now possible to reconstruct acceptable-appearing breasts, the concept of surgical prophylaxis may be not as radical as it once seemed."[139]

Hoffman and Pressman end their discussion with the suggestion that the prophylactic removal of breasts offers the least traumatic solution for a woman with a family history of breast cancer, with lumpy breasts, or with a diagnosis of LCIS: "The alternative to surgery is a lifetime of frequent physical examinations and mammography, watching and waiting for an invasive cancer to become apparent. Bilateral total mastectomies offer the certainty of a cure with minimal deformity."[140] Anthropologist Sandra Gifford proposed a different view of prophylactic mastectomy: "while doctors treat risk through a physical removal of part of the body, risk for women has been transformed into a new state of physical ill-health."[141]

CHAPTER FIVE

The Origins of Screening

"Be Quick!" The Call for an Early Detection of Cancer

In the first half of the twentieth century preventive treatments of premalignant lesions was the exclusive domain of the clinician. Doctors detected suspicious changes in a person's body and decided (sometimes together with individuals and their families) what to do about these changes. After the Second World War, with the development of mass screening campaigns, preventive treatments of precancerous lesions became closely intertwined with public health interventions. The growing popularity of these campaigns led in turn to a significant increase in the number of people (nearly exclusively women) diagnosed with precancerous changed in tissues and advised to undergo a preventive treatment.[1]

Screening for cancer is a voluntary measure that has to be accepted by those being screened, hence the central role of education of the public in its promotion. Also by the first half of the twentieth century, experts and cancer charities already enthusiastically advocated early detection of malignant tumors, presented as the most efficient way to reduce cancer-related mortality. This approach was summarized in a title of a 1928 leaflet of Massachusetts Department of Public Health: "Cancer. Be Quick! Cancer Control Is a Race against Time."[2] Only rarely one could hear dissenting voices, such as the opinion expressed by James Ewing in 1926: "It appears more and more evident that early diagnosis alone is not capable of accomplishing the desired reduction in death rate. Every experienced observer(s) knows that the patient coming with an early diagnosis all too often fails completely of a cure . . . I think it should be frankly recognized in all public propaganda that the intelligent use of all present knowledge of prevention, early diagnosis and modern treatment, will still leave cancer the greatest of all natural hazard in the adventure of living."[3]

Ewing's skeptical evaluation of the practical value of early detection of cancer was at odds with the view that dominated twentieth-century discourse on this disease.[4] The main educational message of the American Society for the Control of Cancer (ASCC), the British Empire Cancer Campaign (BECC), La Ligue Franco-Americaine Contre le Cancer was the importance of early detection of malignant tumors. This message, it is true, was often conveyed through careful wording. The heir to La Ligue Franco-Americaine Contre le Cancer, La Ligue Française Contre le Cancer had a slogan: "cancer can be cured if detected early" (detecté tôt, le cancer peut être gueri). This slogan could be interpreted in two ways: as accentuating "cure" (of all the cancers that were detected early) or "can" (some cancers can be cured if detected early, but others cannot).[5] Physicians knew that the "early detection" principle was valid in selected tumors only. Malignancies of internal organs (such as the lungs, stomach, liver, and pancreas) were nearly always detected at a stage at which medical intervention was of little value. Professor Jean Firket from University of Liège, warned that "one should be very careful when organizing popularization and education campaigns. When calling the public to have regular medical check ups in order to detect cancer, one should always make it clear that while some cancers can indeed be cured if detected early, this is not the case for many other malignancies. Many cancers are beyond the pale of our therapeutic means."[6]

Specialists were also aware of the fact that early (that is small and localized) tumors were sometimes borderline or slow-developing growths and thus very different from aggressive cancers.[7] Some pathologists and surgeons criticized accordingly the indiscriminate use of the term "early tumor." The French surgeon Amadé Baumgarten explained in 1908 that the clinical entity of breast cancer lumped together fast-growing and highly malignant tumors and slow-growing, less malignant ones. A small tumor is often also a slow-growing one, with a low capacity to spread in the organism. When detected, it has a favorable prognosis not because it was caught early, but because it belongs to a less virulent type.[8] Massachusetts General Hospital surgeon Robert Greenough proposed in 1935 clarifying the meaning of the term *early diagnosis* in connection with breast malignancies to eliminate the confusion between early in time and early in a natural history of the clinical disease cancer: " 'early diagnosis' of breast cancer means early in the course of disease, rather than early as measured by the duration of the symptoms in point of time . . . taken in this sense, few of us will deny that 'early diagnosis' is by far the most significant factor in prognosis of cancer of the breast."[9]

Then again, the lumping of two distinct meanings of the term *early tumor—*

"early on an absolute time scale" and "early in disease's trajectory"—facilitated the educational activities of cancer experts and cancer charities, the diffusion of the "do not delay" principle, and the promotion of therapeutic optimism.[10] These trends were amplified after World War II, when the efforts to promote an early detection of cancer were incorporated into public health policies.

Between Triumphal Vision and Scare Politics

The "do not delay" campaigns were driven by doctors' and activists' sincere desire to reduce cancer-related suffering and, in the early twentieth century, also by the wish to eliminate the frightening physical disintegration linked with this disease. William Sampson Handley's notes from 1894 describe the malignant tumors he encountered as a medical student: extended, necrotic, and foul-smelling lesions, akin to chronic ulcers, syphilitic and tubercular lesions, or diabetic necrosis.[11] Doctors who work in Western hospitals today—with a possible exception of those who treat homeless and marginal people—rarely see cancerous lesions like those depicted by Handley. Such lesions can, however, still be seen in developing countries. Handley's notes illustrate the usual context of cancer diagnosis in the late nineteenth and early twentieth centuries. Critics of Halsted's radical mastectomy sometimes evaluated technologies of the late nineteenth century according to criteria of the late twentieth century and forgot that in an earlier period a radical breast surgery was often a palliative measure. Women who underwent a large excision of the breast and of pectoral muscles frequently did not escape death from disseminated cancer, but at least they did not end their life with a painful and smelly extended necrotic tumor that was destroying their body. It is not very surprising that Halsted and his colleagues counted women who did not have a local recurrence of the tumor but died from distant metastases (with luck, rapidly and without excessive pain) among the successes of their method.[12]

The first call to create a cancer charity in France linked an argument in favor of an early detection of uterine cancer with detailed descriptions of prolonged, abject suffering of women with advanced disease.[13] The aim of the fight against cancer, French cancer expert Gustave Roussy explained in 1929, is not only to cure people with this pathology, but also, and perhaps above all, to attenuate their suffering: "Isn't cancer one of the most horrid diseases, one that leads to death after terrible agony?"[14] In the interwar era cancer charities oscillated between optimistic representation of the progress in the "war against cancer" and scare strategies that accentuated the devastation induced by this disease. The American

Society for the Control of Cancer sometimes employed such scare tactics, as did the French Ligue Française Contre le Cancer.[15] For example, in 1931, the Ligue's bulletin, *La Lutte Contre le Cancer* (The Struggle against Cancer) published an article on the cancer of the tongue, destined to encourage people to be watchful for early signs of this disease. If they failed to do so, they might develop a disease that is "very serious from its very beginnings, and becomes intolerable with time." Cancer was depicted as extremely painful, to the point that some people committed suicide to put an end to their suffering. In addition the tumor secretes a foul-smelling liquid: "the smell is so repulsive that one says that even the most devoted friend or the most faithful spouse refuses to come near the patient."[16]

People might very well have had good reasons to delay the diagnosis of cancer. Many saw cancer treatment as "worse than the disease,"[17] dreading the consequences of surgery: drastic disfigurations linked to large excisions of face and neck tumors, reduced mobility and chronic pain induced by radical mastectomy, or colostomy bags employed after the excision of the colon or the rectum. Radiotherapy could also induce severe and lasting mutilations. For example early attempts, made at the Curie Foundation in Paris, to treat breast cancer with radiotherapy alone produced often extensive and painful scarring or inflammation (radiodermitis) that refused to heal.[18] Radiotherapy of uterine cancers occasionally induced chronic pain and deformations such as vaginal fistula. The latter complication led to chronic incontinence pain and frequent infections. Vaginal fistula was also one of the complications of hysterectomy for uterine tumors. Historian Barbara Clow quotes a Canadian woman who wrote to the Ontario Department of Health in the 1930s to explain why she refused radiotherapy for cervical cancer: "Three of my friends had similar treatment and they told me they were dying a death of a fiery infernal furnace. Knowing of their untimely death and awful agony, I was determined to die comfortably, if need be, by the inroads of cancerous growth."[19]

Cancer charities employed the fear of cancer—and probably also the fear of treatments for advanced cancer—to promote early detection. A Toulouse chapter of the Ligue Française Contre le Cancer issued in the spring of 1929 a poster that asked local politicians to support the fight against cancer. With a better public understanding of the nature of malignancies, the poster claimed, "90 percent of the patients will see the doctor with cancers that can be cured." This message is accompanied by photographs that graphically illustrate the gradual aggravation of untreated cancers. The poster depicts an extended, ulcerated cancer of the head "that started with a small wound made by a comb," a cancer covering half of the person's face, "that has begun as a small lesion behind the ear," another head and neck cancer that covers the eye's socket, the nose, and part of the face and described as "cancer that started near the nose," a breast cancer en cuirasse (in amour) that covers most of the chest, and a huge "ulcerated tumor of the dorsal region."[20]

The 1929 poster of the Ligue Française Contre le Cancer is probably an extreme example of this scare policy. Educational materials diffused by cancer charities seldom displayed images of extended cancerous lesions. The usual place of such images was not on the city's walls but within specialized journals and textbooks where their purpose was to teach professionals and students what advanced cancer looked like. The aim of the Toulouse poster was different. The main message it conveyed was not that cancer is a frightening disease—one may assume that people did not need explicit photographs to be afraid of cancer—but that it gradually evolves from small, insignificant, and seemingly harmless changes in tissues. The poster stressed the direct continuity between a "small lesion made by a comb" and a frightening tumor that "eats away" half of the person's face and stated that experts are able to spot the malignant potential of innocent looking lesions. Such small, insignificant lesions, the implicit connotation was, were as threatening as the extended tumors that destroy the person's body. Images of advanced tumors legitimated mutilating treatments that eliminated such lesions.

Early Detection of Female Malignancies

The educational activity of the French Ligue Contre le Cancer was frequently directed to both sexes. The Ligue's main publication, *Lutte Contre le Cancer,* stressed the importance of early detection of uterine and head and neck tumors. The latter, linked with tobacco and alcohol consumption, were more often found in men. The choice of these two malignancies as main targets of the Ligue's public campaigns was probably related to the importance of radiumtherapy and radiotherapy in the development of French oncology. The key role of radiotherapy in establishing departments and institutions specialized in cancer therapy in France contributed to the visibility of these types of cancers, which were treated mainly by this approach, and lesser visibility of breast cancer, which were seen as a surgeon's disease.[21]

By contrast, early detection campaigns conducted by British and U.S. charities were focused on female cancers.[22] At first the early detection campaign of BECC covered all the malignant tumors. Doctors who worked with BECC acknowledged, however, in their internal publications that an indiscriminate use of the

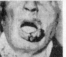

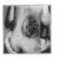

A poster illustrating advanced cancers disseminated by the Toulouse chapter of La Ligue Contre le Cancer, 1929. *La Lutte Contre le Cancer* 24 (Apr.–June 1929), Archives, Ligue Nationale Contre le Cancer. Used by permission.

early detection slogan might be problematic. An outline of a public conference "Cancer and the Needs of Research" proposed to BECC lecturers in the 1920s explained that the speaker should avoid the word "cure." Expressions such as "arrest of growth," "disappearance of growth," "apparent restoration of health," "satisfactory treatment" and such were much safer. A government memorandum from 1923 appended to this document explains that "most medical authorities believe that in cancer an early operation affords the best chance for the patient, although they would not feel justified in saying that all risk of recurrence is necessarily removed by operation, even if undertaken in an early stage of the disease."[23]

Janet Lane-Claypon's finding that small, localized breast tumors had excellent cure rates probably helped to shift the attention from early detection of all malignancies to a concentration on female cancers. In the 1930s, BECC documents argued that between 80 and 90 percent of individuals diagnosed with very early stages of breast or uterine cancer were alive five years after their treatment (as compared with 20 to 30 percent five-year survival of individuals diagnosed in later stages of the disease), conveying the implicit message that early detection would transform these cancers into curable diseases.[24] Lecturers for the BECC campaign were told to focus on breast and uterus cancer, especially if the public is feminine, with these words: "By contrast, it is a poor idea to speak about stomach cancer. There is no early diagnosis, and people with slight indigestion will believe they have cancer."[25] In the United Kingdom, the advocacy of early diagnosis became increasingly understood as a call for the detection of women's malignancies.

The publications of the American Society for the Control of Cancer (ASCC) were from the very beginning (the 1910s and 1920s) mainly dedicated to female cancers: breast and uterine.[26] U.S. governmental agencies conveyed a similar message. A poster produced in the framework of the Federal Arts Projects in 1939 boldly stated "More women die of cancer than do men. 70 percent of the 35,000 women who die annually from cancer of the breast and uterus could be saved if treated in time."[27] One of the goals of ASCC's educational campaigns was to fight the false modesty that prevents women from consulting doctors with signs of a gynecological disease. In 1930 Joseph Colt Bloodgood founded the "Amanda Sims Memorial Fund" (ASMF), named after the wife of the donor who helped to establish it, carpenter John E. Sims. This fund was dedicated nearly exclusively to raising women's awareness about cervical cancer. ASMF's director, Florence Becker, a nurse and public health activist, efficiently diffused the message about the need to pay attention to gynecological symptoms among women's organizations and women's clubs. ASMF was one of the sources of inspiration of ASCC's

Women's Field Army, dedicated to the spreading of educational messages about female cancers, especially through networks of women's clubs.[28] The educational campaigns of both ASCC and ASMF (the two organizations collaborated frequently) were at least partly successful. While Bloodgood complained in the 1930s that less than 10 percent of women visited their gynecologist regularly, in the 1950s newspapers reported that women then went for their pelvic examinations as casually as they went shopping.[29] ASCC's and ASMF's campaigns were aimed at the detection of already existing, symptomatic, cervical malignancies, but they familiarized women with the idea of frequent gynecological examinations and opened the way to screening for asymptomatic (silent) cervical lesions.

Cervical Cancer: From Early Detection to Screening

Early detection of malignancies was advocated already in the 1910s, but the rise of mass screening for cancer is a post–World War II story. It is related to the development of epidemiological studies of cancer, a greater awareness of "health risks" in general, and, in Europe, also with a shift to national health insurance.

In the 1950s, cancer prevention was divided into primary prevention—measures that should prevent the appearance of the disease—and secondary prevention— the elimination of already existing tumors and premalignant lesions. Primary prevention of cancer included some lifestyle-related measures—avoidance of mechanically induced chronic irritations, sunburns, and cigarette smoking—but this term was used mainly in debates over the prevention of occupational cancers, especially those linked with radiation and the manipulation of chemical carcinogens. Primary prevention was thus seen above all as the responsibility of the government and public health authorities.[30] Secondary prevention of cancer, defined as "finding cases in early stages and treating them promptly" was focused, especially in the United States, on regular annual or biannual check-ups made by a family doctor and was presented as the individual's responsibility. Such check-ups were not a new invention. Linked with the movement for preventive medicine, they became popular among middle-class Americans in the 1920s.[31] American Cancer Society, or ACS (which replaced the ASCC in 1945), attempted to transform such check-ups into the main site of an early detection of cancer. Physicians were encouraged to check systematically for hidden cancer signs, especially those of tumors of the breast, lung, and cervix. The ACS energetically promoted the slogan "every doctor's office is a cancer detection center."[32]

The development of the Pap smear accelerated the promotion of early detection of cervical tumors. Describing his "exfoliative cytology," George Papanicolaou stressed that this method can be employed for large-scale detection of malignancies:

> The present difficulty in accomplishing early diagnosis lies in the fact that we must depend on subjective symptoms of the disease to bring the patient to the physician, and by the time the patient becomes sufficiently aware of symptoms to seek help the disease is far advanced. . . . if by any chance a simple, inexpensive method of diagnosis could be evolved which could be applied to large numbers of women in the cancer bearing period of life, we would be in a position to discover the disease in its incipiency much more frequently than is now possible, that is, detect this cancer at a stage shown to be highly curable by the existing therapeutic methods.[33]

Papanicolaou's claims were confirmed by other investigators, and the Pap smear was adopted rapidly by gynecologists.[34] A 1945 text explained that the new test would radically change the story of pelvic carcinoma in women.[35]

The idea to systematically look for signs of beginning cervical cancer in symptom-free women was not entirely new. In the interwar era, many gynecologists had noted that the perfection of therapies for uterine cancer, coupled with women's greater awareness of warning signs of this malignancy, did not lead to a significant increase in survival rates. After an initial progress, the five-year cure rate of cervical malignancies stabilized in the best centers at approximately 40 percent of "treatable" malignancies (the "untreatable" malignancies, those too extended for surgery or radiotherapy, were always fatal). Failing to treat the majority of cervical tumors was attributed to the difficulty of detecting truly localized cases of this pathology. When women noticed the first symptoms of a cervical malignancy, such as irregular bleeding, the disease was frequently already well advanced. Some cancer experts, such as Claudius Regaud, proposed therefore the introduction of a systematic gynecological examination of all women in order to detect beginning cervical tumors before they produced clinical signs.[36]

Viennese gynecologist Walter Schiller, who was among the first to observe superficial proliferative lesions of the cervix, developed a rapid method of visualizing such lesions by staining them with diluted iodine (called the Lugol stain). Normal cervical cells contain glycogen and adsorb iodine, while transformed cells do not store glycogen and remain white. The method was not sensitive enough to provide a firm diagnosis, but it gave a first indication of potential trouble. Schiller proposed in 1933 the use of the Lugol stain for a routine detection of beginning cervical cancer. The unstained areas of the cervix could be observed with a colposcope, a variant of binocular microscope designed by Hinselmann in 1925 to examine the cervix and adopted by numerous gynecologists in German-speaking countries. The colposcope facilitated both a direct visual observation of the cervix and biopsies of suspicious areas. According to Schiller, if every woman would have a routine Lugol test two or three times a year, it would be possible to identify very early stages of nearly all cervical carcinomas and to increase the percentage of cures of this malignancy to 95 or 100 percent.[37]

Schiller reiterated his proposal five years later. At that time he came to the conclusion that cervical cancer was often a slow-growing malignancy, with an especially long stage of superficial (noninvasive) growth of transformed cells. This view of the natural history of cervical tumors reinforced the argument in favor of a periodical testing of all women.[38] In January 1937, Schiller presented this idea at the meeting of the American Society for the Advancement of Science at Atlantic City. *Time* reported that "Dr. Walter Schiller of the University of Vienna offered a simple new way of determining whether or not a woman has cancer of the cervix. He paints it with iodine. If the cervix is healthy, the iodine makes the surface turn blue. If there is the slightest trace of cancer, the spot will turn white. Dr. Schiller urged all women to have the iodine test every six months, or at least once a year."[39] Schiller's proposal could have led to development of an alternative method of screening for cervical cancer.[40] The choice of exfoliative cytology rather than the Lugol test was probably related to the proposal that such test had to be made by a gynecologist. Gynecologists (with the exception of those in Germany and Austria) were not familiar with the use of colposcope, and they might have resisted the performance of time-consuming routine tests. By contrast, the Pap test dissociates a vaginal smear—a rapid and simple act that can be made by a general practitioner or a nurse—from the more tedious and time-consuming analysis of collected samples, made in specialized laboratories. In addition, the late 1930s and the 1940s were probably not the best time for diffusion of methods that originated in German-speaking countries. The Pap smear had a double advantage: simplicity of sampling and U.S. origins.

Pap Smear: From Diagnostic to Prediagnostic Test

One of the key questions opened by the generalization of the Pap smear and consecutive cervical biopsies was the percentage of in situ lesion that progress to cancer, compared with those that remain stationary or regress. Forty-eight among the seventy U.S. gynecologists, who in 1951 answered a questionnaire on the detection and treatment of cervical cancer, declared that they had never observed spontaneous regression of in situ cervical cancer; four answered that they had seen such a regression, and eighteen did not answer this question. When they were asked, "do you believe spontaneous regression of 'cancer in situ' occurs?" fourteen answered yes, thirty-four no, and twenty-two were not sure.[41] At that time, epidemiological data, which juxtaposed the prevalence of in situ tumors and invasive malignancy, pointed to discrepancies between the detected rate of cervical dysplasia and the prevalence of cervical malignancies. Such discrepancy strongly suggested that the majority of cervical lesions did not progress to malignancy.[42] A 1953 estimate made on the basis of population data proposed accordingly a 7 percent to 15 percent progression rate.[43]

One should be very careful with the interpretation of the results of a Pap smear Georges Gricouroff that warned of in 1954, because a cytological diagnosis alone cannot predict the future of a given lesion. Even a result of a cervical biopsy does not provide such information: "It is rather obvious that all cancers have an initial pre-invasive phase; for example all the epitheliomas pass thorough a stage of intra-epithelial cancer. Nevertheless there is an important danger of error because a microscopic aspect of a lesion does not allow distinction between a temporary, benign proliferation, and a permanent, malignant one."[44]

Leopold Koss and his colleagues attributed the differences between the number of women diagnosed with superficial lesions of the cervix and those who developed invasive malignancies to the fact that biopsy, the technique that makes cervical lesions visible to doctors, usually destroys these lesions. It is possible, they argued, that cervical lesions never regress spontaneously, but it is impossible for us to know what their "true" natural history is.[45] The semi-accidental observation that carcinoma in situ of a cervix can be readily eradicated by a variety of minor procedures led nevertheless to the conviction that local treatments of cervical dysplasia may be sufficient to avert the danger of cervical cancer and to the generalization of such treatments.[46] The initial aim of screening for cervical tumors was the cure of a potentially aggressive early cancer with an equally aggressive surgical approach. Later, however, the aim of the screening was redefined as the identification and elimination of weak, poorly established cervical lesions.[47]

Early promoters of the Pap smear hoped to extend this method to all women. Boston physicians Daniel McSweeney and Donald McKay, who pioneered the massive use of the Pap smear for early cancer detection and were the first to call the process "screening," believed that symptom-free women could be convinced to undergo regular testing.[48] Other specialists were not sure if "the womanhood of America can be enticed into the laboratory for routine vaginal smears at regular intervals."[49] They pointed to another obstacle for the generalization of de-

tection of proliferative lesions of the cervix: lack of agreement among pathologists about the classification of such lesions.[50] In 1956, twenty-five pathologists
were sent twenty identical borderline slides and were asked to determine how
many of the lesions were precancerous and how many should be classified as true
malignancy. The results displayed a perfect Gaussian distribution: three pathologists found no cancer, three a single case of malignancy, and, on the other end,
four had found nine cases of true cancer, one found twelve cases, and one found
thirteen such cases.[51] Because pathologists were not able to agree what pre-
invasive lesion of the cervix was, they provided widely disparate estimates on the
occurrence of such lesions in the general population. In the 1950s such estimates
varied between 0.02 percent and 3.5 percent.[52]

At first sight, disagreements of that magnitude between the specialists should
have become an insurmountable obstacle for the development of mass screening
campaigns. This was not the case, however. The absence of homogenous diagnostic and prognostic criteria did not hamper a rapid diffusion of the Pap test and
the generalization of screening for premalignant cervical lesions.

The reading of vaginal smears, like other cytological diagnoses, relies on experts' interpretation of visual evidence. It is therefore very difficult to standardize.[53] In the 1950s and 1960s, one of the main objections to the generalization of
Pap smears was the impossibility of training—and paying—a sufficient number
of specialists to do this work. A possible solution could have been an automatic
reading of slides.[54] It was hoped that machines would eliminate all the obviously
normal slides, greatly reducing the number of preparations that needed to be
seen by a specialist. In the 1960s and 1970s, with the beginning of the development of automatic analysis of blood cells, this seemed a feasible approach. Ulti-
mately, however, the Pap test resisted automatic execution.[55] The only alternative
solution was the recruitment and training of a sufficient number of cytology
technicians (mostly women) able to perform routine examinations under the
supervision of competent pathologists (in the 1950s and 1960s, mostly men), a
costly and complicated arrangement that nevertheless became the standard way
of detecting cervical lesions.

In the United States, ACS, committed to the early detection of cancer, strongly
supported the diffusion of the Pap smear.[56] ACS sponsored the First National
Cytology Conference (Boston, 1948) and funded the training of pathologists by
George Papanicolaou. The generalization of exfoliative cytology was also supported by the National Cancer Institute and the U.S. Public Health Service.[57] An
efficient institutional backing and the engagement of many public figures in favor
of screening helped to overcome the difficulty of homogenizing diagnoses. The

Pap smear was never truly standardized or made fully reliable. It was also never tested in randomized clinical trials.[58] It became, however, as Monica Casper and Adele Clarke put it, "the right tool for the job."[59] The criteria of differentiation between dysplasia and in situ cancer remained fluid, and in the 1970s, too, pathologists readily acknowledged that "one man's dysplasia is another man's carcinoma in situ" and that the progression of a precancerous lesion to invasive cancer is an unpredictable process. They proclaimed nevertheless their confidence in the efficacy of screening for cervical malignancies.[60]

Casper and Clarke explain the practical success of exfoliative cytology as a result of the development of efficient division of labor between cytotechnicians and pathologists, the replacement of attempts to create universally valid classifications by a locally negotiated order and the regulation of laboratories.[61] One can add two additional elements: the role of colposcopic examinations and cervical biopsies and the acceptability of a high level of overtreatment. The Pap smear became gradually perceived as a prescreening rather than a true diagnostic test. A positive result was seen above all as an invitation for a further exploration, usually by colposcopy, and if necessary, cervical biopsy. In the interwar era the colposcope was seen mainly as a research tool.[62] The diffusion of the Pap smear led to a wider use of colposcopic examinations, often coupled with a cervical biopsy, and led to the development of a new group of specialists: gynecologists who specialized in colposcopic diagnosis of cervical lesions.[63] As one expert stated: "colposcopy, the stereoscopic magnification of the cervix, can give the gynecologist a clinical understanding of carcinoma in situ of the cervix which is not otherwise possible."[64] The routine use of colposcopy following an abnormal Pap smear reduced the need to make the Pap test accurate. It also eliminated the objection that exfoliated cervical cells are not representative of the tumor. The presence of such cells was transformed from a demonstration of a malignant transformation to a warning sign that something may be wrong.[65]

An additional element in the success of the Pap smear as a screening tool was the relative ease of elimination of suspicious cervical lesions. Surgical pathologists agree that a fine-grained cytological diagnosis of such lesions has a restricted role in their management: "If one accepts that the cervical intraepithelial neoplasia [in situ lesions] is a continuous process, then the grade of de-differentiation is principally a statement of probability of development of an invasive carcinoma, but such an aggregate probability statement is meaningless for the individual patient. The important element for a women diagnosed with a proliferative lesion of the cervix is the ease of elimination of a suspicious lesion and not details of its histological diagnosis."[66]

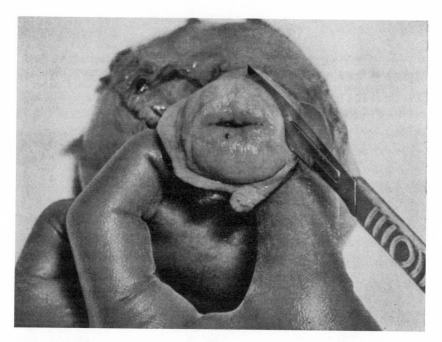

Conization biopsy—excision of large portion of the cervix. Hugh McLaren, *The Prevention of Cervical Cancer,* London: The English University Press, 1963, 53. Reprinted by permission of Hodder & Stoughton Ltd.

The demonstration that destruction of cervical lesions was as efficient as hysterectomy in eliminating the danger of malignancy led to a greater acceptability of overtreatment. This development in turn decreased the need for an accurate diagnosis of cervical lesions even more.[67] With the generalization of the conservative therapies, the main problem of screening became to reduce the number of false negative diagnoses. An unnecessary minor surgery following an incorrect diagnosis of proliferative lesion of the cervix is less distressing than a failure to detect a potentially lethal disease. Accordingly, screening techniques (reading of Pap smears and biopsies) were calibrated for high sensitivity (low number of false negative results) and low specificity (higher number of false positive results).

The transformation of the Pap test into the "right" tool for the diagnosis of pre-invasive cervical lesions—or rather the right tool for the selection of women who need to be seen by a specialist—did not put an end to debates on the natural history of cervical lesions or the scope of desirable medical intervention. Debates on this topic continue in the early twenty-first century. Evaluations of the rate of progression of premalignant lesions to cancer continued to differ widely, and the distinction between dysplasia and in situ cancer remains fluid.[68] A 1996 pathology textbook acknowledged that it is not possible to predict what the future of a given cervical lesion will be. The definition of a given lesion of the cervix as premalignant is an act of faith: "Dysplasia is an imprecise but practical term: pathologists see it when they have to give a name to cellular changes that are too irregular to be called hyperplasia and not irregular enough to be called neoplasia. This is a compromise and an admission of ignorance, but there is an excuse; according to current theories of carcinogenesis, some in-between changes *should* exist."[69]

Clinical guidelines that reinforced the principle of physical elimination of every suspicious cervical lesion diminished even more the practical importance of an accurate classification of these lesions. Such guidelines accentuate the importance of careful colposcopic evaluation of every doubtful case. The slightest suspicion of anomaly should lead to a further investigation, and when the doubt persists, to an excisional procedure, preferably a cold knife conization.[70] Diagnostic uncertainty was transformed into therapeutic certainty, and highly heterogeneous diagnostic categories became manageable thanks to the homogenization of good practice rules.

Pap Screening in the United Kingdom: Between Activism and Public Health Policies

Pap screening has a unique history in the United Kingdom. The initiative to start such screening did not come from gynecologists, cancer experts, or health administrators but from women themselves. BECC's director, Malcolm Donaldson, visited the United States in 1950 and was impressed by the ACS-sponsored network of 125 cancer detection clinics, dedicated mainly to the diagnosis of cervical malignancies.[71] He believed, however, that such an initiative was not possible in Britain because the National Health Service (NHS) could not be persuaded to make a substantial investment in cancer screening. He was overly pessimistic. A grassroots initiative of a group of women led to the establishment of a national screening program in the United Kingdom.

The group who spearheaded Pap screening in Britain, the Medical Women Federation (MWF), was founded in London in 1879 to promote women in medicine. By 1910, what was then called the Association of Registered Women Doctors had branches in all major British cities. In 1916, it took on its current name. MWF's activities were focused on making women's specific health problems visible. In the 1960s, MWF became the main organized force behind Women's

National Cancer Control Campaign. The idea to start such a campaign emerged from a meeting of Stoke Newtington Liaison Committee of Women's Peace Group in 1964. The Stoke Newtington group—a progressive and antimilitarist organization—previously promoted banning tests of nuclear weapons. After the Test Ban Treaty was signed, the group was looking for another activist cause. They invited, partly by chance, a doctor interested in screening for cervical cancer to their February 18, 1964, meeting. One of the women present at this meeting, a physiotherapist, was strongly impressed by this doctor's statement that three thousand women die yearly in the United Kingdom from an easily preventable disease and decided to found a committee dedicated to the promotion of the Pap smear. She contacted MWF, who was immediately interested. A Labor parliament member, Joyce Butler, joined the MWF's committee for cervical cancer screening and helped to put this issue on parliament's agenda.[72]

The National Cervical Cancer Prevention Campaign was founded in January 1965. It was sponsored by MWF and also supported by the National Council of Women and the Women's British Legion. Joyce Butler was named the Campaign's president. MWF had links with multiple political associations: the Labour Party, Association for Maternal and Child Welfare, the Family Planning Association, National Council of Women, British Society for Clinical Cytology, and the Communist Party's Women Committee. One of the Campaign's first successes was to promote debates on screening for cervical cancer in the Parliament and the House of Lords. One of the arguments used in these debates was that the introduction of a contraceptive pill may increase cancer risk, "because we are tampering in the dark with a very delicate piece of machinery."[73]

Preliminary debates on screening for cervical cancer often evoked the difficulty of recruiting a sufficient number of qualified cytology technicians. It was automatically assumed that these technicians would be female, and the issue was reformulated as the training of women and the establishment of conditions that would allow married women with children to work in a cytology laboratory.[74] Additional issues were the frequency of screening (every five, three, or two years) and the fear of inaccurate results. False negatives may lull women into neglecting symptoms, while false positives may lead to unnecessary hysterectomies. The British government decided to encourage screening through providing financial compensation for doctors who collect samples and the opening of cytological laboratories. The number of screened women tripled between 1964 and 1966, as did the number of technicians who read cervical smears. In 1966, screening for cervical cancer was proclaimed a national service by the British government, and the NHS established local co-coordinating committees to implement such screening. In parallel the NHS decided to promote the establishment of regional screening centers that centralized the collection of vaginal smears and their reading.[75]

By around 1968 it became clear that the proposed approach was not working well. The report of the British Women's National Cancer Control Campaign (previously Women Cervical Cancer Control Campaign) for that year explained that facilities established at great cost were not being fully used. Highly skilled technicians were underemployed, and clinics had begun to close. There is a need, the campaign activists argued, to make the services better known through educational activities addressed to specific groups, especially working-class women and migrant populations. Educational materials should disseminate hopeful news about cervical cancer.[76] One of the problems, the committee's report proposed, may be a lack of attention to women's priorities. Behavior that may seem unreasonable from a doctor's point of view, such as not consulting promptly for suspicious gynecological symptoms or refusing screening, "may be perfectly reasonable from the point of view of a outwardly healthy woman who worries about her work, her mortgage, her family, and does not have much faith in doctor's efficacy."[77] NHS developed mobile gynecology units to limit difficulties in scheduling appointments and to bring screening to women who needed it most. Initial experience with such units revealed, however, that women who visit them were mainly interested in obtaining treatment for already existing gynecological problems.[78] Finally, British health authorities decided that the most efficient solution would be to switch the responsibility for Pap screening to general practitioners (GPs), who would be supervised by public health physicians.

In the early 1970s, screening for cervical cancer was redefined in the United Kingdom as a community service. Educational leaflets on Pap smears stressed that it was a painless, simple procedure and presented the treatment of abnormal lesions as an equally unproblematic intervention. A follow-up of reactions of GPs who collected vaginal smears revealed a more complicated image. The insertion of the speculum was sometimes painful, GPs were not always familiar with the range of variation in cervical anatomy, some of the samples they obtained were inadequate, and not all the doctors were happy to perform this task. Nevertheless, the NHS was able to stabilize the uptake of cervical screening tests and to construct a reliable network of GPs, public health doctors, cytology laboratories, gynecologists, and oncologists. Screening for cervical cancer never became entirely problem free. It became, however, a reasonably efficient public health intervention credited with an important decrease of mortality from cervical tumors in the United Kingdom.[79]

Teaching British Women about Screening for Malignancies

In the 1960s, the Women's National Cancer Control Campaign sponsored a series of short films on screening and early detection of female cancers. Some of these short films, destined mainly to be projected in movie theaters, linked the call to undergo Pap smears with an injunction to see a doctor rapidly when noticing suspicious symptoms. Eight scenarios were selected by the Campaign. One was a short humorous cartoon calling all women to get tested. Seven others tell short stories that illustrate the need to be screened for cancer.[80]

1. "Calling All Women." Story of Mrs. Jones, a young mother, who undergoes screening for cervical cancer. The film stresses that examination with a speculum, which makes women especially anxious, is not painful. Mrs. Jones has suspicious cells, and she undergoes a conical biopsy, described as a "cancer treatment." Her doctor tells her that "the cancer was localized in the cervix." After she comes back from the hospital, Mrs. Jones is helped by a health visitor to cope with her household duties. She is reassured by her physicians that in spite of the treatment she can have children and sex ("it won't make any difference to your married life"). An animated insert explains the danger of cancer and methods of eliminating this danger. In the last shot, the heroine is playing with her children "to look at her now, you'd never believe she'd ever had a thing wrong with her, let alone cancer."

2. "Take Action." Cartoon situated in a production plant with female workers, among them an Indian woman, Amina. One of the women says that she learned about cancer screening (Pap smear) and that they all have to have it. The shop steward, Peg, goes to the (male) plant manager, telling him that other workplaces, like Marks and Spencer, had organized testing for their female workforce. The manager immediately agrees to do the same and calls the local Officer of Health. The latter explains that in order to send health workers to the plant, they need to organize a full session. Peg and her friends produce posters and leaflets. They also provide information to men, because, "while they do not get it, they need to be concerned. Cancer hit them where it hurts: no more nights out at the pub, no more football on Saturdays, just staying home with all these grizzling kids." Amina volunteers to translate the posters into Hindi. Men indeed became concerned, fearing the loss of their spouses. The screening session is a big success, with 95 percent attendance.

3. "Cancer Control." Interview of health visitors with uncooperative men in a working-class neighborhood. At first the workers resent the "meddling" visitor. An offscreen voice comments that "if a working class 'mum' falls ill, the husband

has almost no chance of keeping the family together." The children are either divided between relatives or looked after by the local authority. The health visitor
adds that if the problem is a short-term one, one can ask neighbors to help. The
film switches to an interview with a young mother who had a "surgery for breast
cancer" five years ago and is fine now: "her life was saved because she went to a
doctor in time." Another interview, with a working-class woman who underwent
screening for cervical cancer, stresses that the test does not take much time and
"a babysitter is easy to arrange." The film ends with an interview with MP Joyce
Butler and one of the leaders of the Women's National Cancer Control Campaign, Lady Donaldson.

4. "Emergency Stop." Three women in a bus, two in their thirties and middle-
aged "Gran," and a small boy. Gran is telling about a friend who luckily went to
the clinics in time and had "the test." She explains that the test is so easy, like a
postnatal exam, and the mother says, "Shh, not in front of the boy." Gran is speak-
ing then about another friend who was lucky, too, because the lump in her breast
was found rapidly, and she was cured. Were it otherwise, "young Bob would've
been lost without her, with all these kids . . . they'd have had to go on the council, I suppose." Mum says, "Shame, lovely kids," but Gran replies, "Do not get
mournful, she is all right, they only kept her a week or so, she says she hasn't felt
so well in years." Mum adds, "Well, it must have pulled her down, having that all
the time." The other woman is convinced now to call the clinics immediately and
schedule a Pap smear and she hurries to do it.

5. "The Building Site." A film aimed at husbands. It attempts to show them the
difficulties they will encounter if their wives became ill. One worker has to cope
with a large family while his wife is spending a few days in the hospital following
a positive Pap smear. His mates are making fun of him and then realize it can
happen to them, too. They start asking questions about the test, the hero is explaining that he is happy that his wife is doing well and ends by saying, "If you
want to know any more, get your old woman to go to the clinics."

6. "Over the Wall." Women discuss the test "over the garden wall." One of their
neighbors had a positive Pap smear and they are waiting for her to come out of
the hospital. The second had the test as matter of course after the birth of her last
child and persuades another woman, who is pregnant, that it is not a big deal. The
third woman has no children and thinks that she is not concerned by this test. In
one case, the husband has not been cooperative. A health visitor who tries to convince him fails at first and then finds an ally—the husband of the woman who
was found to be positive. The latter is going to persuade his mate to get his wife
to be tested.

7. "Stay Young, Stay with Us." A girl got married in her teens and faced multiple disasters because she had not heard about prevention. The water pipes in her house burst, she accidentally sets fire to the neighbor's house without being insured, her children are not vaccinated and have had to be put in quarantine. Finally she reforms and does all the necessary preventive actions, including a test for cervical cancer that will keep her healthy.

These educational films, like other propaganda materials on cancer screening, convey an infallibly upbeat message. They even present the treatment for cancer as unproblematic—a woman after a mastectomy "never felt better in her life." They affirm in parallel that screening saves lives of mothers of young children, conveying the implicit message that it's the mothers' duty to undergo screening for cancer, otherwise their children will end in state-sponsored institutions. These movies were explicitly directed to working-class women. Cervical cancer was linked to low socioeconomic status, and the Women's National Cancer Control Campaign aspired to reduce cervical cancer deaths among lower-class women, seen as especially endangered by this disease. Similar movies destined to the American public, and, inspired by experts' rather than activists' point of view, emphasized personal happiness and the freedom from cancer threat. They did not stress the mother's responsibility for her children and did not attempt to redress class-related inequalities in access to medical information.[81]

Pap Smears and Public Health Considerations

Even a highly efficient screening test, Louise Russell had shown, can have a negative cost-benefit ratio. Screening for cervical cancer may be efficient in principle, but if it is poorly distributed, with some women "overscreened" and overtreated, with others lacking access to screening services, it is not efficient in practice.[82] British, French, and North American public health experts discussed cost-benefit of screening for cervical malignancies. In the United Kingdom experts recommended three-year intervals between vaginal smears. The existence of NHS-monitored programs (first a regional ones, and, from 1988, a national screening program) did not put an end to controversies on classifications of cervical lesions, quality of cytological services, or the global efficacy of screening.[83] In a widely discussed 2004 article, Julian Peto and his colleagues affirmed that screening for cervical cancer in the United Kingdom was an impressive success. It prevented up to five thousand cancer deaths per year, especially among young women.[84] Other epidemiologists argued that these evaluations were too optimistic. Deaths from cervical cancer undoubtedly went down as did the prevalence of this disease, but this did not mean that the only reason for this decrease was the introduction of the Pap smear. Other factors—such as better hygiene, the use of oral contraceptives, changes in sexual behavior and probably other, unidentified environmental or lifestyle-related elements—might have contributed to the reduction of the prevalence of cervical cancer in the past twenty years.[85] British experts agree that screening is efficient, but they propose divergent views on its contribution to the epidemiology of cervical cancer, and have different opinions on its cost-benefit ratio.

In France, debates on a national program of screening for cervical cancer started in the 1970s at the initiative of the Health Ministry. A 1975 report of the Ministry's Cancer Commission advocated a nationwide campaign for the screening of cervical cancer destined to cover 50 percent of the target population in its first year. The proposed periodicity of screening was every five years. The report modeled the costs of such a nationwide screening campaign, compared it with the burden of cancer, and concluded that the screening was cost-effective.[86] An additional report discussed the training of cytology technicians. It stated that training in this area was insufficiently regulated and proposed opening a state-sponsored school that would provide one year of training to become a technician, with a possibility of studying another year for a diploma of higher rank technician. Cytology technicians (the document did not mention their sex) would provide only a true screening, that is, a distinction between normal and abnormal slides. Diagnostic tasks should be exclusively reserved to physicians specializing in cytology.[87] The conclusions of these two reports were never implemented. A national program of screening for cervical cancer in France started only in 2003, with the introduction of the National Cancer Plan.

Screening for cervical cancer in France was nevertheless strongly encouraged by gynecologists' associations and the Health Ministry, and its costs were fully reimbursed by national health insurance. The ministry promoted several pilot projects in selected regions. These projects proposed a thirty-month interval between screenings.[88] Elsewhere the Pap smear was diffused through the education of gynecologists and then by GPs.[89] The latter played an important but uneven role in the propagation of cervical smears outside major cities. Intervals between screenings were left to the discretion of individual doctors, and practices varied greatly.[90] The 2003 national cancer plan adopted the principle of triennial screening for women with two consecutive normal annual smears, a recommendation conforming to the opinion of many European experts.[91] The use of the Pap smear in France is still uneven. According to data published by the French Institut du Cancer, 35 percent of French women have never had a Pap smear, while many others—women with higher level of education, those who live in cities, those who are followed by a gynecologist rather than a GP—probably overuse the test.[92]

In the absence of national health insurance, screening for cervical cancer in the United States is the responsibility of individual doctors. The result is the promotion of frequent screening for affluent women and a paucity of programs that support screening of underprivileged populations.[93] The majority of U.S. gynecologists were in favor of annual Pap screens, and 80 percent of women who underwent regular screening were tested every year.[94] Cost-effectiveness analysis revealed that this was a wasteful strategy. It saves very few additional lives, greatly increases the overall cost of screening, and amplifies the danger of overtreatment. Some U.S. experts proposed therefore the adoption of standard European recommendations: women with three consecutive negative annual smears should be then tested every three years.[95] A 2004 editorial of *Diagnostic Cytology* strongly criticized this strategy. Women, this text claimed, should manage their "health capital" using the same logic they employ to manage their stocks and increase their gains: "Investment in annual cervical cancer screening is in many ways like investing in diversified funds for the long term: not very exciting but very effective way to lower your risk of cancer over lifetime. . . . It is important for women investing in their own health to have their investment choices appropriate for their goals of cervical cancer prevention for their entire life, and not just one 3-year window in time. A more efficient but less effective Pap test may not be the best way to meet these investment goals."[96]

The recent demonstration of the role of human papilloma virus (HPV) in the genesis of cervical tumors changed the screening for cervical cancer and modified the overall perception of this disease. Doctors who studied prevalence of female cancers noticed that cervical cancer is more frequent in married women and is very rare among virgins. By contrast, breast cancer was more often found in unmarried women. Nuns were considered to be virtually free from cervical cancer and especially prone to breast malignancies. Some authors linked cervical cancer with lacerations produced during childbirth, while others connected it with women's sexual activity and then with an excess of such activity.[97] A 1975 study connected the prevalence of cervical cancer to ethnic origins and the age of first sexual relationship and stated that "cervical cancer has certain characteristics of a venereal disease; in particular the risk has been associated with sexual promiscuity."[98]

At first the infectious agent responsible for "sexually transmitted malignancy" was thought to be the herpes simplex virus, a frequent sexually transmitted infection, associated in the early 1980s with the newly described acquired immunodeficiency syndrome. In 1983, thanks to improved methods of DNA-based diagnosis, cervical cancer was linked by several groups with another virus frequently found in sexually active women, HPV.[99] In the early twenty-first century, women with abnormal Pap smears continued to undergo colposcopy, but they were also tested for the presence of "carcinogenic" HPV strains. Some experts proposed (in 2007) replacing Pap smears with the search for such HPV strains.[100] HPV strains are diagnosed with molecular biology techniques that identify DNA variations. The switch to a systematic search for carcinogenic HPV strains can facilitate homogenization of screening (it is easier to standardize molecular biology techniques than the detection of abnormal cells in a smear) and make its automatic execution possible (DNA sequencing is often made today by fully automated machines). If adopted, this approach—still seen as problematic because of its low specificity—will probably end difficulties linked with the calibration of the reading of Pap smears.[101] Such a change (if it happens) probably will not eliminate the need for HPV-infected women to undergo colposcopies and biopsies and will not solve dilemmas linked with the definition of the threshold and magnitude of therapeutic interventions.

The redefinition of cervical cancer as a sexually transmitted disease occasionally led to the stigmatization of women who tested positive and were suspected of "promiscuity" and to a parallel fear of stigmatization.[102] It included men in the circle of people concerned about cervical cancer, because male partners of women infected with HPV may be invited to be treated, too. Finally, the new understanding of cervical cancer extended the definition of risk of cervical tumors. Only a small portion of HPV-infected women develops cancer of the cervix, and the majority of women diagnosed with potentially dangerous HPV strains spontaneously eliminate the infection in one or two years. Nevertheless, a diagnosis of infection with a "carcinogenic" strain of HPV is seen by some women as a disturbing and potentially life-threatening event, adding an additional layer of complexity to an already complicated testing for cancer risk.[103]

The Price of Screening

In the second half of the twentieth century, screening for cervical cancer was transformed into a demonstration of the validity of the early detection principle. "Low cost" therapeutic interventions—in monetary terms but also in terms of their consequences for screened and treated women—efficiently reduced the danger of malignancy. The low cost of elimination of cervical lesions is not, however, a zero cost. Conization biopsy or a laser therapy of cervical lesions may be experienced as traumatic events even when the individual receives efficient anesthesia, good postoperative follow-up, and an adequate explanation of the whole process. In addition, the elimination of cervical dysplasia has a nonnegligible complication ratio and may occasionally induce sterility or problems during pregnancy.[104] Some experts criticize an indiscriminate use of a not-entirely-benign surgical procedure, a practice fueled, especially in the United States, by doctors' apprehension of litigation.[105]

In a culture with a high level of fear of cancer, especially among women, screening for cervical cancer may have an important psychological cost as well. One of the rarely discussed drawbacks of such screening is an irreversible generation of uncertainty.[106] The detection and the elimination of cervical lesions greatly reduces a danger of a future malignancy and is therefore highly beneficial for women with proliferative changes in the cervix. Such an individual benefit has, however, a collective price. Screening provides important advantages for a small number of women—those who escaped cervical cancer—but it may change the sense of body and self of many other women who do not personally benefit from the screening. It may also unsettle those who find themselves with unclear diagnosis, prognosis, and future.[107] Women who received abnormal results of a Pap smear described themselves as being in a liminal situation. Diagnosed with a potentially threatening condition with an uncertain meaning, they are not sure if they should see themselves as sick or as healthy.[108] This is especially true for women diagnosed with ACUS—atypical cells of unknown significance. Submitted to an intensive medical surveillance (frequent colposcopies, smears, HPV tests, sometimes biopsies), they may remain for a long time in a limbo produced by medical technologies.[109]

The great majority of the experts, but also of activists, enthusiastically endorsed screening for cervical cancer. Their point of view was sustained by epidemiologic data. This does not mean, however, that such screening is problem-free. A positive result of a screening test, medical sociologist Nicky Britten proposed, may radically change one's view of the body. When she learned about the presence of abnormal cells in her cervical smear, she was unable for several days to think about anything but death. And, she adds, "the experience has not left me unchanged. It is as if, having allowed the possibility of one disease to enter my body, a host of other conditions have crowded behind it. . . . I lost an innocence of outlook."[110]

Britten believes that screening for cervical cancer is a good and necessary public health measure. She wished only to attract attention to some of its more problematic aspects. The important point, she argued, is to inform women about the hazards of screening to one's mental and physical health, in order to allow them to make truly informed choices. Sociologist Naomi Pfeffer agrees. She believes that since health promotion interventions such as screening for cancer are neither neutral nor innocuous, they should be submitted to the same informed consent rules as other medical acts.[111]

Other researchers are less sure that all the problems raised by the generalization of screening for cancer and cancer risk can be solved by providing more accurate information about procedures and outcomes and explaining more clearly individual choices. Living in a screening culture limits the possibilities of opting out of it and increases the price of such "irrational" behavior for those who choose to do so. Screening for cancer focuses attention on selected elements and makes others less visible. The English word for a search for hidden cancers—screening—and the metaphor of a sieve it evokes conveys the idea of capturing something of particular interest, while enabling irrelevant entities to fall through the sieve's holes.[112] The selective grid of cancer screening often "screens out" uncertainty about medical interventions and the unique experience of screened people. The latter are invited to perceive themselves at the same time as healthy and complete, and as (potentially) unhealthy and (de facto) flawed. The French term "dépistage" (tracing) conveys a similar meaning. An exclusive interest in traces of early malignant and premalignant changes in the body may lead to a neglect of "untraced" entities such as side effects of biopsies (pain and postsurgical complications), overtreatment, or psychological consequences of coping with an ambivalent diagnosis.[113] In an optimistic appreciation of a "bio-risk culture," the new focus on embodied risks opens spaces for the shaping of new identities, responsibilities, alliances between people, social links, and creative ways of being in the world.[114] In a more pessimistic view of such a culture, the new accent on the management of cancer risk may also undermine people's—and especially women's—confidence in their bodies.[115] Partial erosion of women's trust in their bodies may be an acceptable price of an effective way to prevent a deadly disease. The great majority of critics of screening for cervical cancer did not question the principle of such screening, only the ways it was implemented, and the tendency to "screen out" of some of its consequences. The extension of screening to other malignancies was a more problematic endeavor.

CHAPTER SIX

The Generalization of Screening

From Cervical to Breast Tumors

The practical success of screening for cervical cancer validated the principle of physical elimination of premalignant lesions and legitimated the extension of this preventive approach to other tumors.[1] The transformation of cervical cancer into a model malignancy was, however, made possible by selective emphasis on some aspects of this tumor. For example, experts brought to the foreground the possibility of displaying of all the stages of transition from a mild cervical dysplasia to a fully invasive carcinoma but did not dwell on the erratic and unpredictable behavior of cervical lesions or the difficulty of correlating cytological diagnoses with outcomes.[2] Their descriptions seldom indicated that cervical lesions have many unusual traits: very slow growth, accessibility to the physician's gaze, and great fragility. A view that accentuated the universality of the "cervical cancer" model and underplayed its particularity facilitated the initial transposition of this model to other tumors. It might have also favored underestimating the difficulties of such transposition.

Many cancer experts were influenced by the debate on the "biological determinism" of malignant tumors. This debate focused on early detection of breast cancer. Surgical pathologist Ian MacDonald, biometrician Neil McKinnon (both were Canadians, but MacDonald worked in at University of Southern California), and their colleagues argued in the 1950s that the "curability" of a given breast tumor depended mainly its biological characteristics. Slow-growing tumors can be cured even if discovered late (on an absolute time-scale), while aggressive and rapidly growing ones cannot be cured even if discovered early. Advocates of this view strongly criticized the "false premises and false promises" that dominated the field of cancer prevention and cure.[3] Their views impressed many practitioners. For example, a young American radiotherapist Franz Bushke wrote in 1957 to his mentor, Maurice Lenz:

> I suppose that you have seen Ian Macdonald's paper in the proceedings of the Third National Cancer Conference, 1957. I thought it was very interesting and it thoroughly fits my philosophy. If his observations stand the test of criticism, I think they should once and *for* all stop our insistence on proving statistically the superiority of one method over the other. If 25 percent have a favorable prognosis, regardless of what is done, and 50 percent have an unfavorable prognosis, regardless of the type of therapy, and only in 25 percent treatment is critical, I do not think that one can ever prove the superiority of one method over the other by statistical methods.[4]

Many doctors, especially in Europe, agreed with MacDonald and McKinnon's views and argued that if a cancer of the breast is growing slowly, a delay in its detection will not make much difference in terms of survival, and if it grows fast, it had already spread at the moment of detection of a lump in the breast.[5] One of the promoters of this view, British surgeon Lester Breslow, explained in 1959 that "the practice of actively looking for lumps in the breast brings to medical attention and treatment nowadays cases of slow-growing cancer that in former years would have been neglected. These should have perhaps never have been diagnosed in the past, and also might have never have advanced to the point of causing death. Tabulating such cases now as cured or as long term survivors may be illusory."[6]

Robert Sutherland's 1960 book, *Cancer: The Significance of Delay*, reflected a similar preoccupation.[7] Sutherland, a senior lecturer in preventive medicine at the University of Leeds and director of British Empire Cancer Campaign (BECC) council in Yorkshire, opens his book with Cicero's quotation, "There are two grand faults to be avoided: the first is an over-great hastiness and rashness in giving up our assent, presuming that we know things before we really do so." A diagnosis of early tumors, Sutherland explained, often relies exclusively on a histological analysis, not on information on the tumor's biological behavior.[8] However, histologically identical tumors can have very different fates: "Surely it would be better to discard the words early and late with their time connotations and their ambiguity, and to replace them with such purely descriptive terms as non-infiltrating, non-infiltrating but metastasizing, infiltrating and infiltrating and metastasizing."[9]

Not only was the biology of a tumor highly variable, but reactions of the person who has the tumor were changeable, too; moreover, both were influenced by environmental factors. Malignant tumors remained latent for long periods of time if they belonged to a slow-growing variety, were kept in check by the person's immune response, were modulated by environmental stimuli, or all of the above.[10] Facing such triple variability, predictions grounded in morphological criteria only were highly problematic. Sutherland did not advocate therapeutic nihilism. The doctors' duty, he explained, is to try to do whatever possible to help their patients. An effort to find malignancies as rapidly as possible may sometimes provide such help. Doctors do not know beforehand who among their patients will benefit from an early diagnosis, he believed, and should do their best to provide such a diagnosis to all. But, Sutherland added, "we should remember that the benefit is statistically moderate: our claims must be modest."[11]

Transparent Breasts: The Rise of Mammography

The success of screening for cervical cancer directly stimulated efforts to find ways to detect premalignant and very early malignant lesions of the breast.[12] From the 1960s on, such efforts focused on radiological detection of breast anomalies. Mammographic screening for cancer became popular in the 1970s, but the principle of radiographic diagnosis of breast tumors was much older. In the interwar era, radiologists had already used x-rays to diagnose breast anomalies, and they improved this technique in the postwar era.[13] The increasing popularity of this approach was probably related to the growing conviction that the rise of "breast cancer awareness" and the intensive propaganda, especially in the United States, in favor of breast self-examinations (BSE), failed to improve the cure rate of breast cancer.

Many practitioners believed, however, that when detected clinically, breast cancer often had already produced micro-metastases. The existence of divergent views about the natural history of breast cancer may explain differences between the introduction of screening for breast and screening for cervical malignancies. Screening for cervical cancer was grounded in experts' quasi-unanimous conviction that the elimination of cervical lesions was an efficient way to prevent cancer. This supposition originated in cytological observations and was partly validated by epidemiological data, but it was never tested in a controlled clinical trials. The physiological logic of elimination of cervical lesions was supported by direct observations of the cervix and by data on the fate of untreated cervical lesions. Such data were either obtained intentionally, in clinical experiments, or because doctors discovered such lesions retroactively when they reexamined slides of a woman who had later developed cervical malignancy. Proliferative lesions of the breast are not directly accessible to clinicians' gaze (at most, they can sample tissue through biopsy), while mammography provides data on changes in architecture of breast tissue that are only indirectly related to malignant transformation. It was therefore important to test the role of mammographic screening in decreasing mortality from breast cancer in clinical trials. The first among them was the systematic screening of women enrolled in the Health Insurance Plan of Greater New York, which was introduced in the early 1960s. This clinical trial demonstrated the feasibility of mammographic screening and indicated that it reduced the occurrence of breast malignancies.[14] Other clinical trials of mammography confirmed these results. Trials conducted in two Swedish counties, Östergötland and Kopparberg, were presented as especially solid evidence of mammography's efficacy. The only exception was a Canadian clinical trial, conducted in the 1980s. This trial failed to demonstrate positive effects of mammographic screening, but the negative results were attributed to methodological problems and the use of inappropriate mammography equipment.[15]

In the 1970s critiques of mammographic screening focused on radiation risk. The development of new x-ray machines with a lower radiation level attenuated these objections. In the United States, experts rapidly adopted the principle of a yearly mammographic screening for women over 50.[16] Such screening was covered by private health insurance, and at first was mainly used by middle-class women.[17] In the 1990s the U.S. government established the Centers for Disease Control's National Breast and Cervical Early Detection Program, which financed mammographic screening of uninsured women and those from underprivileged social strata.[18] Nearly all the specialists agreed that regular mammograms in women over 50 reduced the number of breast cancer deaths. By contrast, the efficacy of screening for women between ages 40 and 49 remained controversial. Younger women have denser breasts, more difficult to examine with x-rays, but they also have a lower incidence of breast cancer. It was not clear therefore if they would benefit from mammographic screening. The National Cancer Institute (NCI) recommended in 1989 starting such screening at the age of 40, and the American Cancer Society (ACS) made a similar recommendation. However, in 1992, following the publication of a large-scale study (the Canadian National Breast Screening Study) that failed to show benefits of mammography in women under 50, the NCI decided to revise its initial guidelines.[19] ACS experts disagreed. They decided to maintain their original recommendation of starting mammographic screening at 40, arguing that even if the efficacy of such screening could not be demonstrated in controlled clinical trials, it could still save the lives of some women.[20]

NCI's position led to a storm of protests.[21] During congressional hearings on this subject, cancer patients testified that mammograms made in their forties saved them from a certain death, and politicians denounced indifference to women's plight.[22] The strong endorsement of mammography for women in their forties was grounded in the assumption that mammograms are always beneficial for women. The only obstacle to the dissemination of this life-saving technology, patients, activists, and radiologists explained, was its cost.[23] Pressured by politicians, eager to show their constituencies that they cared about women's health, the Committee on Government Operation of both houses stated that NCI failed to examine objectively scientific evidence on mammography.[24] In an attempt to justify its position, the NCI established in 1997 a consensus conference on mammographic screening of women aged 40 to 50. The panel concluded that the evidence on efficacy of mammography in this age group was weak, and it did not justify a recommendation of systematic screening of all women. Radiologists immediately protested, as did politicians. The Senate voted a resolution supporting mammography for women in their forties. The advisory board of NCI bowed to the political pressure and recommended starting mammographic screening at the age of 40.[25]

In Western Europe, the great majority of experts recommend starting mammographic screening at 50 and proposed longer (two or three years) intervals between mammograms.[26] In the United Kingdom, the Medical Women Federation (MWF) developed interest in breast cancer screening and the promotion of mammography in the late 1960s. However, while MWF enthusiastically supported the generalization of Pap screens, it had a more reserved attitude towards a systematic use of x-rays to diagnose changes in the breast. MWF's secretary Jean Lawrie explained in 1968 that it was not yet proven that screening for breast cancer increased life expectancy. She added, however, that even if early detection did not save lives, it may have a positive psychological effect:

One group of specialists says that the outlook is better if the cancer is found when it is small, and another equally respectable group says that it is the type of cancer that matters, not the size of the lump when originally detected. Therefore it is impossible to say confidently that the outlook is better when the lump is small. However, I think that a woman's fears may be relieved if the lump is treated when it is small, because she may probably take comfort from the feeling that she has not neglected herself.[27]

In the 1970s, British radiologists and gynecologists introduced mammographic screening in selected clinics. At that time (1975), the British Breast Group declared that more research was needed to ascertain if there was a place for a national program.[28] Ten years later, a commission headed by Patrick Forrest estimated, on the basis of analysis of Swedish and Dutch clinical trials, that such evidence existed already. The Forrest commission recommended in 1986 a triennial screening of all British women between the ages of 50 and 69, covered by the National Health Service (NHS). A national plan, the report claimed, is the precondition not only for maintaining high clinical standards but also for an effective evaluation of the efficacy of screening.[29] NHS continued to monitor the quality of screening centers and established national standards of good practice for radiologists, pathologists, and oncologists. British experts justify longer intervals between mammographic screenings (three years, instead of the one year in the United States) by the argument that such intervals greatly reduce the proportion of false positive results without compromising the rates of cancer detection.[30]

Until 2003, France did not have a national coordination of mammographic screening. A few regional programs were introduced in the 1990s, but by and large mammography was promoted by individual gynecologists and occasionally by general practitioners (GPs). It was reimbursed by the national health insurance (Sécurité Sociale).[31] The French situation was described in the late 1990s as chaotic. In spite of the existence of a national health system, mammographic screening was characterized by a multiplication of small centers and highly heterogeneous, unsupervised screening practices.[32] Moreover, each radiology practice purchased and calibrated its own apparatus. Worries about the quality of such privately acquired equipment led in the 1990s to a government-sponsored campaign of checking and homogenizing mammography machines.[33] In 2003, the French national "Cancer Plan" proposed a free, biannual screening for all the French women aged 50 to 75 and fixed the goal of coverage of 70 percent of the target population. According to Institut du Cancer data, mammographic coverage of French women increased from 33 percent in 2003 to 49 percent in 2006.[34]

Attitudes towards mammography screening can be related to those toward BSE. BSE was energetically advocated by the ACS. In 1950 ACS and NCI jointly produced a film, "Breast Self-examination." ACS propaganda leaflets and posters explained that BSE saves women's lives and that its neglect is an irresponsible behavior. This argument was reinforced by testimonies of women who attested that BSE saved their lives or, occasionally that they were dying from cancer because they failed to regularly perform BSE. The implicit message transmitted by these educational materials was that an advanced breast cancer is a self-inflicted disease.[35] BSE was also promoted in the United Kingdom and in Canada, and, to a lesser extent, in continental Europe. Its popularity was sustained by the belief that early detection of breast tumors saves lives, but also by the observation—valid today, too—that the majority of breast cancers are discovered by the women themselves or by their partners.

Attitudes towards BSE continue to vary greatly. A European survey indicated a relatively low level of use of this method: between 6 and 15 percent women practiced self-examination of the breast.[36] In the early twenty-first century, a series of controlled studies indicated that not only does BSE not improve survival but that it also may be harmful. It induces higher rates of unnecessary biopsies and increases women's anxiety.[37] Many women resisted these conclusions. Some remained attached to the idea that they could do something to protect themselves from a dreaded disease. Others believed that they were able to save their lives thanks to this practice. The continuing endorsement of BSE by many breast cancer advocacy groups may mirror faithfulness to a practice that may still be beneficial for some women, in spite of its negative effects on the population level.[38] It may also reflect the power of cancer schemata and the success of a century of efforts to persuade women that early detection is a necessary and sufficient condition for breast cancer cure. This conviction permeates the lived experience of disease. Women with advanced breast cancer often believe that at some point their disease could have been prevented and blame (mostly) themselves and (sometimes) their doctors for their poor prognosis. At a retreat for women with cancer, "the discussions about 'how could I' and 'how could they' were intense expressions of grief, anger, betrayal, and regret; a yearning for a different story that offered better odds."[39]

Mammography: Consensus and Questions

In 1989 one of the main promoters of mammography in the United States, Philip Strax, wrote a poem to the glory of the early detection of cancer:

Let's seek out the foe when it starts its ills
And not be mislead by false cries of alarm
Let's ferret him out with our newly found skills,
And destroy him before he can do any harm.[40]

Strax's poem transmits a clear message: early detection is a decisive weapon in the war on cancer. Not all the specialists agreed. In spite of the large consensus on benefits of mammography, dissenting voices pointed to residual problems. One such problem is high rates of false positive results. In the United States, one third of women who have a yearly mammogram for ten years will be confronted with a "suspicious mammogram," and 18 percent will undergo either a needle biopsy or a surgical one (the removal of the lump or suspected area of the breast). The great majority of such biopsies do not reveal malignancy, but even a negative result is linked with stress, fear, and pain. In addition, surgical biopsies induce scarring of the breast, making consecutive detection of tumors more difficult.[41] Another problem is the difficulty of correlating morphological parameters and outcomes, especially when dealing with lesions detected only by mammography.[42] Mammographic screening was linked with an overtreatment of in situ tumors and unnecessarily aggressive treatment of minimal, slow-growing invasive cancers. Many years ago, Rose Kushner was already concerned by this issue: "The question of what to do when X rays of the breast find something that might be cancer is an enormous problem for women. For some doctors, it seems simple. They have named these little things 'minimal' or 'stage o' breast cancer and they recommend the same kind of treatment for these as they do for large, definitively invasive cancers . . . the problem is aggravated by the fact that many doctors propose mastectomy for such minimal cancer, insisting that an extended surgery can guarantee 100 percent cure."[43]

Kushner drew, among other things, on a 1979 paper that argued that the disease "breast cancer" covers in fact two very different clinical entities. Analysis of survival curves of women with breast cancer suggests that two populations exist: Forty percent have a rapidly metastasizing, incurable disease that drastically shortens their life span. The remaining 60 percent have a much less aggressive pathology and exhibit a relative mortality only modestly different from that of women of similar ages without evidence of disease. In their early stages, the two forms of breast present, however, identical radiological and cytological images.[44] Early detection of breast cancer, Kushner stressed, is not a panacea, because a tumor's size is not a perfect indicator of degree of malignancy or dissemination. In 23 percent of women with non-palpable tumors detected by mammography, the tumor had already spread to lymph nodes: "small does not always mean early, and large does not necessarily mean late."[45] Doctors and cancer charities, she argued, should not promote the unproven claim that early detection always saves lives but rather the more modest one that an earlier detection may allow less drastic breast surgery.[46]

Kushner's worries echoed the 1950s debates on danger of a too-eager search for small and slow-growing breast tumors that might have never advanced to the point of causing death in the patient's lifetime.[47] This debate reemerged in the context of discussion on advantages and disadvantages of mammography.[48]

Reevaluation of early clinical trials of mammography, critics of this screening method argued, failed to show net benefit in overall survival, while the decrease in breast cancer deaths recorded by these trials may reflect a better access to health care and better treatment, rather than a direct effect of radiological screening.[49] Moreover, while women whose cancers are detected by mammography have indeed better survival rates than those diagnosed with clinically visible cancers, this observation, some critics had pointed out, does not necessarily mean that mammography saves lives.[50] According to an alternative explanation, mammography picks preferentially slow-growing—and thus not very dangerous—breast tumors, because such tumors more often produce microcalcifications visible on x-ray film.[51] Mammographic screening favors therefore an aggressive therapy of lesions that are not very malignant and that do not endanger the women's life.[52] While few experts adopt such a pessimistic view of mammography, more agree that a precise evaluation of the positive effects of this approach is very difficult.[53]

In Situ Tumors of the Breast and the Sensitivity of Detection Techniques

Critiques of large-scale screening for cancer argue that such screening often reveals "non-disease": conditions that will not produce clinical disease in a given person's lifetime. This argument is grounded, among other things, in the observation that autopsies of people who died from cancer-unrelated causes reveal a high proportion of small tumors and premalignant lesions.[54] Approximately one-third of men aged 40 to 50 carry in situ prostate cancers (this proportion increases with age), and virtually all people aged 50 to 70 carry in situ cancers of the thyroid gland.[55] Search for in situ cancer of the breast among women who died from a wide range of tumor-unrelated causes also uncovered numerous malignant and premalignant lesions. Among seventy-seven cadavers of women (mostly over age 50) analyzed in one series, fourteen were diagnosed with an in situ carcinoma of the breast (LCIS or DCIS), and one with an invasive cancer.[56] In another series of 110 cadavers of relatively young women (ages 20–54), two were diagnosed with invasive tumors and twenty with in situ cancers.[57] A third study had found severe atypia or in situ cancers in 26 percent of dissected female breasts.[58]

Taken together, these results indicate that autopsies reveal a much higher prevalence of invasive and in situ tumors of the breast than the prevalence rate calculated from epidemiological data.[59] This discrepancy between findings in living and dead female bodies can be explained by the observation that the number of proliferative lesions found in autopsies was directly proportional to the number of examined breast sections.[60] Pathologists who examine a breast biopsy as a part of a routine diagnostic procedure look at a few sections only and often analyze a small part of the breast tissue, whereas when they analyzed cadaver breasts for research purposes, they made numerous thin sections through the whole organ. Such an intensive search greatly increased their chances of detecting small in situ or invasive lesions.[61]

The whole concept of cytological diagnosis of malignant changes in tissues is brought under scrutiny by the proposal that the more the pathologists look for cancer and precancer, more likely they are to find it. As a 1958 editorial of *Lancet* put it: "the startling discrepancy between the clinical and the postmortem prevalence of carcinoma virtually demolished ideas of cancer as an essentially killing disease."[62] It also raises the question of optimal sensitivity (detection power) of cytological methods that make in situ and minimal cancers visible. Should pathologists be encouraged to increase the sensitivity of such techniques and augment the danger of overtreatment, or should they decrease their sensitivity and accept the risk of overlooking dangerous lesions?

The role of resolution of medical imagery techniques in detecting premalignant changes in the breast raises similar questions.[63] Some experts wish to increase the sensitivity of mammography and to introduce techniques such as NMR (nuclear magnetic resonance) able to detect additional breast tumors. Early debates on mammographic screening implicitly assumed that a better quality of x-ray images improved the capacity to detect hidden tumors. The negative results of the Canadian National Breast Screening Study of 1980 were discredited with the argument that the mammographic equipment used in this trial was not sensitive enough and did not produce reliable results.[64] A similar argument was used to refute a more general criticism of mammography screening. The impression that screening for breast cancer is not very efficient, some experts claimed, is grounded in analysis of aggregate data that combine results obtained in good centers with those obtained using inferior equipment and poorly trained radiologists. When performed by competent specialists in well-equipped facilities, mammography is a truly efficient diagnostic tool, the argument goes. To put it otherwise, mammography is perhaps not perfect for underprivileged women or those unable to visit a good radiology center, but it works well for educated, discriminating, and affluent consumers of medical technologies.[65]

Experts in medical imagery attempt to increase the capacity of mammograms to capture minimal changes in the breast and to transform them into meaningful clinical signs. Scientists from Oxford University's engineering department constructed mathematical models able to enhance specific visual signals in the mammogram.[66] Their model filter removes noise that may mask "interesting" items on the radiography film such as microcalcifications, allowing the translation of confused images into a unambivalent visual representation of a tumor. The result is truly impressive. Diffuse patches of white spots are organized into a readily recognizable image that makes sense for a nonexpert too.[67] But an enhancement of radiologists' capacity to see tiny clusters of microcalcifications does not automatically produce a more desirable outcome for the patient. Excessively sensitive image-generating machines may identify more precancer, and thus produce more clinically ambivalent results. And vice versa: less sensitive radiology equipment can produce a lower proportion of false positive results and detect less "pseudo-disease" (that is, changes in tissues that will not produce clinical symptoms of cancer in the woman's lifetime).[68]

Another autopsy study that used cadavers of women who died in accidents illustrates the latter point. This study compared mammographic images made on cadavers with systematic cytological investigations of the x-rayed breasts. It has shown that mammography detected only 18 percent of the tumors—both invasive and in situ—found by pathologists who analyzed numerous thin slices of the breast.[69] Had mammograms been sensitive enough to pick out all the "silent" tumors uncovered by pathologists, a much higher proportion of women would have been classified as cancer patients and would have been invited to undergo either a partial mastectomy with radiation or a surgical ablation of their breast.

The repeated finding of unexpectedly elevated rates of "silent" breast cancer in women who died from cancer-unrelated causes inspired a mathematic model of breast cancer growth. The authors of this model start with two simple assumptions: breast tumors are highly variable in their rate of growth (some double their volume in a few days and some in a few years) and all pass through an obligatory DCIS stage. Their model also postulates irreversibility: given infinite time, all the DCIS lesions will progress to malignancy. The authors of this model calculated that for each clinically visible breast tumor there are roughly fifty to sixty invisible ones, either invasive or at a DCIS stage. Without medical technology, the great majority of such tumors will remain invisible during the woman's lifetime. Mammography and other medical imagery approaches can display some of these invisible tumors, but many others will be not visible even with these techniques and can be discovered only by chance.[70] Or perhaps by misfortune: once an invisible tumor becomes visible, a woman has a high probability of undergoing a treatment that produces undesirable side effects and a quasi-certainty of losing her peace of mind.

Mammography and the Management of Fear

Until recently, controversies about mammography remained confined to specialists. In the early twenty-first century, selected breast cancer advocacy and consumer groups became interested in problematic aspects of this technique. The
websites of these groups provide information about benefits of mammography
but also about its disadvantages: false negative and false positive results, unnecessary biopsies, overtreatment, and psychological harm.[71] The majority of
women, and the majority of breast cancer activists, continue, however, to support
mammographic screening and view it as a life-saving practice. Surveys on both
sides of the Atlantic have shown that women between ages 40 and 50—a group
for whom the benefits of mammography are especially contested—have high
hopes that mammography will protect them from cancer.[72]

In the United States, the introduction of mammography was the driving force
behind the establishment of specialized breast care centers.[73] These structures
were relatively late offshoots of Women Health Centers and were linked with the
activism of the Women's' Health Movement in the 1970s. These centers dealt with
controversial aspects of women's reproductive health such as contraception and
abortion, and their practice often incorporated critique of overmedicalization of
normal events in women's lives such as menstruation, childbirth, or menopause.
Later, however, many Women's Health Centers were transformed into purveyors
of medical services that competed for a specific segment of the market.[74] Specialized breast care centers were part of the latter trend. According to a 1995 survey,
82 percent of these centers were hospital sponsored, 20 percent provided only
mammographic screening, while 80 percent supplied additional breast-related
services such as biopsies and ultrasounds. Thirty-seven percent of centers also
provided treatment of breast cancer. Some of the breast care centers maintained
a feminist commitment to women's health but the majority were commercial en-
terprises that drew on the market potential of women's health and promoted the
rhetoric of responsibility for one's health that included the consumption of risk-
reducing medical technologies.[75] Breast health centers stressed their pro-woman
attitude and presented screening for cancer as an empowerment strategy. Searching for early signs of malignancies allows women to control decisions concerning their health, and to become knowledgeable, well-informed consumers of
medical services.[76] In the meantime, critics of this approach pointed out, the existence of breast health centers may also increase women's dependence on a med-
icalized management of health risks.[77]

Epidemiologist Kay Dickersin deplored requiring women under 50 to undergo mammography because she believed that screening women of that age is costly and inefficient and can induce harm. In spite of these beliefs, she insisted on the necessity of taking into consideration the opinions and feelings of mammography users. Breast cancer is a very frightening disease. Such fear—of the disease itself but also of its treatment—needs to be addressed through education as well as through interventions that reduce cancer-induced suffering.[78] Mammography gives women the impression that they can do something to avert the cancer threat. Such a feeling is summed up in a testimony of a woman quoted in the 2006 report of the French Institut du Cancer: "Cancer is the disease that scares me most, especially women's cancer: breast and uterus. I know that screening can help catch breast cancer early. If the cancer is caught on time [pris à temps] the surgeons takes out the lump, sometimes prescribes a few sessions of radiotherapy or chemotherapy. But if one waits too long, it's immediately an amputation of the breast, a horribly mutilating intervention!"[79]

Other Screening Campaigns

Women were the main targets of the twentieth-century screening enterprise. A 1988 review explained that "screening has proved effective for only two cancer sites, the breast and the cervix. Only for these, therefore, should screening be a part of routine clinical practice."[80] Experts proposed, however, mass screening for three other cancers: lung, prostate, and colon: one (lung) at first predominately found in men, one (prostate) found in men only, and one (colon) found in both sexes.

Lung Cancer Screening

The issue of "pre-cancer" never truly arose in lung cancer because putative histological changes in the bronchi conducive to development of an invasive lesions are not (as of now) accessible to medical gaze. Accordingly, the goal of screening for this pathology was an early detection of already malignant nodules. It was hoped that such detection would transform lung cancer from a nearly invariably fatal to a curable disease.[81] In the 1950s, cancer specialists proposed searching for tumor cells in the sputum, a variant of exfoliative cytology used to diagnose malignant and premalignant changes in the cervix. In parallel, they suggested looking for signs of cancerous transformation on chest x-rays.[82] Thanks to a combination of these two approaches, they believed that "malignant lesions of the lungs can be found several months before the appearance of the symptoms . . . it therefore seems desirable to encourage frequent examinations, every 6 months, or even every 3 months, among persons likely to develop lung cancer, such as men over the age of 40 who have been cigarette smokers."[83]

ACS leaders were startled in the early 1950s by evidence of a sixfold increase in the incidence of lung cancer in the preceding 20 years. As a consequence of this, they launched a nationwide campaign of early detection of lung cancer through radiological screening and sputum cytology. In 1954 the ACS produced a movie called *The Warning Shadow* on the life-saving potential of screening for lung cancer and a pamphlet with the same message. This propaganda material aimed "to shock the readers and to prompt them to visit the doctor's office for the mandatory yearly check up and bi-annual x-rays."[84] ACS's publications emphasized individualized management of cancer risk. Environmental pollution, a 1956 article stressed, may perhaps account for some cancers, and legislation may be needed to regulate polluting industries, but for the man in the street concerned about cancer, "no amount of congressional legislation will free him of his own personal responsibility. Knowledge of cancer and its symptoms, and the awareness of necessity of early protection and prompt treatment will still be his first safeguards against the disease"[85]

The enthusiasm for early screening for lung cancer decreased when epidemiological studies made in the 1950s and 1960s indicated that the proposed screening procedures were unable to identify individuals able to benefit from a therapeutic intervention. Only a small portion (20 to 30 percent) of people included in these studies were classified as "operable" and, even among these individuals, life gains obtained by surgery were modest.[86] At the same time, the description of causal links between smoking and lung cancer shifted the emphasis to the prevention of this malignancy and led to a perception of lung cancer as a self-inflicted disease. The shift in the understanding of causes of the sharp rise of incidence of lung cancer, especially among men, probably affected the search for early detection tests.

Some experts continued nevertheless to argue that while the overall therapeutic gains in lung cancer are low, early diagnostic procedures may still help to identify subsets of individuals who will benefit from the surgical excision of their tumors. In the 1990s, researchers developed new tests for the early detection of lung cancer, such as spiral computed axial tomography (CAT) scans and multisliced CAT-scanning, able to detect localized tumors that can be definitively eliminated through surgery. They claimed that five-year postsurgery survival of persons with stage I-A non-small lung tumor is 60 percent, a significant improvement over the low survival rates in lung malignancies. Moreover, because the most important risk group for lung cancer—cigarette smokers—is well identified, advocates of this method argued that screening could be targeted to people who had high chances of developing this pathology.[87] In spite of the high prevalence of lung cancer and high mortality from this disease, and thus of potentially important benefits in terms of years of disease-free survival, the investment in screening for this pathology remained low. Health policy makers have consistently recommended against such screening. The relative lack of interest in early detection of lung cancer may reflect technical difficulties in developing a reliable and inexpensive test that will not lead to unnecessary biopsies and surgeries. It may also mirror a widespread lack of enthusiasm for investing money and efforts in a disease perceived mainly to be the result of irresponsible behavior.[88]

Prostate Cancer Screening

Screening of lung cancer was often perceived as inefficient, because many doctors did not believe in the possibility of a cure for this pathology. A similar skepticism about the efficacy of therapeutic interventions affected the development of screening for prostate cancer. Such skepticism was not, however, grounded in a pessimism about outcomes, but in uncertainty about whether a treatment was going to do more good than harm. Histological changes in the prostate can be studied by biopsies, an unpleasant but relatively simple procedure. The meaning of positive biopsies is, however, unclear, because proliferative lesions of the prostate are found in many healthy older men and probably in the majority of those over age of 70. Aware of the high incidence of such lesions, doctors separate the clinical disease "prostate cancer" from the presence of cancerous changes in the prostate.[89] This rule does not only apply to pre-invasive lesions but to invasive ones as well. Prostate cancer is usually a slow-growing tumor and is detected mainly in elderly men. Patients diagnosed with an invasive prostate malignancy have thus a reasonably good chance of dying from an unrelated cause, even in the absence of all treatment.

In the 1970s scientists described a specific protein secreted by prostate—the prostate associated antigen, or PSA. In the early 1990s they linked the rise of levels of PSA in the blood with prostate cancer.[90] The PSA test provides a first indication of a possible prostate tumor. The presence of malignancy is then usually confirmed by a series of random needle biopsies. While imperfect, the PSA test is seen as reasonably reliable. It is also relatively cheap and painless, although the calculation of its true costs needs to also take into account the cost—monetary and otherwise—of multiple biopsies of men who test positive. Doctors tend to view biopsies—especially "minimal" biopsies such as needle biopsies of breast lumps, prostate, and cervical biopsies as entirely benign procedures. Patients may, however, have a very different opinion.[91] The PSA test was rapidly perceived as mixed blessing, mainly because of the danger of overdiagnosis and overtreatment. Surgical therapy of prostate cancer may lead to impotence and incontinence, a high price to pay for the treatment of a condition with unknown potential to harm the patient.[92] Similar issues were evoked during debates on the introduction of tests for hereditary susceptibility to prostate tumors.[93] An additional complication was a growing awareness of the link between the number of biopsies and the number of diagnoses of prostate cancer. Doctors found out that the more one looks for prostate cancer, the more one finds it.[94] Limiting the number of biopsies, including in men already diagnosed with malignant lesions, may reduce the danger of treatment of a pseudo-disease. An author of a 2006 review on this topic explicitly stated that he "does not recommend a routine repeat needle biopsy within the first year following the diagnosis of high grade prostatic intraepithelial neoplasia."[95] U.S. clinical guidelines for prostate cancer screening stressed that because of these problems, PSA testing seems to mandate more clinician-patient discussion than other routine tests.[96]

PSA screening remains controversial. Some specialists continue to oppose screening for prostate malignancies and perceive it as inconsistent with current scientific evidence.[97] The test is, however relatively well accepted in the United States, where the recommendation, "each man should discuss the advantages and the drawbacks of screening with his doctor," led to an increased use of tests. Approximately one-third of American men over 50 underwent this test. This was true also for men over 75, less likely to benefit from screening for prostate cancer.[98] The relatively high use of PSA testing in the United States, in spite of controversies about the heuristic utility of this test, may reflect the North American patients' "enthusiasm for screening." It may perhaps also mirror North American doctors' tendency to promote activities that reduce the patient's risk of "anticipated regret" for inaction, while limiting their own risk of medical error.[99] The great majority of European experts were opposed to systematic PSA testing in healthy men. The use of this test, they proposed, should be limited to men who manifest symptoms of prostate tumor, to those who are classified as being at high risk (usually on the basis of family history), and to those who are especially worried about this pathology.[100] Their views were translated into public policies that discourage systematic testing of healthy men in Europe.[101]

The immediate visibility of difficulties linked with screening for prostate cancer can be contrasted with the slow and uneven diffusion of debates on overtreatment induced by mammographic screening.[102] The difference between the widespread adoption of mammography and the more complicated trajectory of PSA testing may be a gendered one. Women are more inclined to discuss their reproductive health than men are, more apt to adopt a screening discipline, and more inclined to accept preventive surgery to reduce cancer risk. It may also reflect differences in the distribution of breast and prostate cancer. Breast cancer is found mainly in older women, but it affects and kills younger women too. The small, but not negligible, fraction of young women with breast cancer is the most visible—and the most frightening—aspect of this pathology. There are not as many young men with prostate cancer who are expected to be saved by an early detection of their tumor from premature death.[103] Another non-negligible element may be the difference in visibility of these two malignancies in the past thirty years. In spite of the attempts of some men with prostate cancer to increase the visibility of this pathology, it is seldom discussed in the media or in public forums.[104] The relative silence about prostate tumors probably affects the popularity of screening but also the channeling of money for prevention and cure. For example, in the United Kingdom, breast cancer was reported to benefit in 2006 from ten times more funding than prostate cancer, with especially significant differences in the distribution of charity funds.[105]

Colon Cancer Screening

Colon cancer is the second leading cause of death from cancer in Western countries (after lung cancer), and it kills not only the elderly but also the middle-aged. In terms of mortality, but also of years of life lost, its consequences are comparable to those of breast cancer. It might have been logical to assume that screening for this pathology would became rapidly popular, even more so because the elimination of premalignant lesions of the colon greatly reduces the incidence of this tumor. Moreover, the elimination of such lesions (usually during a colonoscopy) is, like the elimination of cervical lesions, a relatively "low cost" procedure for the patient. Nevertheless, screening for colon cancer did not achieve—until now—the widespread diffusion of screening for breast and cervical cancer.

Surgeons suspected for a long time that polyps of the colon and the rectum may become cancerous in the long run. Studies of a hereditary condition— familial adenomatous polyposis (FAP)—confirmed that suspicion: people with multiple polyps of the colon nearly always develop colorectal cancer.[106] Doctors were unable to assess what percentage of adenomatous polyps that became malignant and whether such polyps had specific morphological traits, but they arrived at the conclusion that the majority of colon tumors developed from such polyps.[107] They focused then on the possibility—and the cost—of detection and surgical removal of all the suspicious intestinal polyps and developed techniques that made the colon accessible to visual examination and biopsy: sigmoidoscopy and then colonoscopy. Colonoscopy, a method first used for detection of colon malignancies, was adapted to allow a removal of suspicious polyps for microscopic examination. If the polyp was malignant, such removal eliminated at the same time the source of danger. The diagnosis—as in conical biopsy of the cervix—was also a cure.[108]

Colonoscopy is, however, expensive, unpleasant (individuals must do a special preparation to "purge" their colons before intervention), not entirely risk free, and has to be performed by a skilled surgeon. In the 1970s and 1980s, its generalization to the entire population was not perceived as a viable option from a public health point of view. The majority of the experts proposed therefore a two-step solution. The first step is a simple and inexpensive test, hemoccult, that displays the presence of occult blood in feces, a frequent sign of the presence of premalignant or early malignant lesions of the colon. People who tested positive with hemoccult (often a self-administered test) would then undergo colonoscopy. This approach is not perfect, because many people with suspicious lesions do not have blood in their feces, but epidemiological modeling indicated that its widespread use should reduce the occurrence of colon malignancies.

The transformation of hemoccult into mass screening tests was, however, more difficult than the seemingly more complex task of large-scale diffusion of exfoliative cytology or mammography. First reports on the search of occult blood in feces were published in the 1950s, and in the 1970s, doctors proposed the use of hemoccult to select candidates for colonoscopy.[109] However, the first randomized trials of hemoccult were not conducted until the 1990s. Their results indicated that the test indeed decreased mortality from colon cancer. The results were far from spectacular (15 percent to 20 percent of reduction of mortality), but they were comparable to those obtained in clinical trials of mammography.[110] The consequences of clinical trials of efficacy of mammography and of hemoccult were, however, different. A 20-percent reduction of breast cancer mortality was seen as sufficient justification for diffusion of a complex and expensive technology. A similar reduction in mortality of colon cancer did not lead to a similar diffusion of an inexpensive test. According to professionals, the main obstacle for mass screening for colon cancer was compliance—that is, the difficulty of persuading people to do the test.[111] Part of the problem might have been the reluctance of some people to manipulate their feces and low-tech aspect of hemoccult that did not fit into the high-tech image of cancer detection and treatment systematically diffused by cancer establishment and cancer charities. Doctors may also be more interested in the diffusion of physician-controlled tests (mammography, Pap smear, colposcopy) than of simple ones performed by the tested people themselves. An additional problem might have been the high rate of false negative results of hemoccult and the sensitivity of the test to variations of diet.

In France and the United Kingdom, both countries with a national health service, debates on the general implementation of screening for colon cancer remained inconclusive for a long time. An advisory group for the French Ministry of Health proposed in 1976 identifying people at a high risk of colon cancer and following them regularly by colonoscopy. The text did not specify, however, how to define a high risk of this disease. This task was delegated to individual doctors.[112] A pilot program of hemoccult, conducted in the Burgundy region, indicated feasibility and partial efficacy of such testing. It also revealed difficulties with patients' compliance.[113] Some French experts continued to contest the efficacy of mass screening and advocated instead targeted screening of specific risk groups and a more efficient follow-up of all people with suspicious symptoms.[114] The screening for colorectal cancer was not included in the French National Cancer Plan of 2003. In the meantime, the French Health Ministry enlarged the scope of departmental pilot programs based on the massive diffusion of the hemoccult test. These programs continued to be hampered by low compliance: only a quarter of targeted people took this test. The 2006 plan included the extension of screening for colon cancer to the entire country. This extension was completed in 2008. The number of people getting tested remained low, however: approximately 40 percent.[115]

U.K. pilot programs demonstrated feasibility but were criticized for their low cost-benefit ratio.[116] British health authorities debated in the meantime the possibility of replacing hemoccult by a "once a lifetime" screening with flexible sigmoidoscopy—a visual examination of the colon that, unlike colonoscopy, can be made in a doctor's office and does not need to be done under general anesthesia. If implemented on a large scale, some specialists proposed, this method can reduce mortality from colon cancer.[117] Finally the U.K. Health Ministry decided to develop a national screening program based on hemoccult. The program started in April 2006 and implemented gradually during the next three years.[118] The debates on screening for colon cancer in the United Kingdom or in France did not mention the possibility of generalizing colonoscopic screening—an expensive and labor-intensive method—to all healthy people. Colonoscopy in these countries is proposed only for people at a higher than usual risk of colon malignancy: those with suspicious symptoms, a family history of the disease, past detection of polyps, or a positive hemoccult test. By contrast, U.S. experts recommend colonoscopy for a routine screening for colon cancer.

Clinical trials in the United States have shown, like the European ones did, a statistically significant reduction of mortality from colorectal cancer by regular use of hemoccult.[119] By contrast, the efficacy of colonoscopic screening of healthy people with no family history of the disease was not demonstrated in clinical trials.[120] Moreover, this test had a small but not negligible risk of anesthetic and surgical complications.[121] Nevertheless, a report by the ACS and the American College of Gastroenterology explicitly stated their preference for colonoscopy for surveillance of colon cancer risk. They grounded their choice in the fact that this method was the "gold standard" of screening for precancerous polyps. If conducted properly by experienced doctors, colonoscopy has the highest sensitivity of detection of premalignant polyps of the colon.[122] The ACS's publicity encouraged all healthy people to undergo colonoscopy every ten years starting at the age of 50.[123] In spite of ACS's efforts, the use of a routine screening for colon cancer was not very high. Even the controversial PSA test for prostate cancer was found to be more popular among elderly North American men than the much less controversial screening for colon cancer. In the years 2002–2004, 32.5 percent of American men over 75 underwent PSA screening, compared with 22.8 percent screened for colon cancer.[124] At the same time, more than 90 percent of American women between 40 and 70 underwent mammographic screening. Like the early years of the twentieth century, in the early twenty-first century women's bodies are more often submitted to a medical gaze than those of men.

Cultures of Screening

Toward the end of his life, Pierre Denoix, a central figure of French and international oncology, questioned the logic of the ever-growing cancer screening enterprise.[125] An advocate of rigorous evaluation of cancer therapies and public health measures, Denoix was skeptical about the efficacy of many of the highly publicized measures designed to prevent malignant tumors. Only two such measures, he explained, are truly efficient: reduction of alcohol use and reduction of tobacco consumption, especially the latter.[126] He also criticized data on the supposed effect of early detection of malignancies of survival. Such data often fail to take into account differences between "delaying" and "non-delaying" populations. The "non-delaying" patient is usually younger, better educated, and more inclined to follow the doctor's advice and has therefore a better chance of being cured.[127] After his retirement in 1982 Denoix wrote a text (which was never published), *Carcinologie Demain: Dictonnaire des Idées Non Reçus* (Oncology of Tomorrow: A Dictionary of Unaccepted Ideas).[128] It starts with a short dictionary of main oncological terms, among them:

"Cancer"—cancer is always invasive.

"Mass screening" [dépistage de masse]—a highly inefficient method, especially if one takes in to account its cost/benefit ratio. Was fashionable for a long time. Is still fashionable among backward people.

"Early" [in English in the original]—an English term that, contrary to what one might think, does not mean "early in time" [précoce].

"Life span"—when doctors are able to make a diagnosis earlier but are unable to cure the disease, the only result is that a patient lives longer under the shadow of fatal diagnosis.

"Emergence"—a moment at which a tumor becomes clinically perceptible. An event that doest not reflect a natural history of the tumor but the resolution power of our investigative tools. In the majority of cases, dissemination takes place before the emergence of a tumor. At the moment of its emergence, the game is already over [les jeux sont faits].

"In situ"—"lapalissade" —a French term for a silly or tautological expression.[129]

The belief that early diagnosis reduces cancer mortality, Denoix argued, is the most prominent among many "oncological myths." The majority of cancer experts enthusiastically adhere to the principle of early diagnosis, in spite of the fact that it has never really been proven.[130] The faith in the advantage of this approach is rooted in a double confusion: between "young" tumors and small, localized ones and between an invasive cancer and noninvasive precancerous lesions.[131] The latter confusion led to the construction of a false analogy between noninvasive lesions of the cervix and the breast. The blurring of the boundary between noninvasive breast lesions and true—that is, invasive—cancers favored unnecessary and mutilating treatments. Surgeons, especially risk-averse doctors on the other side of the Atlantic, promoted a drastic treatment of noninvasive lesions of the breast.[132] When he tried to convince an American colleague that one should not use an aggressive surgery to treat in situ breast tumors because in at least 85 percent of the cases such tumors will never became invasive, he was told ironically: "this is a purely logical argument—well, you are a Frenchman."[133]

Oncologists, Denoix explained, work in a "viscous" domain, characterized by an unusually high level of uncertainty. The combination of a frightening disease and a difficulty in predicting who among the patients will benefit from therapeutic intervention may lead either to an excessive inaction or a slippery slope that leads to overtreatment. A doctor's duty is to resist such trends, Denoix said: "each time you should ask yourself: is the result you get worth the price paid by the patient? Did you think sufficiently about the consequences of an absence of intervention that will put some members of this group at a greater risk? And are you ready to impose to all members of a group a treatment that, because of our ignorance of the future of cancerous lesions, will help only a few and will have no effect on other members of this group?"[134]

Denoix was one of the rare cancer experts who argued that screening for cancer may be a double-edged sword. It can prevent a deadly disease but can also induce fear, anxiety, stigma, and overtreatment.[135] Many people harbor undetected and clinically silent tumors.[136] They are not made to feel that they carry ticking bombs in their bodies and do not need to face difficult decisions. Should they be better informed? Some doctors believe that ignorance may be a blessing. A review of the history of medical screening ended with Henry Thoreau's quotation: "If I knew for a certainty that a man was coming to my house with the conscious design of doing me good, I should run for my life."[137]

The majority of people in the United States, a recent study indicated, seem to have a different attitude. They support enthusiastically and without discrimination screening for cancer even in people over age 80 and are in favor of a search for malignancies which would not produce disturbing symptoms in the individual's lifetime.[138] Fervent advocates of screening for cancer seldom mention problematic consequences of such screening, especially for tumors for which doctors were unable to develop a "low cost" method of elimination of precancerous lesions. People diagnosed with proliferative changes in breast or prostate are invited to choose between a permanent threat of cancer and an aggressive surgical solution. Once defined as being at a high risk of malignancy, they are denied the option of life in a "silence of the organs."[139]

The popularity of screening for cancer was linked to the rise of a "risk society."[140] In the second half of the twentieth century, biomedicine became deeply intertwined with technologies of the self. Politics that aimed at improving the nation's body (or the body of a given racial, ethnic, or religious group), sociologist Nicolas Rose proposed, were replaced by an individualized governance of health. Every citizen is expected to make well-informed, rational choices. Biological identity became bound up with more general forms of enterprising, self-actualizing, and responsible personhood, achieved mainly through an enlightened and active consumerism.[141] An appropriate management of embodied health risks is seen as a moral duty, amenable to judgment. People defined as being at risk are expected to obtain an accurate assessment of their health risks, to find specific ways to reduce these risks, and to adopt a behavior compatible with risk reduction.

The "risk society subjects" are expected to submit themselves to a double discipline: self-examination and external controls.[142] They are keen to eliminate every possible risk of impaired health while being blissfully oblivious to the risks of medical information.[143] They are attuned to their bodies and turn the clinical gaze on themselves; as sociologist Ann Robertson puts it, they "swallow the panopticon."[144] At the same time, they delegate an important part of management of their risk to professionals. They are enlightened and well-informed consumers of medicine who nevertheless faithfully follow their doctors' recommendations. They possess the right level of fear of disease: not too high, otherwise they may be driven to denial or avoidance, but sufficiently elevated to accept experts' advice.[145] Such ideal medical subjects can be found in publications of cancer experts and cancer charities, in health education materials, posters, films, and popular press. An "enthusiasm for screening" was not generated in a void.

Critics of screening for cancer point to problems of false negative results, false positive ones, and, more rarely, dangers of overtreatment. One can argue that such problematic outcomes of screening are relatively rare. The great majority of screened people are reassured about their health. A negative result of a screening test may be presented as a nonevent, a "nearly nothing." [146] But the very fact of looking for hidden malignancy can, by itself, create indelible meanings. Its effects can be compared to efforts to physically erase a bothersome inscription. The more one tries to erase such an inscription ("this is nothing") the more it may acquire a strong physical presence ("this is something").[147] Publicity for mammography that explains that one hundred ninety-nine out of two hundred mammograms do not find cancer also proclaims forcefully that one out of two hundred healthy, symptom-free women who visit a radiology center will discover that she has breast cancer, changing her life forever.[148] Each time a woman undergoes a routine mammogram, she is reminded of the danger lurking in her body and is introduced to a culture of fear.[149] The persistent "something" of the "nearly nothing" of a routine screening for malignancies produces a setting that favors an aggressive management of cancer risk, be it expressed as the presence of abnormal cells, as some suspicious shadows on an x-ray film, or as changes in DNA sequences.

CHAPTER SEVEN

Heredity

Familiar Adenomatous Polyposis: Hereditary Predisposition and Precancerous Lesions

Screening for cancer is grounded in the principle that everybody is at risk of this disease. Search for the hereditary tendency to develop malignant tumors is grounded in the opposite supposition. It assumes that some people run much higher risk than others and that preventive interventions should selectively target these people. Precancerous lesions and hereditary predisposition to cancer came together for the first time in the 1920s in a study of a rare condition: familiar adenomatous polyposis (FAP). FAP, one may propose, was a "demonstrative disease." It made visible the possibility of hereditary susceptibility to cancer, the role of premalignant lesions in the genesis of a malignant tumor, and the efficacy of preventive surgery. It was also, to an important extent, a "biomedical disease." People with FAP were often diagnosed and treated preventively, before they displayed symptoms of their condition. In spite of its pioneering role, FAP was seldom mentioned in the late twentieth century debates on hereditary malignancies, testing for such malignancies, and the role of prophylactic surgical interventions.

In the late nineteenth and early twentieth centuries, the prevalent view of cancer experts was that this disease ran in families and was invariably lethal. Such a fatalistic outlook did not encourage a search for early signs of malignancy and a prompt visit to a doctor for people who discovered such signs. The promotion of the "do not delay" message by cancer organizations was accompanied by an affirmation that malignant tumors were not hereditary. One of the arguments employed to support this view was the observation that cancer-free "primitive people" became cancer prone when they adopted the lifestyle of "civilized" societies. For example, specialists claimed that while native Africans rarely suffer from cancer, this disease became a common disease among American blacks, probably for the same reason it is widespread in the white U.S. population.[1] Researchers continued nevertheless to look for hereditary factors that may influence the development of malignant tumors. Such studies developed along three lines: investigation of hereditary tumors in laboratory animals, survey of racial susceptibility to cancer, and studies of rare familial malignancies.

Scientists who studied cancer in the laboratory—Maud Slye, Clara Lynch, Nathalia Dobovoskiaïa-Zawadzkaïa—produced "cancer-prone" lines of mice to conduct experimental studies on the role of heredity in development of malignancies. This approach was however problematic, because clinicians viewed these experimental systems as totally artificial and disconnected from the human disease of cancer.[2] The second approach—study of relations between "racial traits" and malignancies—was also problematic, because it was difficult to define what such racial traits were and how they should be studied. This difficulty is illustrated by the study conducted by the Sub Committee on Statistics of the Cancer Committee of the League of Nations, which explored potential correlations between physical type ("race") and the prevalence of cancer.[3] The authors of this study, Alfredo Niecefore and Eugène Pittard, attempted to correlate physical traits of "anthropological types" (color of eyes and of hair, skeletal structure, form of the skull) with susceptibility to malignancies. They concluded in 1927 that the dark, brachycephalic Mediterranean "race" seemed to be less subject to cancer than the blond, dolichocephalic Alpine "race" but added that their result was tentative only, because their study suffered from the absence of accurate data on the racial composition of studied populations.[4] However, the collection of such data became difficult in the 1930s when race became a politically sensitive topic.

The third approach—search for "true" hereditary malignancies—was grounded in clinical observations. Cancer specialists noticed that a few rare childhood tumors, such as glioma of the retina (later retinoblastoma) and Wilm's tumor of the bone, ran in families.[5] They also recorded the presence of families with an exceptionally high prevalence of malignant tumors and cancer-related deaths.[6] Insurance company examiners explained that if all the cancer cases occurred in elderly people, the presence of several cases of cancer in the same family was usually a coincidence. By contrast, families with an unusual number of malignancies in young people should be viewed as true "cancer families," and their members could be asked to pay a higher life insurance premium.[7]

FAP was the first well-studied hereditary cancer. A paper reported in 1882 the concomitant presence of multiple intestinal polyps and colon cancer in a brother and sister.[8] In 1904, John Percy Lockhart-Mummery, a surgeon from the St Mark

Hospital, London (an institution specialized in diseases of the rectum and colon), adapted the sigmoidoscope—a tubelike instrument equipped with a light bulb, which is used to view the inside of the lower colon—to the diagnosis of tumors of the upper rectum.[9] Using this instrument, he was able to diagnose rectal tumors before they became generalized and thus inoperable. The possibility of looking directly at changes in the rectum led Lockhart-Mummery to propose a causal link between intestinal polyps and cancer in 1925:

> Simple adenoma of the rectum is often a forerunner of a cancerous growth. A simple adenoma has a marked tendency in time to undergo malignant change which eventually involves the whole tumor. . . . A careful examination of specimens of cancer of the rectum show that in quite a number, part of the tumor is simply non-malignant adenoma, though the remainder may be typical adeno-carcinomata, and still further, that simple adenomata are frequently to be found growing from the mucous membrane of the bowel either above or below the position of carcinomatous tumor. . . . One cannot help wondering what proportion of the cancers of the rectum and colon start as simple adenomata, and even whether it may not be possible that in all cases a simple adenoma is the starting point of a cancerous growth.[10]

Lockhart-Mummery developed this hypothesis through analogy with adenomatous tumors of the breast. He explained that Sir Lenthal Cheatle had demonstrated that duct adenocarcinoma of the breast (a malignant tumor) is often preceded by duct adenomas (benign growths) and argued that developments in the colon and rectum point to a very similar pattern.[11] This view became more accepted in the 1920s and 1930s. Some adenomatous polyps observed with sigmoidoscope (in symptomatic patients) and removed surgically displayed intermediary, partly malignant traits. The observation of direct relationship between colon polyps and malignancy reinforced the cancer schemata and linked precancerous lesions more firmly with invasive tumors.

In 1925 Lockhart-Mummery published three pedigrees of patients with an extensive polyposis and showed that this condition ran in families. At the same time he demonstrated that the presence of multiple polyps invariably led to the development of cancer. FAP can be therefore defined as a "predisposition to cancer that may be transmitted by heredity." The relationship between heredity and disease, Lockhart-Mummery added, "is one of the most interesting and, at the same time, one of the most difficult problems of modern medicine. The causes at work are very obscure, and the laws governing heredity are but imperfectly understood, though no one can doubt that hereditary predisposition to disease is a most important factor; *indeed it is so recognized by insurance companies.*"[12]

The description of FAP-linked colon cancer as a hereditary condition reflected Lockhart-Mummery's general understanding of the origins of cancer. In the interwar era, the majority of cancer experts believed that malignant tumors were produced by chronic irritation. Lockhart-Mummery believed, however, that cancer was a result of a mutation. The common denominator between all the irritating agents that induce cancer, he argued in 1932, is their ability to produce mutations.[13] Lockhart-Mummery and his colleagues established that polyposis is transmitted as a single dominant Mendelian trait (half of all the children of a parent with polyposis inherit this condition) and proposed in 1939 that, in all probability, cancer arises among the polyps as a consequence of an additional, independent event: "The more rapid growth of the intestinal mucosa increases the possibility of a further gene mutation responsible for malignancy . . . our explanation suggests therefore that familial adenomatosis is the result of inherited instability of epithelial cells of the large bowel."[14]

Lockhart-Mummery then initiated systematic studies of pedigrees and the establishment of a registry of FAP cases. The latter was funded by the British Empire Cancer Campaign, or BECC (Lockhart-Mummery was one of the leading experts of that organization). The establishment of FAP registry, historian of science Paolo Palladino has explained, was a direct continuation of Lockhart-Mummery's effort to make cancer and precancerous conditions visible. Pedigrees enabled the surgeon "to extend the clinical gaze beyond the reach of the sigmoscope."[15] Lockhart-Mummery and his colleagues proposed to prevent cancer through prophylactic removal of the colon (colectomy). They recommended this preventive surgery to all the patients diagnosed with polyposis. Ablation of the colon induced permanent digestive problems but was an efficient way to prevent the development of a potentially fatal malignancy. Lockhart-Mummery's discussion of FAP contained all the major elements that shape the understanding of hereditary susceptibility to cancer in the early twenty-first century: a unique combination of a sophisticated biological explanation and a radically simple solution—a surgical excision of a dangerous part of the body.

People who inherit a predisposition for polyposis develop multiple polyps of the colon, usually in their teens or early twenties. Lockhart-Mummery and his colleagues strongly recommended an annual sigmoidoscopy to people from FAP families from their early teens on and, if polyps were detected, a colectomy. The development of genetic tests for FAP in the 1990s freed half of the children from FAP families—those who did not inherit the mutation—from an obligation of frequent, unpleasant, and somewhat risky medical procedures: sigmoidoscopy or colonoscopy (a more thorough visual examination of the colon made under general anesthesia). However, for people who inherit the predisposing gene, genetic testing did not provide information inaccessible by other means. The principles of management of familiar polyposis were established well before the molecular biology era, together with the conviction that FAP was a rare and unusual cancer.

Cancer and Heredity in the Post–World War II Era

After the Second World War, discussions on links between race and cancer disappeared from scientists' agenda. Scientists continued to investigate hereditary susceptibility to malignant tumors in mice, but these studies were not linked to practical considerations. Danish cancer expert Johannes Clemmesen noted in 1952: "It will be up to the medical profession, especially in the field of pathology and clinical medicine, to claim their reasonable shares of the means available for research on human cancer, and to go ahead with the skill and courage displayed by experimental workers in their gigantic struggle to fight the cancer in mice."[16]

Heredity was seen as irrelevant in common human malignancies, with one exception: breast cancer. In late nineteenth and early twentieth centuries, doctors noticed a higher frequency of breast cancer in first-degree relatives of women with the disease and high prevalence of this malignancy in selected families.[17] A 1908 study had estimated that between 5 and 10 percent of breast tumors were hereditary.[18] Nevertheless, until the 1940s, data on links between breast cancer and heredity remained anecdotal. To display such links, it was important to separate breast cancer from other malignancies. At first, investigators such as Janet Lane-Claypon interrogated breast cancer patients about "cancer in the family" and not "breast cancer in the family."[19] Moreover, researchers initially confused two distinct phenomena—a relatively moderate (two- to threefold) increase of incidence of breast cancer of cancer in daughters or sisters of women diagnosed with this disease and the existence of "breast cancer families" with an exceptionally high frequency of this pathology.

In 1946 a large-scale Danish epidemiological investigation formally confirmed the strongly suspected assumption that breast cancer occurred more frequently in first-degree relatives of women diagnosed with this disease.[20] The same results were displayed by a 1948 British study, conducted by the geneticist Lionel Penrose. Penrose's investigation also indicated that the excess of breast cancer in relatives of women diagnosed with this disease cannot be attributed to a general hereditary tendency to develop malignant tumors: the effect was specific for breast cancer only.[21] Additional epidemiological studies confirmed these conclusions.[22] In the 1950s and 1960s, family history of breast cancer became one of the main elements that prompted doctors to propose a preventive mastectomy.[23] In the early 1970s, cancer experts switched to the probabilistic language of risk and included family history among risk factors for breast cancer. Women with several first-degree relatives with this disease were then automatically included in the high risk group.[24]

One of the main difficulties when studying links between heredity and cancer, David Anderson explained in 1975, stemmed from the coexistence of nonfamilial forms of cancers and morphologically identical familiar forms of same malignancy.[25] Scientists were finally able to disentangle these two forms using pedigree studies. They concluded that all malignancies had familial and nonfamilial forms but in very different proportions. Tumors that were first defined as hereditary, such as Wilm's tumor and hereditary retinoblastoma, have a very high proportion (around 40 percent) of familial cases. Other tumors, such as esophageal cancer, seem to have a very low percentage of familial forms. Breast and colon cancer occupy an intermediary place, with an estimated 10 to 15 percent of familial forms of the disease. Such familial forms are transmitted by autosomal, dominant genes. They usually appear in much younger individuals than the nonfamilial forms of the same malignancy and have a tendency to be multifocal (the tumor develops in several places at the same time).[26]

The investigation of familial forms of common tumors relied to a significant extent on pioneering work of a physician from Omaha, Nebraska, Henry Lynch.[27] Lynch, a family practitioner with a strong interest in cancer, started to construct such pedigrees in the 1960s. At that time, cancer heredity was seen as a marginal research subject, remote from cutting edge investigations in oncology. In the late 1960s Lynch identified a family with a large excess of several types of cancer, especially of the colon and endometrium. Inspired by treatment of people with FAP, he recommended treating the members of this family with preventive colectomy and hysterectomy.[28] He started his argument in favor of prophylactic surgery with the statement: "Euphenics is a term proposed by Lederberg to describe the treatment of hereditary disorders by alteration of genotypic expression through dietary measures, drugs, surgical procedures or other special measures. Certain familial cancer problems lend themselves well to such a "euphenic" surgical management."[29]

Joshua Lederberg, a leading expert in bacteriology and molecular biology, coined the term *euphenics* in 1963, probably as a reaction of what he saw then as new, exciting possibilities opened by the transplantation of organs and tissues.

Euphenics, Lederberg explained, is related to eugenics in the same way as a phenotype to a genotype. At this point, in his view, heredity is not well enough understood to manipulate it at will and provide an efficient eugenic intervention. Luckily, in the meantime doctors can use shortcuts, such as the physical modification of the body. Thanks to the infinite possibilities of grafting body parts, humanity may achieve the goal of changing human biology without tinkering with genes.[30] Lederberg's "euphenic" dreams of replacing defective organs by grafts resonated with Lynch's aspiration to correct hereditary defects through the elimination of dangerous body parts.

In the 1970s geneticists noted that hereditary forms of breast cancer are characterized by an early age of onset of the disease and a high frequency of bilateral breast cancer.[31] Some geneticists also proposed counseling services for women from cancer-prone families. It was not certain, however, what the right preventive approach should be. The standard recommendation was a close surveillance through mammography, clinical examinations, and breast self-examination, but the efficacy of such surveillance in preventing cancer-related deaths remained unknown. The same was true for ablation of the breasts with immediate reconstruction, a drastic solution with a high frequency of postsurgical complications. Some doctors were reluctant to recommend such operations to patients and agreed to perform it only if a woman was truly determined to get rid of her dangerous breasts.[32] Henry Lynch believed that such hesitation was not justified. Cancer experts, he argued, are not sufficiently knowledgeable about genetics and seldom ask geneticists' help. They continue therefore to propose mammographic surveillance to women who should be encouraged to undergo prophylactic removal of the breast. Among these are women from families with numerous cases of breast cancer, especially those who combine family history of this disease with pathological changes such as fibrocystistic disease of the breast. This disease increased cancer risk and made mammographic surveillance difficult. Lynch also argued that when women with a family history of breast cancer are diagnosed with a malignancy in one breast, they should be systematically advised to undergo a prophylactic ablation of the other breast.[33]

One way of making prophylactic ablation of healthy breasts acceptable was to define the excised tissue as precancerous. Such a definition, Robert Hutter proposed, can be extended to familiar predisposition to malignancy: "In the broadest context, we must regard the female breast as a premalignant target organ when exposed to the physiological milieu of the female organism . . . a cancer in one breast is a premalignant condition for the opposite breast . . . a family history of breast cancer is a premalignant condition.[34]

In the 1970s investigation of familial forms of cancer was limited to a small group of specialists. Many doctors continued to resist the definition of cancer as a hereditary pathology. A comment on Henry Lynch's 1978 paper explained that "in this age that emphasizes the individual, equality, and the present, there is a reluctance to think in terms of genetic inheritance as determining our future."[35] Geneticist Walter Bodmer stated in his preface to a book on cancer and heredity that "cancer is essentially a genetic disease on the cellular level, but not a disease with a major inherited component."[36] In the 1970s and 1980s, scientists believed that the solution to the "cancer problem" would come from new developments in immunology and virology. Immunotherapy of cancer was expected to put an end to mutilating and toxic cancer treatments, while scientists hoped that studies of cancer viruses would lead to an efficient prevention of this disease.[37] Compared with the intellectually challenging and technically sophisticated immunological and virological studies, a painstaking construction of family trees and pedigrees could have been viewed as scientists' equivalent of stamp collection. The fate of this presumably backward domain changed radically, thanks to the development of new techniques of molecular biology.

Hereditary Susceptibility to Cancer in the Genomic Era: Dangerous DNA

In the late 1980s advances in molecular biology made the cloning of human genes possible. Genes responsible for hereditary forms of cancer became obvious targets of cloning efforts. Many scientists hoped that the cloning of these genes would open the way for an early diagnosis of cancer and development of new, efficient therapies. Lynch's impressive collection of pedigrees of "cancer families," seen by many of his colleagues as a mere curiosity on the fringes of science, became a rare resource at the cutting edge of developments in biology and medicine overnight.

The race to clone the breast cancer gene became emblematic to the newly revamped domain—oncogenetics (genetics of cancer). Genetic studies established that a hereditary susceptibility for breast cancer is transmitted as a dominant trait and is related to mutations in two genes, named *BRCA* (for BReast CAncer) 1 and *BRCA2*. Women who inherited *BRCA* mutation have a high probability (50 to 80 percent) of getting breast cancer in their lifetime and often develop a tumor at an early age (before 40) and bilateral tumors (malignancies in both breasts at the same time).[38] In addition, *BRCA*-positive women, especially those with mutations in the *BRCA1* gene, have a higher than average chances of developing ovarian cancer. Collections of sera from families with high incidence of breast cancer became a coveted resource in the race to clone the *BRCA* gene. This race was won by the American company Myriad Genetics, which obtained patents for *BRCA1* and *BRCA2* genes. Myriad Genetics decided then to centralize *BRCA* testing at its Utah site and to capture the market for such testing worldwide.

Myriad's commercial strategy was unusual. As a rule, holders of patents for diagnostic procedures commercialize diagnostic kits or sell licenses. Myriad's decision to centralize *BRCA* testing and to construct a "test factory" was partly driven by technical reasons. The *BRCA* gene is very big, about ten times greater than average, and the majority of its mutations are "private," that is, found in a single family. These elements complicate the manufacturing of kits. The decision to centralize testing was probably also influenced by Myriad's leaders' wish to make their expensive automated equipment (purchased during the race to clone the *BRCA* gene) for gene sequencing profitable. Also, while the Food and Drug Administration (FDA) supervises diagnostic kits, it does not regulate the supply of services.[39] In 1997, Myriad Genetics started an aggressive promotion of tests for *BRCA* mutations in the United States. Its campaign included direct marketing of tests to potential users, under the slogan "understanding your risk can save your life." Myriad was criticized for underplaying the uncertainties of genetic testing. In about a third of the families with high prevalence of breast and ovarian cancer, no *BRCA* mutations were found. Moreover, there are no clear-cut data on the efficacy of preventive strategies in reducing hereditary risk of these malignancies.[40] Nevertheless, Myriad's commercial strategy worked well; between 1996 and 2006, the company steadily increased its volume of *BRCA* testing.[41]

Myriad Genetics' patents made it the sole owner of all routine *BRCA* tests. In 2001, the European Patent Office (EPO) granted the U.S. firm three patents on procedures for diagnosing *BRCA1* mutations. The EPO's decision ran counter to the opinions about ownership held by a majority of the French oncologists who participated in the International Consortium. It directly challenged their interests. In summer of 2001, the Curie Institute, a leading cancer genetics center in France, initiated legal proceedings to oppose the first patent taken out by Myriad Genetics in Europe. Later it extended its proceedings to cover the second and third patents. Other French and European cancer genetic centers joined Curie's action. In May 2004, the EPO decided to support the plaintiffs. It denied Myriad Genetics the right to extend its patent to the European Union and canceled Myriad's patent EP 699754, a decision motivated by insufficiency in gene sequencing (Myriad's method accounts only for point mutations, not for larger deletion) and "excessive monopoly."[42] While Myriad's aspiration to control all the uses of *BRCA* sequences worldwide failed (as of now), the EU decision was grounded in technical considerations and did not undermine the principle of patenting DNA sequences that reveal susceptibility to a disease.

Myriad's only method of testing for *BRCA* mutations is a complete, automatic sequencing of the *BRCA* gene. Myriad's monopoly on the U.S. market weakened the perception of hereditary predispositions for breast cancer as a family issue and favored individual decisions. American women who wish to know their *BRCA* status can learn it without informing other members of their family, if they can afford it (or have an insurer that agrees to pay for the test, if they do not mind that their insurer will know their genetic status) and if they can persuade a physician to write them a prescription. By contrast, geneticists in Europe had a strong preference to start tests with a probable mutation carrier, that is, a woman who was already diagnosed with the disease. The tests are expensive and covered by national health insurance. It is thus logical to start testing in a family with a woman who has a higher probability of being a mutation carrier. Once a familial mutation is identified, other members of the family can be tested for a fraction of the cost, since Myriad technicians do not need to sequence the whole *BRCA* gene, only a tiny fragment of this gene. Moreover, the structure of genetic registries in the United Kingdom strongly encourages circulation of information in families, as does to a lesser extent collaboration between French oncogenetics laboratories. In a state-sponsored health system, circulation of knowledge about kinship saves public money.[43]

Debates on testing for hereditary susceptibility for malignancy presented the dilemmas generated by such testing as an entirely new development. Such a claim was inaccurate. People usually want to know whether they have a high probability of developing a malignant tumor, not if such a probability is calculated by looking on cytological preparations or by studying DNA sequences. A detection of a hereditary susceptibility to cancer has, it is true, additional consequences, such as the reinterpretation of family history, changes in family dynamics, or worries about the fate of one's children. On the one hand, classical genetic tools such as pedigrees had already displayed hereditary predispositions to cancer. On the other hand, some important variables, such as the key role of the biotechnology industry or intellectual property issues, were genuinely new. Moreover, the availability of genetic tests led to an extension of the notion of hereditary cancer risk.

Until the late 1990s, people mainly discovered by chance that they had a higher than average risk of malignancy. Cancer-free people often learned about their risk either when they received abnormal results of screening for cancer and underwent additional tests or when precancerous changes were found during a testing for a different condition. One important exception was people from families with an unusually high occurrence of a specific form of cancer, often aware of their high probability of developing this disease. This was certainly not true for all the "cancer families." Some such families were too small or too scattered to notice an excess of cancer deaths, others elected to deny the existence of a "family malediction," others still did not view the high number of cancer cases in their family as being exceptional.[44] The development of genetic testing allowed a systematic testing of healthy (asymptomatic) people for increased susceptibility for malignancies, including those who were not aware of a family history of this disease. The key term is here *systematic*. Knowledge of existence of hereditary forms of cancer preceded the development of genetic tests, but the introduction of these tests increased the number of people who would live with a fear of a malignancy.

Hereditary Risk of Breast and Ovarian Cancer: The Universal and the Local

Between 1995 and 2005, debates on the use of genetic tests for cancer focused on the first, and most visible, test, the search for mutations in *BRCA* genes.[45] The media dedicated numerous reports to the cloning of "breast cancer genes" and to the development of tests for hereditary susceptibility to this disease. Consequently, more women wanted to know their genetic status, a pressure encouraged by Myriad Genetics, but also by experts in cancer genetics, interested in the diffusion of their skills. The access to tests is justified by a woman's right to know, the presumed benefits of early detection of malignancies in high-risk women, and a better targeting of preventive measures. Tests for *BRCA1* and *BRCA2* mutations are expensive, and, in absence of large-scale aggregated data on physiological and psychological effects of testing, it is not known (yet) what their cost-benefit ratio is. In a state-sponsored health system, it may be important to establish that only women in the high-risk category will be tested. This preoccupation is also shared by private health insurers that agree to pay for these tests. The debate on *BRCA* testing was displaced toward the definition of high risk and conditions of access to tests that reveal such risk.

Statisticians developed several mathematical models to calculate the hereditary risk of breast cancer. Experts disagree about the validity of such models, but even if one assumes that a perfect model exists and is able to accurately predict the chances of developing cancer in a given time period—say a 22 percent chances of developing a malignancy in the next ten years—such a model is not sufficient to determine whether the calculated risk is low, moderate, or high and whether the level of risk should lead to testing for *BRCA* mutations. The definition of thresholds of interventions reflects professional and lay concerns, organizational considerations, and budgetary issues. Unsurprisingly, it strongly depends on elements such as the division of medical labor, organization of health care in a given country or region, and structure of health insurance. These elements account for the existence of important national differences in definition of high hereditary risk of breast and ovarian cancer.

Who Controls Testing and Determines Risk?

In the United States, the definition of cancer risk—and means proposed to limit this risk—are entirely privatized. Every doctor can prescribe a *BRCA* test. There is no need to consult a professional specializing in genetics or in cancer genetics. Even in this relatively free structure, the majority of women who undergo *BRCA* testing belong to more privileged social strata and usually see a specialist and not just a general practitioner. Cancer geneticists usually recommend testing when the calculated lifetime risk is higher than 20 to 25 percent, but doctors are free to propose such testing to any woman who wishes it. Prescription practices accordingly vary greatly. Moreover, as U.S. experts have noted, "the current medical-legal environment encouraged clinicians in the United States to use the models that give the highest sensitivity but at a cost of decreased specificity." In plain language, doctors may elect to avoid the risk—for themselves—of being sued by a patient told he or she does not need to undergo a genetic testing and then is found to be a mutation carrier, by recommending such testing each time they uncover even slight suspicion of a hereditary predisposition to malignancy. Such a trend may put more people at risk of anguish over the financial and psychological costs of testing.[46]

In Europe, national health systems control the use of tests and the definition of risk. Access to tests reflects concerns about costs to the community, while liability issues did not appear in debates on *BRCA* testing. In spite of many shared traits, the precise modalities of exercise of such control in Western Europe mirror national differences. In France, *BRCA* tests are performed exclusively by laboratories within the nationalized health system. Women are usually directed to cancer geneticists by their doctors (mainly gynecologists); some are, however, self-referred. A collective expertise conducted by the Institut National de la Santé et de la Recherche Médicale (INSERM) in 1998 outlined rules for the implementation of genetic tests for *BRCA* mutations in France and for the follow-up of individuals at risk.[47] French experts agreed to the use of a single model of risk calculation and recommended the proposal of genetic tests only to women whose lifetime risk of cancer exceeded 25 percent. Cancer geneticists are not obliged, however, to follow these rules. A geneticist can decide to accept a woman's demand to be tested even when her calculated risk is lower than 25 percent (e.g., if she is very anxious or had a traumatic experience of the disease in her family) or discourage testing when the calculated hereditary risk is higher than 25 percent (e.g., if she is over 60 or in poor health).

French oncogeneticists aspired to reach significant segments of women at risk. During the first years of the introduction of *BRCA* tests, they actively sought the attention of the media. Their aim was to inform women about hereditary susceptibility to cancer, and, if they had a family history of this pathology, to encourage them to discuss this issue with their doctor. Simultaneously, these oncogeneticists attempted to educate gynecologists about hereditary susceptibility to cancer and the criteria for a referral to a specialist. The role of gynecologists was seen as crucial, because in France, women's reproductive health—including screening for breast and ovarian cancer—is within the jurisdiction of medical gynecologists, a medical subspecialty dominated by female doctors and distinct from the surgical specialty of gynecological obstetrics. In a parallel development, the decision to place French cancer genetic services within cancer treating centers favored close links between geneticists and oncologists. Oncologists direct people who have a family history of breast cancer or with a kind of tumor frequently linked with a *BRCA* mutation (cancer before the age of 35, bilateral breast cancer, breast and ovary cancer in the same person, estrogen-receptor-negative tumor in a young patient) to a cancer genetics service.[48]

Tests for hereditary susceptibility to cancer were defined as an experimental procedure, regulated exclusively by the experts. French health authorities did not express concerns about the increased influx of women to cancer genetics consultations, assuming that this is a relatively marginal activity of cancer clinics. Moreover, cancer genetic consultations in France are at the same time diagnostic and research related. Oncogeneticists are interested in increasing the volume of tests performed in their laboratory, because this improves their chances of finding "interesting" mutations and developing new directions of research. The lack of formal rules of access to genetics services in France favors a less instrumental approach to the hereditary risk of cancer. Geneticists tend to accept a certain level of "useless" referrals and view dealing with women's' anxieties as a part of their task. However, the French health care system does not actively promote a reduction in inequalities in access to genetics services. Women from an underprivileged background have lower chances than those from more privileged social strata to become aware of an increased hereditary risk of breast cancer and to receive advice about the management of such risk.

The process of *BRCA* testing becoming routine in the United Kingdom was driven by the double need to provide fair access and to keep costs under control.[49] The pyramidal, carefully balanced referral system places issues of hereditary predispositions to cancer in the intersection of two nonoverlapping networks: the cancer network and the genetics network.[50] A regional cancer center provides specialized care to all cancer patients in a given geographic area, while a regional genetics center provides specialized care to all the people with hereditary diseases. Cancer is much more common than hereditary pathologies; the "capture area" of a regional cancer center is therefore much smaller than the one of a regional genetics center.[51] Several regional cancer centers are affiliated with a single regional genetics center that serves a population of 4 to 5 million people and provides clinical molecular genetics services to an extended geographic area. With the availability of tests for *BRCA* mutations, the immediate concern in the United Kingdom was a fear of clogging medical genetics services by excessive demands for these tests. Health administrators assumed that the bottleneck of the system was the capacity of the regional genetics center—and of the single cancer geneticist in that center—to handle cancer genetic testing. Such testing was usually performed in laboratories that handled several other tests and that dealt with routine diagnoses of genetic diseases only. The uncoupling of research and diagnostic activities lessened the geneticists' interest in the increase of volume of diagnostic tests.

The capacity of a given British cancer genetic center to handle *BRCA* testing was constructed as a fixed entity. To prevent excessive use of costly tests, regional health authorities predetermined an "acceptable" volume of these tests. The starting point was the evaluation of the manageable size of population at risk in a given capture area of a regional medical genetic center. The experts then proposed arbitrary definitions of levels of hereditary risk of breast cancer: "low risk"—less than threefold increased risk (age corrected), "moderate risk"—three- to sevenfold increased risk, and "high risk"—more than sevenfold increased risk. These definitions are grounded in simplified—and rigid—criteria: number of relatives with cancer, woman's age (below 40, 50, or 60 years), and nature of the tumor (bilateral cancer, breast and ovarian cancer, breast cancer in a man).[52] The definitions of levels of risk were calculated to generate a "yield" of a few hundred high risk families and few thousand moderate risk families per capture area, that is, a population that can be followed by the single consultant in the cancer genetics center of that area. Only women in the high-risk category are offered frequent mammography, clinical examinations, and access to *BRCA* testing. The role of testing was limited, because women were classified as high risk above all on the basis of their family and personal history. General practitioners were selected as gatekeepers of the system and received appropriate training and educational packs.[53] The system is far from perfect, but it does attempt to achieve a fair access to consulting and testing for hereditary predispositions.

What Is Done after Risk Is Assessed?

Organization of health care and structure of health insurance affected the management of already diagnosed hereditary risk of breast and ovarian cancer. Unsurprisingly, national variables played an important role in this domain, too. One of the important innovations introduced by the generalization of genetic testing was the establishment of the principle of collective management of cancer risk in mutation carriers. The pioneer of oncogenetics in the United States, Henry Lynch, had already introduced the idea that a familial cancer risk should be managed by a group of experts by the 1970s.[54] This concept became more popular in the 1990s. At that time U.S. cancer clinics increasingly proposed team management of breast cancer, a development that reflected the growing specialization in oncology, the increase in number of discriminating and well-educated patients, and the multiplicity of therapeutic options for dealing with malignancy. The team approach to the treatment of breast cancer was extended to the management of cancer risk. Selected U.S. cancer hospitals opened "breast cancer risk clinics," which gather a group of specialists: gynecologists, oncologists, genetic counselors (usually not MDs), nurse-practitioners, and social workers. Such clinics—a variant of the more broadly defined breast care centers—are frequented mainly by middle-class, educated women. The breast cancer risk clinics deal with all the aspects of an embodied breast cancer risk: heredity, suspicious mammographic images, and precancerous lesions of the breast. They provide advice about women's financial options and help them to negotiate with their insurance company or HMO. U.S. experts encourage proactive management of risk: "breast cancer risk assessment and appropriate counseling became standard components of breast cancer screening and overall health maintenance."[55]

In France, genetic counseling is done exclusively by physicians who often have a double training: in a traditional medical specialty (often, pediatrics or oncology) and in medical genetics. These physicians are often simultaneously involved in genetic and genomic research and in genetic counseling and tend to be highly specialized. They are seldom involved in the management of women with proliferative lesions of the breast. The surveillance of women with hyperplasia, ductal carcinoma in situ (DCIS), lobular carcinoma in situ (LCIS), clusters of calcifications, very dense breast tissue, and other cytological and anatomic risk elements is delegated to radiologists, oncologists, and breast surgeons. A decree of June 20, 2000, on testing for late onset genetic disorders states that tests made on asymptomatic individuals should be conducted in multidisciplinary units that include clinicians, geneticists, and psychologists or psychiatrists.[56] This decree deals exclusively with hereditary risk, strengthening the separation between a hereditary and a morphological risk.[57] Women diagnosed with *BRCA* mutations are followed by specialized clinics linked with oncogenetic centers, their gynecologists, or both.

In the United Kingdom, women defined as being at high risk of breast and ovarian cancer are seen by a consultant specialized in oncogenetics (as a rule a physician specialized in clinical genetics), who provides services for several regional genetic centers. During such a meeting, the consultant discusses risks for the woman and her family and establishes a surveillance plan. Such a plan usually does not rely on results of *BRCA* testing, which is seen as a confirmation of a diagnostic of hereditary risk, rather than as its starting point. High-risk women can also see a genetic counselor at their regional genetic center (usually not an MD) and can receive additional counseling, especially about risks for their children, siblings, and other family members. The medical supervision of high-risk women is then confined to their general practitioners, who coordinate the prescribed surveillance and schedule clinical visits and laboratory and radiology appointments. Psychological counseling and team work are not mandatory. Consultants in oncogenetics and counselors who work in regional genetics centers are, however, expected to collaborate with the high-risk woman's physician.[58] Decisions about genetic testing and level of surveillance are made by experts, but the routine follow-up of women at risk belongs to the jurisdiction of the general practitioner.

Taken together, comparative data indicate that in spite of high level of homogenization of research methods in molecular biology and molecular genetics, standardization of definitions of *BRCA1* and *BRCA2* mutations, the meaning of hereditary breast cancer risk is shaped locally, through the intersections between scientific and medical cultures, intellectual property rules, professional division of labor, and the organization of health care on a local, regional, and national level. These variables define who had access to testing, under which conditions, and what the consequences of the testing will be.

Testing for Hereditary Risk of Colon Cancer

In many ways, the story of people with FAP parallels that of carriers of mutation in the *BRCA* gene. In both cases, a mutation carries a high probability of malignancy and a preventive surgery reduces, but does not totally eliminate, cancer risk. However carriers of mutation in *APC* gene (the gene responsible for development of familial polyposis) did not attract the attention bestowed on those who carry *BRCA* mutation, while discussions of management of *BRCA* mutation carriers did not mention the experience accumulated during the treatment of people with polyposis. In the mid- to late 1990s, hundreds of articles written by oncogeneticists, psycho-oncologists, and sociologists dealt with the putative and actual effects of the introduction of *BRCA* testing. As far as I know, none of these articles attempted to gather information from people with FAP and to learn from their experience of life with a permanent risk of hereditary malignancy and with consequences of a preventive surgery. This absence on interest in an "old" hereditary malignancy may reflect a tendency to focus on novelty and to forgo continuities, especially if the latter may dim an optimistic image of a new technology.[59]

Geneticists stress that *APC* mutation is different from *BRCA*, because *APC* mutation induces cancers in practically all of its carriers, a good reason to promote a preventive ablation of the colon. Moreover, people with FAP usually develop cancers earlier than *BRCA* mutation carriers do, another justification for preventive surgeries. The difference between the two hereditary malignancies, however, is not of nature but rather of degree. FAP-associated cancers often appear in people in their thirties. However, in some families with this condition cancer develops much later. For example, in one familial form in which polyps do not extend to the rectum, the median age of diagnosis of colon cancer was 58 years. Other familial forms behave in an opposite way, and people in these families develop cancer at a very young age.[60] Familial forms of breast and ovarian cancer are also variable. Some mutations are associated with a higher probability of cancer than others, and some tend to induce malignancies in younger women.

In the 1970s, thanks to the improvement of surgical techniques, systematic colectomy became the standard treatment of FAP.[61] This surgery remains, however, problematic. It condemns people who elect this therapy to life with digestive problems of variable and unpredictable severity. A colectomy that conserves part of the rectum (illeorectal anastomosis) produces less distressing digestive symptoms, but it increases the risk of cancer in the remaining rectal stump.[62] People with polyposis had also increased tendency to develop tumors of the upper digestive tracts, especially of the small intestine, stomach, and the duodenum. They face, therefore, a lifetime of intensive and only partly efficient medical surveillance.[63] Moreover, 10 to 20 percent of people with FAP who underwent colectomy developed desmoid tumors. These fibroid tumors of the abdominal wall are technically defined as benign (they are not very aggressive and do not metastasize), but they can nevertheless be lethal. Their usual treatment is chemotherapy with or without tumor resection, repeated if these tumors return (as they often do). Desmoid tumors are seen as the main reason for the degradation of the quality of life of patients who undergo colectomy.[64]

People who underwent preventive surgery for FAP usually described their quality of life as reasonably good. However, nearly half of the persons surveyed had a major disturbance of digestive functions, such as incontinence or chronic diarrhea.[65] These individuals are submitted to intensive medical surveillance and usually follow a medical treatment to attenuate digestive symptoms. They also engage in an elaborate set of self-surveillance practices. Such practices combine the management of symptoms (especially those induced by colectomy), the anticipation of life-threatening complications such as the development of desmoid tumors, and the need for control and understanding. Self-surveillance also produces a high level of anxiety. Such anxiety, sociologists stated, usually does not diminish with time. Recently diagnosed patients and those diagnosed a long time ago have similar behavior patterns, and both groups engage in self-surveillance behavior that fails to diminish their level of worry.[66] Attuned to signs of their bodies and constantly aware of the presence of a cancer threat, the behavior of people with FAP is akin to that of people whose cancer is in remission, an observation that highlights the fluidity of boundaries between cancer and cancer risk.

In the 1970s, Henry Lynch and his colleagues described a different familial form of colon cancer, hereditary nonpolyposis colon cancer (HNPCC, or Lynch's syndrome).[67] People from families with this condition were advised to undergo frequent colonoscopies and ablation of suspicious adenomatous polyps. Following the cloning of genes responsible for HNPCC, colonoscopic surveillance was restricted to mutation carriers. HNPCC was also linked with a higher prevalence of endometrial cancer (cancer of the lining of the uterus). Consequently, women diagnosed with these mutations were advised to undergo a hysterectomy after completing their family. Today, people with a family history of colon cancer are usually first given a relatively inexpensive test for microsatellite instability. If the test is positive, they are then tested for the presence of mutations.[68] Tests for mutations that increase HNPCC's risk (the main are *MLH1, MSH2, MSH6,* and *PMS2* mutations) were patented, but the patent owners had chosen the more usual pattern of selling licenses to laboratories that wish to perform genetic testing.[69] People with identified mutations are urged to undergo frequent colono-scopic examinations. Colonoscopy is bothersome and costly and carries some risks. But, while the efficacy of mammography and nuclear magnetic resonance imaging in *BRCA*-mutation carriers remains unproven (as of 2009), specialists agree that colonoscopic surveillance works. The surgical removal of intestinal polyps, like the surgical elimination of cervical dysplasia, decreased the preva-lence of malignant tumors in mutation carriers.[70]

Informed by the experience of FAP, experts discussed the advisability of pre-ventive surgery for HNPCC. Advocates of this intervention explained that the es-timated lifetime probability of a mutation carrier of developing colon cancer may be as high as 80 percent, odds that may justify a preventive ablation of the colon.[71] Comparative studies indicated that preventive surgery does not totally abolish cancer risk but does decrease it greatly, a situation that can be compared to a prophylactic mastectomy.[72] For some specialists, colectomy is seen as no more efficient in preventing HNPCC than a good quality supervision by colonoscopy would be. For others, colectomy is seen as providing a long-term advantage in terms of survival.[73] A 2005 international survey of eighteen centers that treat people with hereditary predisposition to HNPCC revealed that nine of these cen-ters included a discussion of preventive gut surgery when counseling gene carri-ers, while the other nine centers did not provide such a discussion. There seems to be a much higher level of agreement on the value of preventive hysterectomy: sixteen out of eighteen surveyed centers discussed this surgery with female mutation carriers.[74] This difference may be related to differential perception of usefulness of the eliminated organ (everybody needs a colon, but a uterus is nec-essary only to produce children and is sometimes considered "useless" in women who have all the children they want), to the long tradition of surgical removal of the uterus and the ovaries for a wide range of "female diseases," for preventive purposes, or both.

Chemoprevention of Breast Cancer: Hereditary and Morphological Risk

In the 1990s, advocates of testing for hereditary susceptibility to cancer advanced two arguments in favor of such testing. The first was that genetic tests free many people from a permanent fear of malignancy. Even in families with an especially dramatic history of cancer, only half of the children inherit cancer-inducing mu-tations, while the others escape the family's malediction. The second was the pos-sibility of using drugs to prevent advent of malignancies in mutation carriers (chemoprevention). Breast cancer was seen as an especially good candidate for chemoprevention, because it is influenced by sex hormones. Surgical ablation of ovaries can slow down the spread of disseminated breast cancer, while the reproductive history of a woman may modulate her cancer risk.[75] From the 1940s on, researchers expressed the hope of preventing breast malignancies through a hormonal manipulation of breast cells. In the 1980s such hope was focused on inhibitors of estrogen receptors—tamoxifen, trademarked by AstraZeneca as Nolvadex, and its analogues.

Tamoxifen—a drug that belongs to the family of SERMs (selective estrogen receptor modulators)—was initially administered to women diagnosed with breast cancer to mimic the protective effect of surgical ablation of ovaries and to provide a nontraumatic way to shut off ovarian function. In the 1980s, a clinical trial (protocol B-14) conducted by the Surgical Adjuvant Chemotherapy Breast Project of the National Cancer Institute (NCI) has shown that women diagnosed with estrogen receptor (ER)-positive invasive breast cancer and treated with tamoxifen after the removal of the initial growth, had much lower recurrence rate.[76] Preliminary findings of another clinical trial (protocol B-17) indicated that women with DCIS who received tamoxifen after their surgery developed breast cancer less often than a control group did. Since DCIS is classified as premalignant lesion, this was the first indication of a preventive role of this drug.[77] The proposal to test if tamoxifen can prevent breast cancer in women at risk of this malignancy was a logical extension of B-17 finding.[78]

The new clinical experiment, protocol P-1, or the Breast Cancer Prevention Trial (BCPT) started in 1992.[79] To recruit high-risk women to the BCPT trial, NCI's experts needed to develop a homogenous and reliable definition of breast cancer risk. A team of statisticians headed by Mitchell Gail developed a mathematical model to calculate women's chances of developing breast cancer in the future.[80] Women who had more than 1.66 percent probability of developing breast cancer in the next five years were defined as high risk and were enrolled in BCPT. The Gail model focused on variables perceived as having the strongest effect on the incidence of breast cancer: age, the number of first-degree relatives with the disease, ethnic origins, age at menarche (first menstrual period), and the presence of morphological risk—that is, abnormal morphological changes in the breast such as LCIS and atypical hyperplasia.[81] In addition, any past breast biopsy was classified as a risk factor, regardless of its results. The inclusion of biopsies as independent risk factors was justified by the observation that women who had negative breast biopsies developed breast cancer more often than women in the general population. Doctors' decision to perform a biopsy is, by itself, an indica-

tion of a perceived danger of cancer, while some negative results are false negatives. Add to this that the frequency of breast biopsies in a given population is directly proportional to the number of mammograms. Women who are submitted
to a more frequent mammographic screening have a higher probability of undergoing a biopsy and a greater chance to be classified as being at risk of breast cancer using the Gail model.[82]

One of the elements that helped to persuade women to enroll in this trial
was a previous diagnosis of proliferative changes in the breast. A BCPT participant, Ms. Helene Wilson, explained that she has a family history of breast cancer,
and, moreover, "the last few biopsies showed signs of atypical hyperplasia and
microcalcifications, both thought to be strong indications of impeding breast
cancer. In my doctor's words, I was a 'walking time bomb.'"

Wilson felt strongly that she could not just sit and wait until she developed
cancer. When she learned that she was eligible for the BCPT trial, she felt as
though she had won the lottery.[83]

Two European trials, one in the United Kingdom (The Royal Marsden Hospital trial) and one in Italy (a multicentric trial) also tested the efficacy of tamoxifen in preventing breast malignancies in high-risk women.[84] The results of all
the three trials were identical. They showed that tamoxifen halved the incidence
of breast tumors in high-risk women but that treatment had numerous side
effects, some mainly unpleasant (hot flashes, insomnia, leg cramps, gynecological problems, and loss of libido) and others more severe (endometrial cancer,
thrombosis, lung embolism, and possibly stroke). The conclusions of the organizers of these trials were, however, very different. In 1998 the FDA approved the
use of tamoxifen for the reduction of breast cancer risk, estimating that the drug's
benefits outweighed its disadvantages. The European experts believed that their
data did not justify preventive use of tamoxifen in women with a low to moderate risk of cancer. They recommended continuing clinical trials of chemoprevention and focusing on women with an especially high risk of breast malignancies,
such as *BRCA*-positive women.

The BPCT organizers were aware of the shortcomings of tamoxifen. In 1999,
the National Surgical Adjuvant Breast and Bowel Project started a large-scale,
double-blind randomized clinical trial that compared tamoxifen with another
SERM, raloxifene (trademarked as Evista by Eli Lilly), a drug used to prevent osteoporosis. The organizers of this trial hoped that raloxifene would have the same
protective effect as tamoxifen did without its drawbacks.[85] The Study of Tamoxifen and Raloxifene (STAR) trial also recruited women who had over 1.66 percent
chances of developing breast cancer in the next five years according to the Gail

model. Again, many women who elected to participate in this trial were diagnosed with abnormal changes in breast tissue, such as atypical lobular or ductal hyperplasia: "High risk women may consider the finding of cellular atypia to be a more reliable measure of risk that many of the other factors that contribute to elevated Gail model score. The data from both BCPT and STAR suggest that atypia affects women's decision to enter a randomized trial to study breast cancer risk reduction. The reason for this finding may be that the presence of atypia influences a woman's perception of the magnitude of her risk for breast cancer."[86]

Observation of STAR participants confirmed that many of them had a history of benign breast disease. Some of the women were offered mastectomy but declined this option and were grateful when a clinical trial open a possibility of an alternative treatment. One participant explained that "the gynecologist that I was going to and my family doctors wanted me to have the breast taken off and have implants put in. . . . They emphasized that they didn't feel comfortable with the lumps that I had," while another told that "I was high-risk because of the family thing, but never really, you know, until I was diagnosed [with atypical hyperplasia] . . . and all of the sudden, all hell broke loose."[87] Women faced with diagnosis of a precancerous condition—and faced with the prospect of frequent breast biopsies and of life in the shadow of a threatening and uncertain diagnosis, felt empowered by their participation in the STAR trial because it gave them the possibility to do something about their condition.[88]

During a press conference in April 2006 that made the results of the STAR study public, the trial's organizers claimed that raloxifene was shown to be as efficient as tamoxifen in preventing invasive breast cancer (both drugs cut in half the number of invasive cancers), while producing less severe side effects.[89] Dr. Judy Garber, an oncogeneticist from the Dana Farber Institute, Boston, expressed the hope that with the new drug, "people will begin to think of breast cancer prevention in the same way they think of taking statin drug to prevent heart disease."[90] Other professionals, but also some breast cancer activists, were less enthusiastic. They pointed out that a 50 percent risk reduction sounds impressive, but in absolute numbers, tamoxifen and raloxifene prevented very few cancers. Moreover, the definitive results of the STAR trial indicated that raloxifene was no better than tamoxifen: both drugs induced serious side effects.[91] As Barbara Brenner from the advocacy group Breast Cancer Action put it: "we are very concerned that treating risk as a medical condition will result in substituting one disease for another."[92]

Brenner's concerns were probably shared by potential users of chemoprevention. In spite of strong support of this approach by NCI experts and an aggressive direct-to-consumer publicity of AstraZeneca, the producer of the trade-marked version of tamoxifen, preventive use of SERMs in the United States was not very high.[93] In one follow-up study, only 4.7 percent of women classified as being at high risk (as defined by Gail's model) and informed about chemopre-vention by their doctors elected to take tamoxifen to prevent breast cancer.[94] In the absence of doctors' explicit engagement in proposing this treatment, only 2 percent of high-risk women had chosen chemoprevention.[95] Or, as a *Time* mag-azine article put it: "what if doctors had a pill that prevents cancer and nobody wanted to take it?"[96] Specialists who found this situation regrettable noticed that women diagnosed with cytological changes in the breast were strongly over-represented among those who had chosen chemoprevention in a routine setting, exactly as they were among participants of clinical trials of this treatment: "Women may regard histological lesions as more valid markers of personal risk than other risk factors, a finding that is consistent with the literature indicating that women undergoing prophylactic mastectomy are more likely to have under-gone benign breast biopsies than those who chose not to have the procedure."[97]

The logical conclusion was that women at high risk of breast cancer should be encouraged to undergo diagnostic tests, such as needle biopsies, which make the presence of cytological abnormalities in their breast visible. The display of such anomalies will transform their statistical risk—that is, an abstract number pro-vided by the Gail model—into an embodied risk—the conviction that they har-bor dangerous entities within their bodies: "Atypia may be identified in asymp-tomatic, high risk women by epithelial sampling, either with random fine-needle aspiration or ductal lavage. . . . Studies of prophylactics mastectomy specimens from high risk women also suggest that clinically silent histological atypia is pres-ent in a significant number of high risk women. The current study findings re-garding the importance of atypia in the decision to undertake tamoxifen chemo-prevention provide a strong rationale for epithelial sampling in the high risk woman who is uncertain regarding tamoxifen use."[98]

In spite of the efforts of tamoxifen and raloxifene producers, the preventive use of these drugs remained limited to a relatively small group of women defined as having an especially elevated risk of developing breast cancer, among them, women diagnosed with mutations in *BRCA* genes.[99] Reluctance to use SERMs to prevent breast cancer did not extend to *BRCA*-positive women. Experts agree that, for women with a very high risk of breast cancer, the advantages of chemo-prevention outweigh its risks.[100] Chemoprevention was initially presented as one of the main justifications for testing for *BRCA* mutations. Dr. Bernard Fisher ex-plained in 1998 that "from my perspective I see a nexus between the two recent developments, the *BRCA1* and *BRCA2* genes and the identification of the alterations which put a woman at high risk for the disease, and the presence of agents which can possibly markedly decrease this risk."[101]

BRCA-positive women usually do develop ER-negative tumors that are less sensitive to tamoxifen and its analogues. Ongoing clinical trials attempt to evaluate preventive effects of ER inhibitors in *BRCA*-positive women. The results of these trials (e.g., branches of International Breast Cancer Intervention Study and the Raloxifene and Zoladex Research Study) are not yet known as of this writing in 2009.[102] In the meantime, experts agree that the most efficient risk reducing strategy is prophylactic surgery. Until an efficient chemoprevention is found, women diagnosed with *BRCA* mutations will continue to face a choice between a constant threat of disease or consequences of preventive ablation of potentially dangerous organs.[103]

Ashkenazi Mutations: Ethnicity and Embodied Risk of Cancer

Genetic tests formally linked predispositions to cancer with ethnicity. The best known example of such a link is Ashkenazi genetic predisposition to certain diseases. The supposition that Jewish women are especially prone to breast (and for some, also ovarian) cancer had already appeared in Janet Lane-Claypon's 1926 questionnaire on breast cancer, which included the question "is the patient of Jewish origins?"[104] However, the supposition of higher prevalence of breast cancer among Jewish women remained unproven. Some studies had found an excess of breast cancer among Jews, but others failed to demonstrate differences between Jewish and non-Jewish populations. Investigations about breast cancer among Jewish women were linked to a more general debate on "cancer and the Jews." Jews were supposed to have a higher overall prevalence of cancer and different rates of malignancies of the breast, ovary, cervix, and penis. The first two malignancies were reported to be more frequent among the Jews, and the last two less frequent. Cancer of the penis is a rare disease, and data on its prevalence were not statistically meaningful. By contrast, cervical cancer was a frequent malignancy, and experts became persuaded that this pathology is indeed more rare among Jewish women.[105] The two alternative explanations of this phenomenon were racial traits (an explanation that implicitly assumes that the Jews are a race or at least a genetically homogenous population) and environmental variables. These hypotheses had obvious political overtones in the 1930s.

Environmental theories attributed a lower rate of uterine cancers among Jewish women to male circumcision and a higher rate of breast cancer to an urban lifestyle. The circumcision argument was developed by Sampson Handley. Handley explained that other populations that practice circumcision, like the natives of Fiji Island, also had lower rates of cervical cancer than populations that shared the same environment but were not circumcised.[106] Georg Wolff agreed with this explanation but added that cervical cancer is the only tumor for which one can display meaningful differences between Jews and Gentiles. If one examines the overall incidence of cancer in a given country and makes the appropriate corrections for age, lifestyle, social class, and access to doctors (the last of these tends to increase the recorded incidence of malignancies, because more people are correctly diagnosed), the prevalence of cancer in Jewish and Gentile populations was similar. The difference, if any, Wolff proposed, may be related to the existence of familial, rather than racial, differences: "It may be that a study of heredity will bring us to clearer conclusions, but tracing the course of events in particular 'cancer families,' is an important but very difficult piece of work. This, however, is a totally different problem from that of a racial ideology which has but little in common with the exact study of inheritance."[107]

Other researchers, among them Clarence Little, president of the American Association for the Control of Cancer, had found an environmental explanation of the lower incidence of cervical cancer among the Jews unconvincing. The most logical explanation for the consistently lower rates of uterine cancer in Jewish women, Little argued, is a true racial resistance.[108]

After World War II, clinical geneticists described numerous hereditary diseases found only or mainly among Ashkenazi Jews (Jews from Central and Eastern Europe). Troy Duster's list of genetic diseases among different ethnic populations highlights this unique status of "Jewish diseases."[109] Jewish populations often remained endogamous and had high rates of intermarriage, facilitating the fixation of disease-inducing mutations. In addition, the high number of hereditary disorders found among the Jews may reflect the fact that they are especially good research material. Jewish communities often keep accurate genealogical records and conserve data on migrations. Jews often live in cities with good hospitals and advanced scientific institutions. Many Jews elect to be doctors and medical researchers, and many among the latter became interested in studying their own families and community. Finally, such studies tend to be self-propelling. A well-studied group is an excellent target for additional studies in the same area. A cascade of contingent developments could therefore have transformed Western Jewish communities into an ideal target for studies of hereditary diseases. Moreover, since research on Jewish diseases was usually made by Jewish scientists, such studies were not seen as an attempt to stigmatize the Jewish population and rarely encountered negative reactions. Just the opposite was true. Highly publicized stories, such as the success of the elimination of Tay Sachs disease in Jewish ultraorthodox communities through a collaboration between religious leaders and scientists helped to shape a positive image of the search for Jewish mutations. [110]

The first reports on the high prevalence of a specific mutation of *BRCA1* gene found in many women of Jewish-Ashkenazi origins (*185delAG*) was published in 1995, and first estimates were that approximately one percent of individuals in this community carried the mutated gene.[111] Another "Ashkenazi mutation" (*5382insC*) was described in the *BRCA1* gene and an additional one (*6174delT*) in the *BRCA2* gene. The initial reaction of the Jewish community was very positive. A National Institutes of Health (NIH)–sponsored study of *BRCA* mutations among Ashkenazi Jews, which enrolled approximately five thousand people of Ashkenazi origins in the Washington, DC, area, was strongly supported by local Jewish leaders. Rabbi Mathew Simon, the president of United Jewish Agency federation of the greater Washington area was reported to say that Jews were often bled for negative reasons; the NCI study was an opportunity for the Jews to give blood for positive reasons.[112]

Studies on prevalence of *BRCA* mutations among Ashkenazi Jews were also conducted in New York City and in the Boston area. Activists of the National Breast Cancer Coalition protested against the design of these studies (for example the participants in the Washington study did not receive the results of their tests), but these studies were nevertheless supported by Jewish organizations. In 1996 the *Jewish Week,* a popular U.S. Jewish newspaper, reported the commercialization of a test for *185delAG* mutation by the Genetics and In Vitro Fertilization Institute in Fairfax, Virginia (for the relatively modest sum of $295) and recommended that women who wanted more information about genetic testing contact this institute. The *Hartford Jewish Ledger* published in the same year an advertisement for competing testing service, stating that "if you carry damaged breast cancer genes and you live long enough, you are almost guaranteed to develop breast cancer."[113] With the establishment of Myriad's monopoly over *BRCA* genes, all the testing for Ashkenazi mutations in the United States was done by this firm. The "multisite 3 analysis" for the Ashkenazi mutations became one of Myriad's more popular products.

BRCA mutations are indeed more frequent among Ashkenazi Jews. Experts estimate that about one in forty in Ashkenazi women carries a *BRCA* mutation, compared with one in 340 in women in the general population.[114] The great majority of breast cancers belong, however, to nonfamilial forms. A higher fre-

quency of *BRCA* mutations among Ashkenazi Jews does not mean that the overall occurrence of breast cancer among Jews is much higher than the prevalence of
this disease in matched non-Jewish population.[115] A population with a high frequency of *BRCA* mutation contains, however, a significantly greater proportion
of "breast cancer families." This may lead to higher probability of hearing dramatic stories of women who came from such families and thus to a greater visibility of breast cancer in the Jewish community. A greater number of "cancer
families" in the Jewish population may also explain earlier inconsistencies in data
on the frequency of breast cancer among the Jews, because the presence of such
families may increase the chances of a bias in a sample originated in a limited
geographic area.

Ashkenazi mutations are present in the United States, France, and the United
Kingdom, but the reactions to such mutations were very different. In the United
States, medical geneticists and genetic counselors view ethnicity as a central issue.
Many health professionals and many spokespersons for specific ethnic groups
believe that attention to biological differences among such groups promotes a
more efficient targeting of preventive and therapeutic strategies to specific populations. In the United States, Ashkenazi mutations are widely discussed by experts and by lay groups. For example, the Zionist women's organization Hadas-
sah developed a program "It's in the Genes." This program discusses concerns
related to the science of genetics, provides counseling for psychosocial issues, debates discrimination and ethics from a Jewish perspective, and promotes "breast
awareness" groups that develop activities targeted toward Jewish women, especially those with a family history of breast or ovarian cancer. Similarly self-help
organizations such as Sharheret (The Chain) deal with specific problems of young
Jewish women diagnosed with a *BRCA* mutation.[116]

This "ethnicization" of breast cancer may be linked with a previous growth of
awareness of the U.S. Jewish community to Ashkenazi diseases, a high percentage
of American Jews in medical and paramedical professions, and the presence of
many women of Jewish descent among U.S. breast cancer activists. It may also be
related to an efficient marketing of testing for "Ashkenazi mutations" by Myriad
Genetics. The fact that one of the main "founder mutations" for *BRCA* (mutations that are shared by a group and not only a single family) were described in
the Jewish population, coupled with the relative wealth of this population, its elevated level of education, and its high level of health consciousness, made it an excellent target for the marketing of tailored services. Moreover, scientists noted
that many Ashkenazi women diagnosed with *BRCA* mutations were not aware of
family history of the disease. A small family size, the absence of daughters, dis-

ruption of family ties by war or migration, can mask the mutation's visibility.[117] The possibility of offering tests for Ashkenazi mutations at a greatly reduced price—approximately one tenth of the price of testing for a *BRCA* mutation in the general population—is an additional marketing argument. Jewish women are invited by Myriad to check whether they are at increased hereditary risk of developing breast cancer even when their family history did not reveal the presence of this pathology, and the moderate price of this service is probably a supplementary incentive to use it.[118] The success of Myriad's marketing strategy reinforces in turn the association between Jewish origins and breast cancer. Being an Ashkenazi Jew is indirectly presented as belonging to an extended family with a higher than average cancer risk and breast cancer, a pathology with a high prevalence in the general population, became partly transformed into another "Jewish disease."

French geneticists tend to downplay the role of ethnicity. It is usually impossible to know the ethnic origins of a person or a family treated in a French hospital solely by looking at the pedigree drawn by medical geneticist, because such pedigree—or the patients' file—does not contain information on ethnic origins or on skin color. This is not an absolute rule. When the link between high frequency of a specific pathology—and geographic or ethnic origins of the patient is well established, e.g., in thalassemia or sickle cell anemia, a patient's files will contain information on ethnic origins. However, in all the other cases, detailed questioning about origins is seen as inappropriate. The invisibility of this topic, and the general reluctance of French geneticists and French administrators to use ethnic categories, may be related to an attachment to universalistic republican values.[119] Breast cancer is not included among diseases linked with specific origins or a given geographical area ("everybody can get cancer"). Accordingly, French breast and ovarian cancer pedigrees do not indicate race, ethnicity, or skin color, and women who consult an oncogeneticist are not asked if they come from an Ashkenazi family. French oncogeneticists do not construct Ashkenazi origin as an independent risk element and do not develop less stringent criteria for *BRCA* testing when dealing with women from Jewish background than with women from other ethnic groups. Nevertheless, if a French woman who was selected for genetic testing does have a typical Ashkenazi family name, the geneticists will usually start by looking for Ashkenazi mutations to save time and money.

In the United Kingdom, epidemiology, including cancer epidemiology, is traditionally linked with preoccupations about social class, rather than with problems linked with ethnic origins. The same is true for medical genetics: while some diseases are linked with ethnic origins (or rather seen as more frequent in specific groups), ethnicity is not presented as a major preoccupation in regional genetic

consultations. British society is more attuned than the French to differences between communities. Genetic counselors are trained to pay attention to ethnic
origins of their clients to provide culturally sensitive counseling. "Ashkenazi mutations" are more visible in the United Kingdom than in France. For example,
epidemiologists investigated the frequency of *BRCA* mutation in areas of London
known to possess a high density of Jewish population. These mutations are, however, less visible in the United Kingdom than in the United States. The difference
among ethnic groups, British cancer geneticists and epidemiologists explain, is
relative and not absolute. More Jewish women have a family history of breast
cancer than Asian ones, but once such history is brought to the foreground, the
preventive measures they propose to a woman identified as being at high risk of
this malignancy will be exactly the same, regardless of ethnic origins. In addition,
the lower importance of results of genetic testing in decisions about medical
supervision of women at risk reduced the role attributed to "Ashkenazi mutations" in the United Kingdom. In spite of greater willingness of British doctors
to include ethnicity among relevant information about a given patient, in the
United Kingdom, too, Ashkenazi origins were not constructed as an independent
risk factor.

Living with a New Kind of Danger

Tests for hereditary predisposition for cancer are legitimated by the principle of
autonomy and the individual's right to know.[120] Genetic counselors are encouraged to promote informed consent and to explain the advantages and the disadvantages of testing. The option of ignoring one's genetic status is perceived as a
valid one, especially when the benefit of such knowledge is not well established.[121] The principle of autonomy does not extend, however, to risk management. Physicians exercise strong pressure on persons at risk to encourage them
to faithfully follow their recommendations. A woman from a family with identified *BRCA* mutation who refuses genetic testing is seen as perfectly rational.
However, her behavior will be seen as irrational if she refuses also to submit
herself to stringent surveillance (frequent clinical examinations, mammography,
and echography) and, increasingly, to undergo a preventive oophorectomy after
the age of 40. Such an attitude is reinforced by a positive result of a genetic test.
A woman who tests positive for *BRCA* mutation is in principle free to decide how
this knowledge will affect her behavior and can thus refuse intensive medical surveillance. In practice, however, such a refusal will often be perceived as a deviant,
pathological reaction. This view reflects a general pattern of use of probabilistic

evaluations in cancer clinics. Such evaluations are employed to convey uncertainty and, simultaneously, to validate clinicians' choices. Patients are told that they can freely elect their preventive and therapeutic options, but they are strongly discouraged from choices seen as excessively risky by their doctors. The latter often interpret their probabilistic data as providing "absolute" clinical recommendations, even when the difference between the evaluated alternatives is not very big.[122]

The right attitude toward management of hereditary risk of breast cancer, the experts explain, steers away from two extremes: a denial of the danger, which may lead to a neglect of monitoring and preventive measures, and an excessive fear, which may be either paralyzing and hamper efficient action or may lead to obsessive testing and too high of a consumption of medical resources. The navigation between these two extremes is not always easy. Frequent monitoring of women at risk of breast cancer automatically increases the frequency of abnormal findings. Consequently,

a substantial proportion of women whose mammograms show abnormalities but no cancer report having significant impairments in mood and daily functioning, and more than one fourth of high risk women may have clinically elevated levels of psychological distress. Such distress may, in turn, interfere with adherence to recommended breast screening and other preventive measures. Because of these psychological effects, it is important to explore a patient's fears about breast cancer and whether they impair her daily functioning. When reassurance and encouragement do not relieve her anxiety and she is too anxious to participate in clinical decision making, psychological consultation is warranted.[123]

Preventive medicine produces the ideal of rational subjects who faithfully follow the expert's' advice: "by being made aware of the risks, the individual is told to provide for and discipline the future, to calculate future actions and dealings."[124] Oncologists and cancer organizations present early detection and careful evaluation of embodied risks for breast cancer as a moral duty of each woman, even more of a woman at increased hereditary risk of this pathology.[125] Women defined as being at high cytological or hereditary risk of breast cancer are assigned to a close medical surveillance. There is general agreement among health professionals about the necessity of such surveillance, in spite of absence of statistically valid proof of its efficacy.[126] Doctors promote at the same time proactive approaches to risk reduction—chemotherapy and preventive surgery.

"Euphenics," Joshua Lederberg proposed in 1963, corrects negative hereditary traits that cannot be eliminated through eugenic manipulation.[127] Eugenics was initially conceived as an effort to improve hereditary traits of a population. The elimination of "faulty" genes will make the nation (or whatever population group seen as relevant) healthier, fitter, and smarter. Eugenic goals were defined on a population level, but eugenic practices were directed toward individuals. In the interwar era, the main eugenic intervention was the sterilization of people defined as "morons" and judged unfit to be parents. From the 1970s on, the development of prenatal diagnosis (analysis of karyotypes and genes and medical imagery) and a parallel legalization of abortion, allowed parents to prevent the birth of severely handicapped children.[128] A judgment about potential offspring (children of "flawed" parents will be flawed too and, therefore, should not be born) was replaced by a techniques that make it possible to probe an already existing fetus and to decide if she or he should be born. The goal of collective improvement of a population was transformed into a striving for an improvement of quality of life of individuals: children to be born and their families. The new way of dealing with collective dangers was to focus on individual risks.[129]

Epidemiology had undergone a similar transformation from collective- to individual-centered interventions. Initially, epidemiologists studied infectious diseases, that is, events that affect a collectivity. Interventions such as isolations of the sick were justified by the fact that an infected person can contaminate many others. In the 1950s and 1960s, the focus of epidemiological investigations shifted from infectious to chronic diseases, that is, pathologies that handicap only people who are ill and not their contacts. Epidemiologists became interested in individualized risk factors, in techniques that make such factors visible, and in the reduction of detected risks.[130] At first, risk-reducing intervention aimed mainly to promote healthy lifestyles (nutrition, exercise, avoidance of harmful habits such as smoking and excessive drinking) for everybody. Later, however, such interventions were increasingly grounded in doctor-controlled practices. Physicians employed tests (measure of blood pressure, of levels of sugars in the blood, of bone density) that displayed individualized risk and proposed medical interventions (e.g., drugs that lower blood pressure and cholesterol levels) to reduce the detected risk.[131] Management of hereditary risk of cancer mirrors this pattern. Such risk is made visible by tools provided by specialists: the construction of pedigrees or the sequencing of genes. People identified as mutation carriers are then advised to be submitted to stringent medical surveillance, take drugs that may lower their risk, and, very often, to undergo an "euphenic" intervention: a surgical elimination of the danger-laden body part.

Discussing the enthusiastic endorsement of testing for the Ashkenazi mutations in *BRCA* genes by some of the U.S. Jewish community leaders, law professor Karen Rothenberg expressed concern about potential consequences of a diagnosis of a hereditary predisposition to malignancy: inequalities of access to testing, insurance discrimination and confidentiality issues, and, for an identified mutation carrier, a life in the shadow of a mortal danger. She proposed that "until we have a better understanding of the benefits and risks of genetic testing and efficient strategies how to best protect the public, we must strive to resist a genetic 'quick fix' mentality that promotes genetic testing in the healthcare market. Obviously there is no 'quick fix' for the ethical, legal and social challenges."[132]

Rothenberg's article was published in 1997. At that time, the race for cloning and patenting *BRCA1* and *BRCA2* genes had ended, Myriad Genetics was on the point of obtaining a monopoly of the testing market in the United States, and genetic tests were about to become a marketable commodity. Their diffusion was driven by professional and commercial interests but also by patients' demands. It was also encouraged by important coverage of the race to clone the breast cancer gene in the media. When Rothenberg wrote her paper, the process was already irreversible. Once these tests were introduced into routine medical practice, it was no longer possible to recover a pretest innocence. People with a family history of cancer can still exercise their right not to know if they are personally at higher than average risk of malignancies, but the existence of genetic tests created a radically new situation. It became increasingly difficult to forgo the awareness of a family history of malignancies, to avoid testing, and—for those who test positive—to escape dilemmas associated with the detection of a "molecular lesion" and knowledge of existence of an embodied risk. [133]

CHAPTER EIGHT

The New Surgical Radicalism

Prophylactic Mastectomy: A Cultural Phenomenon?

The recent focus on dilemmas experienced by women diagnosed with *BRCA* mutations and facing decisions about prophylactic mastectomy have deflected attention from the peculiarity of a comeback of radical surgical solutions. For more than eighty years the accepted view on cancer surgery—and by extension, on surgical treatment of precancerous conditions—was that more is better. This view was challenged, however, in the late 1960s and the 1970s by the rise of a more physiological understanding of cancer. Thanks to the new emphasis on the role of the immune system in the elimination of residual malignant cells, cancer experts increasingly abandoned the view that the only way to eliminate a malignant growth was to cut it out or to burn it with rays.[1] Immunotherapy of cancer did not produce efficient cures for common cancers, but it favored the diffusion of other systemic approaches to cancer treatment, such as adjuvant chemotherapy and hormonotherapy.[2] In 1977, Bernard Fisher, one of the main promoters of the conservative treatment of breast cancer in the United States, presented surgical radicalism as a hopelessly outdated approach. The belief that cancer can be cured only if extirpated sufficiently early, Fisher argued, belongs to the dark ages of pre-scientific past. With the recent understanding of breast cancer as a systemic disease, "we are witnessing now the end of an era of surgery which must be viewed as incredible in terms of both its longevity and its freedom from criticism."[3] In 1996 Fisher reiterated his opinion that new biological understanding of malignancies was rapidly making surgical radicalism obsolete. The improvement of drug therapies of malignant tumors would probably soon lead to a complete disappearance of breast surgeries, he argued.[4] Three years later Fisher noted that instead of disappearing, mastectomies had become more frequent, for him a very disturbing trend. The combination of enhanced tumor detection and new uncertainties brought by progress of scientific research, such as data on hereditary susceptibility to malignancies, had led to a partial reversion to Halsted's old dogma. The result is, he proposed, a growing regression to the "non-science" of anecdotalism and classical inductivism that threatens to nullify the progress that had been achieved earlier.[5]

Stories of those confronted with the possibility of cancer seem to confirm Fisher's impression that American cancer experts changed their attitude toward surgical ablation of breasts in the late 1990s. In the early 1990s, Anne-Marie de Grazia, traumatized by a family history of breast cancer, looked for a U.S. surgeon willing to remove her breasts. She had found that surgeons were reluctant to amputate healthy breasts, fearing that she would sue them if the surgery went wrong or that she would change her mind.[6] As recently as 1997, in an episode of the CBS TV series *Chicago Hope,* a woman with a strong family history of breast cancer asked for a preventive mastectomy. The young surgeon who examined her was horrified by the idea of cutting off healthy breasts.[7] By contrast, more recent accounts stress doctors' active involvement in the promotion of preventive mastectomies. An advertisement for the Mayo Clinic tells the story of four sisters Vittone who had a strong family history of breast cancer but no mutation in the *BRCA* gene. All the sisters, those diagnosed with cancer and those without malignancy, underwent a prophylactic ablation of breasts and ovaries, and they praise the Mayo clinics doctors for helping them to reach this decision, then rapidly performing prophylactic surgeries.[8]

Preventive ablation of the breast is a controversial surgery, and doctors are expected to objectively present arguments for and against this intervention. Nevertheless, many have strong opinions on this topic and find ways to make it known. Bianca Kennedy's breast tumor was initially treated with lumpectomy and radiation. When she learned that her sister had a recurrence of her cancer, she told her doctors that she wanted both her breasts removed: "they had not tried to push me into doing it, but after I said what I wanted they told me that they thought it was the wisest thing to do."[9] Jerome Groopman—a physician, book author, and writer for the *New Yorker*—described in 1998 a case of a *BRCA*-positive woman, "Karen," a patient and friend, whose mother died from breast cancer and whose twin sister was diagnosed with the same disease. Groopman explained to Karen that her options were waiting under surveillance or prophylactic removal of breast and ovaries. He added then that prophylactic surgery eliminated most, but not all the risk, since it is impossible to excise all the breast or ovary cells. Karen's first reaction was that something should be done: "You want to do something for yourself, something proactive, and not just live under surveillance. It seems like passively waiting in the ghetto for being selected." Nevertheless, she felt unable to accept prophylactic surgery. When Karen finally said, "I cannot do it. I cannot get rid of my breasts and ovaries," Groopman was taken aback by Karen's reaction: "Above all I wanted Karen to be saved. Surely that imperative overrode the loss of breast and ovaries, of self-image and libido."[10] He was relieved when, a week later, Karen returned with a firm decision, "I'm going to have my breasts and ovaries removed."[11]

The level of enthusiasm for prophylactic mastectomy is, however, far from being uniform. French oncologists were reluctant to recommend this treatment, an attitude that can be related to their preference for a conservative treatment of breast cancer. A 2006 French study revealed that more than three quarters (77.5 percent) of people diagnosed with invasive breast cancer were treated with a breast-conserving surgery. French surgeons' unwillingness to amputate breasts that actually contained cancer probably influenced their reluctance to excise healthy breasts of women at increased risk of breast malignancy.[12] In 1998, when I started a study with two of my colleagues on the use of newly developed tests for the detection of *BRCA* mutations in France, I did not encounter a single case of preventive mastectomy.[13] At that time, a panel of experts named by INSERM (Institut National de la Santé et de la Recherche Médicale, roughly the French equivalent of the U.S. National Institutes of Health) discussed the practical applications of the new technology. The group's debates led to the publication of national guidelines on management of women diagnosed with *BRCA1* or *BRCA2* mutations. These guidelines recommended frequent clinical examinations and mammography, outlined experimental protocols of surveillance of *BRCA*-positive women by other medical imagery techniques (e.g., nuclear magnetic resonance, breast and ovarian echography) and, potentially, chemoprevention. The INSERM guidelines also suggested discussing preventive oophorectomy with mutation carriers, especially if they had a family history of ovarian cancer. By contrast, prophylactic mastectomy was mentioned only briefly and was not presented as a valid therapeutic option.[14] For the French, the only candidates for such surgery were high-risk women who strongly insisted on having their breasts removed, either because they were particularly anxious or because they came from families with an unusually high incidence of breast cancer and cancer-related deaths. All the other women, including those with confirmed *BRCA* mutations, were expected to keep their breasts until a diagnosis of a malignant tumor. The rationale behind such advice was that a mutation carrier could hope to escape cancer altogether or at least to avoid this disease until an advanced age.[15]

In the late 1990s, specialists estimated that approximately 20 percent of American and British women at high hereditary risk of breast cancer had undergone prophylactic mastectomy, while the rate of such surgery among high-risk French women was well below 5 percent.[16] Intrigued by the variable rates of preventive mastectomy, French and American experts at first proposed an explanation grounded in broad cultural differences. Women in Latin and Catholic countries, they claimed, are more attached to their body integrity and less inclined to make decisions grounded in probabilistic evaluations than women in Nordic and Protestant ones.[17] Sociologists confirmed the existence of national differences in attitudes toward prophylactic mastectomy. French women were reluctant to undergo this surgery, and French doctors were reluctant to recommend it. By contrast they saw preventive ablation of ovaries as an acceptable option for women with *BRCA* mutations despite of the fact that this operation is seen as a less efficient way to reduce cancer risk than prophylactic mastectomy. The authors of these studies concluded that the French do not seem to have a rational attitude toward the management of health risks.[18]

The presumed difference between Catholic and Protestant cultures cannot, however, explain all the differences in the diffusion of prophylactic mastectomy among *BRCA*-positive women. It does not elucidate, for example, why more than half (54 percent) of women diagnosed with *BRCA* mutation in Rotterdam elected a preventive mastectomy, but only 4 percent of mutation carriers in Melbourne made the same choice. Cultural factors are even less well adapted to explain important differences between hospitals in the same country; such differences are frequently more important than those between countries.[19] One survey compared practices in five U.S. hospitals that proposed prophylactic mastectomy to *BRCA*-mutation carriers and found that the percentage of *BRCA*-positive women who underwent this surgery were, respectively, 3 percent, 13 percent, 15 percent, 27 percent, and 51 percent.[20] The great variability in among hospitals (probably related to differences in approaches of leading experts in these hospitals) may point to the role of doctors in shaping the choices of a mutation carrier. When high-risk women and health professionals were questioned in 1998 about their putative reaction to a diagnosis of a *BRCA* mutation, only 6 percent of American women said that they would like to undergo a prophylactic mastectomy, while 34 percent of American doctors (and 12 percent of nurse-practitioners) said they would recommend it to their patients.[21] It is reasonable to assume that broad cultural factors affected a patient's choice of preventive surgery, but clearly such factors are not the whole story. Other elements were probably at least as important: organization of health services, division of medical labor, and professional traditions.[22]

There are important national differences in doctors' choices. For example, high rates of hysterectomies in the United States attest to surgical activism of gynecologists, their aversion to risk (including the risk of being sued for malpractice), and their preference for radical solutions. Lower rates of hysterectomy in France may reflect a professional culture that valorizes medical rather than surgical solutions to gynecological problems and sees the doctor's capacity to provide a more conservative—and efficient—treatment as a hallmark of professional skill.[23] It is entirely possible, however, that aggregated national data often hide important disparities between treating centers. Such disparities may reflect site-specific traditions and contingent elements. A close cooperation between plastic surgeons and oncologists may encourage the latter to propose mastectomy with an immediate reconstruction more often, while strong charismatic leaders may influence therapeutic trends among their followers.[24] Variations between local medical cultures are probably as important, and sometimes more important, than those between national ones.

Preventive Mastectomy and the Visualization of Embodied Risk

Medicine is at the same time a local and a global practice. Doctors are influenced by their training and work environment but cannot disregard reliable and persuasive evidence. In the 1990s preventive mastectomy for *BRCA*-mutation carriers was seen as a logical but unproven—and for some, extreme—choice for a woman at a hereditary risk of cancer. The attitudes toward this preventive approach changed in 2001, following the publication of studies that demonstrated the efficacy of preventive mastectomy in reducing breast cancer risk of *BRCA*-positive women.[25] This conclusion was confirmed in 2004 by results of the Prevention and Observation of Surgical Endpoints study group. Nearly half of the *BRCA*-positive women in this study who kept their breasts (48.7 percent or 184 participants) developed malignancies, while only 1.9 percent women (two participants) in the mastectomy group were diagnosed with cancer. The authors of this research concluded that "for those women who chose bilateral prophylactic mastectomy, this study provides definitive evidence that they have chosen an efficient prevention strategy."[26] In absence of proof of the efficacy of alternative solutions—chemoprevention and mammographic surveillance—the ablation of cancer-prone organs increasingly appeared as the only truly efficient way to keep in check a hereditary predisposition to cancer.[27] French experts could not ignore these new findings. The French National Ad Hoc Committee on Hereditary Breast and Ovarian Cancer changed its guidelines in 2004. The new document states that since the effectiveness of prophylactic surgeries is now well established, doctors should discuss this possibility with *BRCA*-positive women and help them to establish whether in their case the expected benefit of such surgery will outweigh its negative aspects.[28] In France, too, preventive surgery became increasingly perceived as a possible answer to some of the dilemmas produced by genetic testing. One of the topics most often discussed in 2005 and 2006 on a French language Internet forum on breast cancer and heredity was prophylactic mastectomy.[29]

The preventive ablation of breasts of *BRCA*-positive women became increasingly viewed by doctors as a rational way of managing hereditary risk of cancer. It remained nevertheless a problematic solution. By contrast, preventive ablation of ovaries of *BRCA*-mutation carriers was universally viewed as an uncontroversial way to reduce a hereditary risk of ovarian cancer, a disease with very low cure rates.[30] In addition, researchers had found that *BRCA*-positive women who underwent prophylactic oophorectomy had a lower probability of developing breast cancer. This observation strengthened the tendency to propose prophylactic oophorectomy to all *BRCA*-positive women, not only those with a family history of ovarian cancer.[31] Surgical ablation of ovaries was used from the late nineteenth century on to slow down the spread of advanced breast cancer.[32] The well-documented efficacy of this approach opened the way to the supposition that removal of ovaries may help reduce the rates of breast cancer in *BRCA*-mutation carriers as well. This hypothesis was confirmed by clinical data.[33] The protective effect of oophorectomy, endocrinologists propose, is not simply related to the elimination of the source of estrogen. *BRCA*-positive women who underwent a prophylactic ablation of their ovaries and then employed estrogen to fight symptoms of early menopause had lower breast cancer rates than those who kept their ovaries.[34]

Debates on preventive surgery for *BRCA*-mutation carriers were, as a rule, focused on the ablation of breasts and ovaries of healthy women. The term *preventive surgery* for *BRCA*-mutation carriers has, however, an additional, and less publicized, meaning: the ablation of the unaffected breast, and often of ovaries as well, of a *BRCA*-positive woman diagnosed with an invasive or in situ carcinoma in one breast. Women diagnosed with breast cancer who have a family history of the disease may be encouraged to immediately undergo testing for the presence of *BRCA* mutations.[35] The rationale of such testing is that the presence of a mutation can influence therapeutic decisions. Moreover, in the United States, a diagnosis of malignancy eliminates one of the main obstacles for *BRCA* testing: the fear that a positive result may lead to a loss of health insurance or a steep increase in its rates. In the majority of U.S. states, the law did not allow the use of results of genetic tests to limit access to health insurance. Insurance is, however, an imperfectly regulated domain, as is the protection of confidentiality of medical data.[36] Genetic counselors often advise women to be tested anonymously without notifying their insurers.[37] This means, however, that they have to pay several thousands of dollars out of their pocket, something that only affluent people can afford. By contrast, once a woman is diagnosed with breast malignancy, secrecy is no longer an issue. She can therefore feel free to ask her insurer to pay for a *BRCA* test, the more so because the result of such test can be presented as an essential element in selecting treatment options.

Mutation carriers diagnosed with breast cancer are frequently advised to undergo a more radical surgery than those without known hereditary predispositions.[38] The rationale for proposing a radical surgical solution—often a bilateral mastectomy with oophorectomy—is that *BRCA*-positive women have higher rates of local recurrence and a higher probability of developing cancer in the contralateral breast. Women diagnosed with *BRCA* mutations often accept their doctors' recommendations. According to a U.S. survey, half of breast cancer patients diagnosed with a mutation in the *BRCA* gene had chosen prophylactic removal of the second breast. A quarter of newly diagnosed breast cancer patients with a family history of this disease who tested negative for *BRCA* mutations made a similar choice. The latter finding may attest to the strength of a fear of breast cancer in these women. It may also point to a growing acceptability of prophylactic ablation of breasts in the United States.[39] This growing acceptance is not universal. An international survey of the frequency of contralateral prophylactic mastectomy in women with *BRCA* mutations, published in 2008, revealed important differences among national practices. According to one study 49 percent of American and 28 percent of Canadian *BRCA*-positive women underwent prophylactic ablation of the contralateral breast when diagnosed with cancer, while only 5 percent of European and Israeli women underwent such surgery.[40] A different sample yielded somewhat lower overall rates of prophylactic mastectomy and confirmed that highest rates of this surgery were found in the United States.[41]

While rates of prophylactic surgeries may vary, *BRCA*-positive women accept as a rule the verdict of hereditary susceptibility and view their options in light of this verdict. The rapid adoption of a DNA-based interpretation of hereditary susceptibility to breast cancer is not self evident. In many complex, multifactorial illnesses, such as Alzheimer's disease, people do not replace an old understanding of "blood" and heredity with a new understanding grounded in molecular biology. New biomedical techniques do not dissociate (yet?) illness and suffering from the messiness of human contingency and biography.[42] The readiness of many *BRCA*-positive women to view their cancer risk through molecular "lenses" and to act upon such an understanding of risk can perhaps be related to the history of making women responsible for breast cancer. The "do not delay" imperative implicitly stated that women who died from breast malignancies brought their fate on themselves, while the long tradition of prophylactic mastectomy following a diagnosis of precancerous lesions might have made preventive treatments of this disease more amenable to decisions that depend above all on results of a laboratory test.

Specialists believe that the principle that women with "good prognosis" breast cancers are the best candidates for a prophylactic ablation of the contralateral breast should be applied to *BRCA*-mutation carriers too. They argue that women whose first tumor was not very aggressive were lucky once but cannot be sure that their luck will hold the next time. The histological type of cancer developed in a contralateral breast is not related to the type of the first malignant tumor; it may be more aggressive and more difficult to treat. Prophylactic mastectomy is an efficient way to make sure that a second round of malignancy will not happen. Not all the *BRCA*-positive women diagnosed with breast cancer followed this logic. A survey of women's decisions revealed that more *BRCA*-positive women diagnosed with stage II cancer (that is, with cancer that had spread to axillary lymph nodes) accepted bilateral prophylactic mastectomy than those diagnosed with in situ cancer or with a tumor limited to the breast only (stage I). This difference was attributed to women's poor understanding of the effects of prophylactic surgery and to a greater willingness of women diagnosed with a more advanced disease to match the aggressiveness of their cancer with an aggressive therapy.[43] An additional reason may be the loss of confidence in medical surveillance. *BRCA*-positive women undergo frequent mammographic and clinical examinations and are told that a stringent surveillance favors an early detection of cancer. Women diagnosed with a tumor that has spread to their lymph nodes in spite of their faithful adherence to surveillance guidelines may fear that this may happen again and may be more willing to get rid of their breasts.[44]

Preventive mastectomy for *BRCA*-positive women—those diagnosed with a tumor who undergo the ablation of the contralateral breast and those with no clinical signs of malignancy—acquired an additional legitimacy through the description of a higher frequency of proliferative lesions in breasts of mutation carriers. Pathologists reported an unusually high levels of histological abnormalities (ductal carcinoma in situ, lobular carcinoma in situ, atypical ductal hyperplasia, and atypical lobular hyperplasia) in breast tissue of *BRCA*-positive women.[45]

They also observed multiple precancerous changes in ovaries and Fallopian tubes of mutation carriers who underwent prophylactic oophorectomy.[46] The argument that *BRCA*-positive women had a higher than average tendency to develop proliferative lesions of breast and ovary transformed a future danger into an already existing one and helped to justify the decision to excise healthy organs by presenting it as the elimination of flawed and diseased body parts.[48] Testimonies of women who underwent prophylactic mastectomy stress this aspect. TV writer Jessica Queller was told by her surgeon after her operation: "You had precancerous changes in your right breast tissue, Jessica. Atypical ductal hyperplasia. . . . If you had any doubt about the course of action you choose, this should dispel it. You did the right thing."[48] Writer Masha Gessen hoped for the same and was disappointed: "I did hope that the pathology will reveal just one cancer cell—or rather a non-invasive, very early-stage cancer—so I would not have to undergo chemotherapy but will still know I had done the right thing. No such luck. The pathology results were clear."[49]

In the mid-1990s oncologists believed that the hereditary forms of breast and ovarian cancer could be aligned with the familial form of colon cancer (hereditary nonpolyposis colon cancer). People diagnosed with this condition (a genetic test for the major mutations that induce this condition, *MLH1*, *MSH2*, and *MSH6* has existed since the late 1990s)—are strongly advised to undergo a regular colonoscopic supervision. Surveys indicate that such a supervision, coupled with a systematic removal of all the suspicious lesions, led to the prevention of 70 to 80 percent of colon tumors.[50] It was hoped that surveillance with medical imaging techniques (mammography, nuclear magnetic resonance, echography), possibly associated with a prophylactic drug treatment, would rapidly lead to a similar reduction of breast and ovarian cancer risk. This did not happen, however. During the first ten years of the introduction of genetic tests for hereditary predisposition to cancer into clinical practice, some hereditary forms of malignancies (colon, melanoma) followed the cervical cancer model. In these cancers, people diagnosed with familial predisposition to cancer undergo a close surveillance that facilitates the detection of premalignant lesions. The surgical excision of such lesions (adenomatous polyps or flat lesions of the intestine, suspicious moles) is not an innocuous procedure, but it usually does not induce major iatrogenic effects.[51] By contrast, during the first ten years of use of genetic tests for susceptibility to breast and ovarian cancers, these malignancies became aligned with a preventive treatment of familial adenomatous polyposis (FAP). For these cancers, for the time being, only drastic, mutilating surgery with lifelong consequences allows an important reduction of the hereditary risk, without eliminating it totally.

The Experience of Prophylactic Surgery: Women with Breast Cancer

Stories collected at Internet sites dedicated to the education of the public about prevention and treatment of breast cancer make visible the fluidity of boundaries between preventive and nonpreventive surgeries and between risk and disease. One may call such stories "pathoblogs," because of their resemblance to "pathographies"—autobiographic narratives of disease.[52] Using pathoblogs to learn how individuals react to diagnosis and treatment has obvious drawbacks. Women who choose to go public with their cancer stories are not, in all probability, representative of the majority of people who have cancer. They tend to be more outspoken, more extroverted, more knowledgeable, and more proactive. They are also distinctly younger than the average person with breast cancer. The average age of diagnosis of breast cancer is mid-sixties, while the majority of the women who publish their stories in specialized blogs are in their twenties, thirties, and forties. The Web seems to reinforce the image of breast cancer as a young woman's disease, a trend already promoted by the media and cancer organizations.[53] Nevertheless, these stories can provide a vivid illustration of data presented in scientific papers.

Pathoblogs dedicated to breast cancer relate relatively frequently the experience of radical surgeries for in situ breast tumors, presented either as a life-saving strategy or as the only way to achieve a peace of mind. Here are examples of typical narratives:

Cindy's mammography revealed a cyst in her breast. The cyst itself was characterized as benign but a needle aspiration revealed DCIS in its vicinity. She underwent ablation of the affected area. However, the margins of the incision remained unclean [not entirely free of transformed cells], and her doctors strongly recommended mastectomy, explaining that otherwise she would have a 30 percent chance of developing an invasive cancer in the next 10 years. At first Cindy resisted this recommendation—then she heard an "inner voice"—which she identified as the Holy Ghost—telling her she had to go ahead and undergo a mastectomy. Three years after her surgery she feels very grateful that her *cancer* was found in such an early stage. She concludes her story: "Get your mammograms! Do your breast self exams! It could save your life!"[54]

Carole had a lumpectomy [the excision of the affected area of the breast] at the end of August 1984 and was diagnosed with hyperplasia, a benign proliferative disorder of the breast. The surgery to eliminate areas of abnormal proliferation of breast tissue was, theoretically, a minor one, but Carole found it very traumatic: "When I had my lumpectomy a hematoma (collection of blood in the tissue) and an infection resulted at the surgical site. The wound had to be reopened and drained. This was both painful and repulsive (smelly, gross stuff came out of the wound and hot compresses had to be applied over several days). Certainly, I did not want to be in the position of having to have repeated lumpectomies, which one of the surgeons felt was a distinct possibility." Carole also feared that because she had lumpy breasts, doctors would miss a tumor, and she would end up having an advanced breast cancer: "it seemed at the time that having my breasts removed would be the best course of action—it would take away all the fear and anxiety." After consulting with her family physician and two surgeons she decided to proceed with bilateral mastectomies and underwent a mastectomy and breast reconstruction with silicone implants.[55]

Sharon was diagnosed with DCIS in one breast and LCIS in the other (both detected through biopsies following an abnormal mammogram). She was treated with a lumpectomy, but the margins were not clean. She was given an option of larger excision of her DCIS, and surveillance, but her two oncologists believed that she should undergo bilateral mastectomy. On the other hand, Sharon felt that they were also respectful of her need to make her own decision. At first Sharon was very reluctant to lose her breasts, but later she learned how problematic a conservative surgery may be: "if I took the cautious approach, my breasts would be deformed by repeated surgeries, probably requiring some reconstruction anyway, and I would have to undergo 6 weeks or so of radiation. In the end, if the chipping away at some point resulted in the need to finally have a mastectomy, I would be forced to have the extensive, time-consuming microsurgery required for latissimus dorsal and/or gluteus maximus free flap surgery, since I am too thin for the abdominal flaps and wouldn't like those scars anyway." After thinking for a few days and reading stories of other women's experiences, she called her surgeons to schedule the bilateral mastectomies and an immediate reconstructive surgery.[56]

Sue's pathology report showed that she had ductal carcinoma in situ (DCIS). She was also diagnosed with severe atypical hyperplasia of the breast. She was at first shocked and confused. She then found out that there was a great deal of debate over how to treat her cancer. The main options were an additional excision for clean margins and tamoxifen, the same with added radiotherapy, and mastectomy. She ended by electing a double mastectomy: "many studies showed this was overtreatment, and my radiologist told me that I was overreacting to my diagnosis. But I just wanted to do all I could to have the least chance of recurrence."[57]

Joanna's mother had a double mastectomy for an early cancer in 1959—and remained healthy since. When Joanna was diagnosed with DCIS, her doctors, in light of her family history, recommended a complete mastectomy. She agreed to the proposal. She was aware of the fact that some women diagnosed with DCIS consider a less aggressive surgery, but she explained that, "in view of my mother's experience, I was not interested in breast conservation. I was not going to cut this dog's tail by inches. By finding the cancer at this non-invasive stage, and by choosing complete mastectomies, I needed no additional treatment: no radiation and no chemotherapy. Most importantly, my choice gave me peace of mind. I have a 99 percent chance of no recurrence. It doesn't get much better than that." Discussing it with family, friends, and health professionals, she realized that although DCIS is increasingly diagnosed, it is not well understood, because people find the concept of non-invasive cancer and malignancy without a well defined lump confusing. Joanna's perception of cancer evolved following her diagnosis: "now I believe that it is imperative that women, and people who love them, become aware that no tumors does not necessarily mean no cancer. Only a mammogram can reveal what cannot be felt—the presence of deadly cancer cells."[58]

When Beth was diagnosed with DCIS, she accepted (gladly) the treatment proposed by her doctors: large excision, radiotherapy, and tamoxifen: "one of the things that led me to my final decision about the radiation and tamoxifen was an exercise that my radiation therapist asked me to do. She said, "Imagine yourself ten years from now. . . . You're in your kitchen on a sunny, summer morning. The breeze gently blowing through your window. As you calmly walk from you kitchen, down your hallway, you think to yourself. . . . I am so glad that I decided to _____. Fill in the blank."[59]

The unspoken subtext is that if Beth did not agree to the proposed therapy, there will be no sunny summer mornings any more, a powerful argument in favor of a preventive surgery.

The Experience of Prophylactic Breast Surgery: Women with *BRCA* Mutations

Rational consumers of medical services are increasingly asked to learn to evaluate probabilistic evidence, to appropriate the managerial language of decision making, and to transform the understanding of their embodied risks into norms of self-understanding and action.[60] This language that stresses multiple possibilities and open-ended decisions often frames more constraining realities.[61] People diagnosed with a mutation in the *APC* gene that induces FAP can theoretically decide to decline a prophylactic ablation of the colon (colectomy). In practice, however, the logic of the medical system does not leave them much choice in the matter. Similarly, *BRCA*-positive women are increasingly encouraged to undergo prophylactic oophorectomy once they have completed their family. The prophylactic ablation of breasts is perceived as a more problematic choice, and women who refuse this solution are not seen as being irrational. Testimonies of women diagnosed with *BRCA* mutations, however, indicate that for many of these women a prophylactic mastectomy is seen as an inescapable consequence of a positive result of the genetic test.[62] This is especially true for women with a past trauma, such as losing a mother to breast cancer at an early age. One of the recurring elements in testimonies of *BRCA*-positive women who elected preventive surgery is that their mother's or sister's experience of breast cancer was so distressing that they were willing to do everything possible to avoid such a fate, a dark side of the upbeat discourse on recent advances in the treatment of this disease.[63]

One of the main arguments in favor of prophylactic breast surgery was the satisfaction expressed by the majority of women that made this decision. Women who elected to remove both their breasts either after a diagnosis of cancer or to prevent future malignancy reported that they were pleased with their choice. The decision to undergo a prophylactic mastectomy, a follow-up study indicated, does not negatively affect the quality of life of women who made this choice. Moreover, while bilateral mastectomy did not entirely eliminate (entirely) cancer worry, it lessened it. Fifty percent of women who underwent bilateral mastectomy after a diagnosis of malignancy continued to worry about a recurrence of cancer, as compared with 74 percent of women who underwent a more conservative surgery.[64] The conclusion of this study—"A large majority of women undergoing this procedure were satisfied with their decision and reported contentment with quality of life comparable with cancer survivors who did not undergo this procedure"—was translated in the media into affirmations like "preventive mastectomy satisfying" or "preventive mastectomy offers women relief."[65] This doesn't take into account that self-reported questionnaires may provide inaccurate data. People who undergo a traumatic experience such as cancer may go through a "response shift." They change their internal standards of what "feeling good" means and adjust their levels of pain and discomfort to this new level.[66] For example, a Dutch study found that women treated for an invasive or in situ breast cancer reported higher levels of well-being and less pain than controls in the general population.[67] Self-reported satisfaction about the outcome of prophylactic surgery may be at the same time a sincere description of one's feeling and a biased answer.

Testimonies of women diagnosed with *BRCA* mutations and undergoing preventive surgery to reduce their breast cancer risk reflect akin attitudes. Women interviewed by sociologists and those who write pathoblogs dedicated to this issue do not seem (to date) to have developed a critical stance toward understanding and treatment of breast cancer risk. They may be dissatisfied with specific doctors or institutions but not with the way the medical establishment deals with hereditary risk of cancer. It is possible that the unconditional acceptance of doctors' point of view will change with time: the development of critical attitude of some activists toward the dominant trends in treatment of breast cancer was a slow process.[68] Pathoblogs that describe prophylactic mastectomy for women diagnosed with *BRCA* mutations reflect the growing consensus that this surgical operation is the most rational attitude to a diagnosis of a mutation. An additional diagnosis of proliferative lesions of the breast, such as atypia or mammary dysplasia, may reinforce the view of one's breasts as "ticking bombs" and prompt preventive action. Mette Nordhal Svensen questioned a Danish woman, Ellen, whose mother and aunt had breast cancer. Ellen was aware of the family cluster of cases and agreed to undergo more frequent mammographic screening but was not pleased to learn that a *BRCA* mutation was detected in one of her cousins. Until then, she hoped that she had already escaped the danger of hereditary cancer. When a mutation was detected in her family, she felt that she could not avoid genetic testing any longer. This conviction was amplified by a recent diagnosis of proliferative changes in her breast:

> Before I was diagnosed with abnormal cells, I kept thinking, one more year has passed without illness. Those family members who have had cancer were all younger than I am when they were diagnosed. Most of them died when young. I had the idea that it was a disease that hit in youth. I thought, one more year has passed and you are probably the one to escape. You are the one who hasn't

got it. After all it is not that hereditary. . . . Knowing that I had dysplasia, and that I had come this far . . . it just felt right to be tested. And then when the result came I was not shocked. The positive test result was just a natural consequence of all the other things that had happened to me.[69]

Knowledge, Ellen stressed, is irreversible. Once the information about the presence of the mutation in the family became available, it was practically impossible to find a standpoint from which she could refuse genetic information or the obligation to act upon this information. Svensen argues that genetic testing provided women with a possibility of becoming moral agents, of making rational decisions based on probabilistic evaluations, and of transforming irrational fear of cancer into a concrete, calculable risk.[70] Such testing allows them "to change from a 'sphere of danger' in which the possibility of future breast cancer is not objectified by science to a 'sphere of risks' in which the possibility of breast cancer is scientifically assessed, and decisions about what to do about it are within their reach."[71] In BRCA-positive women, one may add, the use of scientific knowledge to reframe the present and to eliminate fear often leads to a physical elimination of a dangerous part of the body. Scientific rationality is directly translated into surgical radicalism.

The personal stories on websites for women with hereditary predisposition to develop breast cancer, FORCE , the forum of a self help group for women with BRCA mutation, Facing Our Risk, and Bright Pink, a site for women at high risk of breast cancer—reflect an aspiration to control one's fate. The motto of the Bright Pink website is "Be Brilliant, Be Bold, Be Bright Pink," and it declares: "Bright Pink believes in the beauty and strength of women. It exists to enlighten and empower high-risk individuals to take control of their breast health by providing education, support and a sense of community for a better, brighter future," a somewhat ironic statement in the light of the observation that nearly all the contributions to this site discuss prophylactic surgery, usually mastectomy.[72] The majority of women who write on the FORCE website define themselves as "previvors," a term coined to describe healthy mutation carriers. The websites movingly document hesitations and misgivings about preventive surgery. However, women who provide testimonies on life with high risk of breast cancer usually conclude their story with a decision to undergo prophylactic mastectomy and with a variant of the affirmation: "I know that I made the right decision for myself."[73]

Dixie was, at the age of 38, cancer-free but worried, because her mother developed a bilateral breast cancer at an early age (and survived it). Being of Jewish ancestry, she underwent testing for the presence of an Ashkenazi mutation.

Both she and her mother tested positive. Her mother was relieved to know that there was a reasonable explanation why she had suffered. Dixie decided then to undergo a prophylactic mastectomy with an immediate reconstruction, for her, a way of fighting back her cancer. She says that she woke from the surgery with a distinct feeling of relief that has never left her since: "A month later I laughed out loud the day I purchased patio furniture that would last a lifetime. And I mean a long lifetime! What a psychological shift! Was this worth losing my breasts? As they like to say in Colorado, YOU BET!"[74]

Tricia, whose mother died from breast cancer and whose sister developed the disease, decided to undergo preventive mastectomy at the age of 28. She felt she had no other choice: "you will do everything in order to save your own life." Her feeling that she was an active participant in the process that saved her from certain death (her story does not mention genetic testing) explains her satisfaction with the process and with its outcome. The title of her story provides its content: "Stopping a time bomb."[75]

Katieb explained that she has always known that she would get breast cancer. There were numerous cases of this malignancy on her mother's side, and, although no *BRCA* mutation was found, experts believed that this was a dominant genetic condition. After living with fear since she was fourteen, Katieb finally decided to do something about it. Three months after her wedding she had a bilateral mastectomy: "That was 6 days ago. The thing is Friday we got the pathology report and there was cystic growth, often a precondition of breast cancer." Katieb's message is entitled: "What a relief!"[76]

Pat was diagnosed with cancer three years after her sister. Their oncologist advised her to undergo *BRCA* testing, and the test came back positive. She educated herself about the meaning of mutations and learned that because she had the *BRCA1* mutation she had a higher risk of developing ovarian cancer and of having a recurrence of her breast cancer. She chose therefore oophorectomy and bilateral mastectomies with immediate reconstruction. The decision to undergo the mastectomies was difficult, but immediately after her surgery she felt liberated: "I no longer feel like I'm waiting for the cancer to come back and can live my life. My husband has been terrific and supportive through the whole thing. I am 16 days post-op and physically feel ugh! But I know that eventually I will feel fine and that's what I hold onto. I'm 44 years old and have a new chance at life. How lucky can you get!!!!"[77]

"Tinker" was less lucky; she developed a breast cancer in spite of prophylactic surgery. She underwent a preventive ablation of the breast in 1989, because of strong family history of the disease, had a breast reconstruction by the TRAM technique in 1994, and was diagnosed with cancer in 1998: "yes, since breast tissue looks like any other tissue they can't tell if they got all of it. I developed the cancer on the chest wall (not a good sign) under my left arm, about level with the nipple. Found it on yearly mammogram, but only one centimeter, and node negative. My daughter had prophylactic surgery also."[78]

BRCA-positive women ("Caro," "Ptiote," "Nene," "Chiffonet," "Marie"), who posted their testimonies about their preventive surgeries on a French language forum on breast cancer and heredity, explain that the decision to undergo prophylactic mastectomy was easy. The stress of surgery and possible complications were relatively insignificant, when compared with the relief from the fear of cancer. They use expressions like "it's the light at the end of the tunnel," "it's a near-definitive way to avoid cancer," "one erases one's risk," "anything is better than cancer," "one needs to put all the chances on one's side," "I cut the claws of this marine beast." They were also frequently reassured by their surgeon's assessment that the amputated breasts contained "some abnormal cells" or "a very beginning cancer." "Caro" added that she considers the discovery of her genetic status as a blessing. She was able to undertake an efficient action instead of living in the dark. Marie was even more explicit: "science at least showed us our enemy: the mutation. And it also provides us with tools to fight it . . . mastectomy. Why not to use it?"[79]

Writer Masha Gessen provides a complex and fine grained testimony of the experience of testing positive for *BRCA* mutation. Gessen has a family history of breast cancer: her mother and aunt died from the disease in their midlife. In spring 2004 she tested positive for one of the Ashkenazi genes. She then educated herself thoroughly about the meaning of this test.[80] The first thing she learned was that a positive test radically transformed her health status. When she asked her doctor not to treat her as a cancer patient because she has no cancer yet, she was told that she has no *detectable* cancer.[81] Reluctant to undergo preventive surgery, she consulted with leading medical specialists (among them Dana Farber onco-geneticist Judy Garber), but also psychologists and experts in a probabilistic decision making. Gessen's story is not typical because, she was even more worried about an artificial menopause at 37 following a prophylactic ablation of her ovaries than about losing her breasts. Finally, after several weeks of hesitation Gessen decided to undergo mastectomy with reconstruction, encouraged by an upbeat attitude of her plastic surgeon. She also decided to delay oophorectomy until she was 40. In spite of her hesitations, she strongly felt that she did not have much choice. Her only rational option, and the one which allowed her to feel on control of her destiny, was a preventive surgery. And she was able to give a positive meaning for the numbness of her postsurgical body: "for now, I felt like I was carrying something like a shield on my front, and this seemed fitting enough."[82]

One testimony, on a blog of "blue gal in a red state" (the blogger is a political activist and a health care professional) stands out, because the author is a woman at high risk of cancer who resists prophylactic mastectomy and frames her opposition to this surgery in feminist terms: "Of course my gentile primary care physician thinks I should have prophylactic mastectomies and surgical reconstructions. 'A new set that will never sag or get cancer.' His pretty blonde nurse, Trish, chirps at me and I grimace. She is 20-something, and does not have my background in Women's Studies; to her it's just a cosmetic surgery. To me this is about politics, and sociology, and gender identity dysphoria."[83] The "blue gal in a red state" blogger is frustrated about her choices—or rather the paucity of such choices. It's either "aggressive monitoring of the high risk patient": endless appointments with oncologists and endocrinologist, repeated mammograms every three months and an MRI of the breasts every six months, or a preventive surgery. She has already had one cancer scare and knows she will probably have other such scares in the future, and that it is probable that she will end up with a cancer diagnosis. Nevertheless, she still wants to be free to frame her difficult options in her own terms: "I have had an 'event' and I am playing a hand with the genetic cards stacked against me. Let's add a couple more descriptions to 'high-risk,' shall we? How about resistant to fad treatments? How about medically literate? How about cautious?"[84]

New Breasts for the Old: Reconstructive Surgery

Masha Gessen's decision to immediately undergo prophylactic mastectomy was influenced by her encounter with an enthusiastic plastic surgeon. Reconstructive surgery of the breast was simultaneously assimilated with cosmetic surgery (dedramatizing this approach) and differentiated from it (to disarm accusation of frivolity and vanity). The assimilation with cosmetic surgery favored a dedramatization of this operation. As Devyn, a 28-year-old *BRCA*-positive woman who accepted her oncologist's strong recommendation of prophylactic surgery explained: "I live in Los Angeles so I guess when the whole process is said and done, I'll fit in nicely with all the women sporting boob jobs."[85] Reconstruction was presented as an equivalent of a minor surgery undertaken by numerous women who wish to improve their self-image and self-confidence. Such comparison is inaccurate, because a reconstructive surgery following curative or prophylactic mastectomy involves building of a nonexistent breast. It has a much higher rate of complication and failure than a cosmetic breast surgery that conserves the basic structure of the breast and only modulates its size. An analogy with cosmetic surgery allowed, nevertheless, the promotion of a more positive attitude toward reconstruction. Many blogs dealing with dilemmas of *BRCA*-mutation carriers and other high-risk women mention the bonus that comes with a decision to undergo prophylactic mastectomy—the possession of good-looking breasts, and, if they undergo reconstruction with autologous muscle and the body's fat (transverse rectus abdominus muscle [TRAM] or deep inferior epigraphic perforator [DIEP] procedure), also the elimination of excess fat from other parts of the body. As Gessen put it: "I am sold. Taking the pound of fat that has stubbornly camped out on my belly since I gave birth, moving that up to my chest, and winding up with a flat stomach, smaller breasts and a vastly reduced risk of cancer, seems worth it."[86]

It was also important to make a distinction between reconstructive and cosmetic surgery to neutralize the claim that women who are asking for breast reconstruction after a mastectomy are vain or frivolous and that they should be satisfied with external prosthesis. U.S. breast cancer activists fought for the reimbursement of breast reconstruction by health insurance. They accentuated the advantages of this surgery and underplayed its more problematic aspects. During the congressional hearing on the Women Health and Cancer Act of 1997, women with breast cancer, such as Mary Armao McCarthy, and activists, such as Frances Visco, the president of National Breast Cancer Coalition, expressed deep concern for insurers' refusal to cover breast reconstruction. They stressed the need to reimburse breast reconstruction as well as surgery that made the breasts symmetrical. These plastic surgeries, Senator Olympia Snowe argued, provide women with physical relief and restore a sense of wholeness to their lives.[87]

Congressional debates on reimbursement of breast reconstruction brought to the foreground the distress of women with breast cancer who wished to have their breasts reconstructed and who faced arbitrary and occasionally incoherent decisions of insurers. Congressional debate accentuated the dichotomy between vital needs of suffering patients and greedy policy of insurers who wish to save money. Such dichotomy deflected attention from a third variable in the breast reconstruction story: professional and financial interests of plastic surgeons. Plastic surgeons undoubtedly believe that their skills help their patients to accept difficult, but necessary, choices. Gessen's surgeon, Dr. Adam Tobias from Boston's Beth Israel Deaconess Hospital (one of the hospitals linked with Harvard), sincerely believes in his mission: "in response to my usual what-would-you-do question, he says that if his wife tested positive for a mutation, he would advise her to have a preventive mastectomy and a DIEP flap reconstruction."[88] But it must be admitted that plastic surgery is a lucrative profession and that a prophylactic breast ablation with an immediate reconstruction, especially of the DIEP flap variety, is a long, complicated, and expensive—and thus profit-generating—operation. Surgeons who encourage women to undergo this procedure are sincerely persuaded that they act in their patient's best interest, but at the same time they improve their own material well-being.

Plastic surgery of the breast had a bad press in the 1990s, following the recall of silicon breast implants in the United States and similar recalls in other countries (in France silicon breast implants were banned between 1992 and 2001) and trials of their producers. The silicone implants were suspected, on the basis of anecdotal evidence, to induce autoimmune diseases such as rheumatoid arthritis, lupus erythromatosus, scleroderma, or myalgia. At the time of the recall, there was no clear-cut proof that linked silicon implants with these pathologies but also no evidence of the contrary. The producers of silicon implants never rigorously tested their safety. Such studies were undertaken only in the aftermath of the implants' scandal. They failed to statistically demonstrate meaningful links between autoimmune disease and silicon implants. In retrospective, it is possible, as Marcia Angel did, to present the recall of the silicon breast implants as an overreaction to insufficient evidence.[89] It is also possible to see this episode as an appropriate application of the precaution principle: consider a device unsafe until proven otherwise. The main point of that story may be, however, elsewhere. Controversy about potential links between implants and autoimmune disease masked a different issue: multiple complications of routine breast enhancement surgeries and breast reconstructions.

Silicon implants—a plastic pouch filled with silicone gel—may leak and may produce local inflammation and distortion of the breast. Moreover, implants often induce the formation of hard, painful capsule; they may also move within the breast and deform it.[90] With the ban on silicon implants, women who underwent either prophylactic or therapeutic mastectomy were offered the choice between saline implants (plastic pouches filled with salted water) and reconstruction with tissues taken from the body: TRAM flap, and more recently the DIEP flap technique. Recently, U.S. doctors were allowed once again to use silicon-filled implants, in the framework of a clinical trial of this device. Sadly, none of these techniques is problem free. People treating their breast cancer, especially those with extended surgeries, may learn that their hope to forget their disease once it is no longer being treated is not a realistic option. As a woman named Donna explained: "slowly I have learned that cancer never really goes away, and I have learned to live with that."[91]

Plastic surgeons tend to be optimistic about outcomes of surgeries. French doctors affirmed that the rates of major complications in breast reconstruction are usually below 10 percent. They also stress the esthetically pleasant results of reconstruction.[92] Studies of long-term outcomes of breast reconstruction present a somewhat different picture. A French survey has revealed that the satisfaction of women who underwent breast reconstruction with implants decreased markedly with time. One year after the surgery 85 percent of the women were pleased with the results, but five years after the surgery, only 52 percent continued to be satisfied. Their dissatisfaction was related to problems with the implants (capsule formation, growing asymmetry between the two breasts) and the persistence of unpleasant and painful sensations in reconstructed breast or breasts.[93] A similar study in the United States found that 30 percent of women who underwent prophylactic mastectomy with reconstruction suffer from severe complications of this surgery. Such complications were more frequent in women who had chosen the TRAM or the DIEP procedure. Seventy-one percent of the women who underwent these reconstruction methods required additional surgical interventions. Implants (either silicone or saline) are less complication-prone, but they are also less permanent. Women who choose implants need to take into consideration the necessity of undergoing additional surgeries in the future.[94] Mastectomy without reconstruction also induces postsurgery complications, such as pain, seroma, and infection, but the rate of complications induced by breast reconstruction was much higher. Moreover, the prevalence of such complications has increased in the past twenty years, a finding that may reflect the growing complexity of reconstruction techniques.[95] *BRCA*-positive women who underwent prophylactic mastectomy had rate of complications similar to women operated on for breast cancer, in spite of the fact that this surgery is not constrained by the anatomical characteristics of the tumor.[96]

Accounts of prophylactic mastectomy seldom discuss one important complication of this treatment: chronic postsurgery pain. Chronic pain is one of the main complications of surgical ablations of the breast, and it is more prevalent in women who underwent breast reconstruction. A long-term study of American women who underwent surgery for breast cancer had found that 35 percent suffer from chronic pain. Another study found an average 30 percent of women with such pain. A British investigation reported that 43 percent of women reported pain three years after mastectomy. In half of those women, the pain was reduced with time; the other half continued to suffer chronic pain nine years after their surgery. Younger women suffer more often from such pain, in spite of their positive attitude and their aspiration to live to the fullest after cancer.[97] Ruth Handler, CEO and cofounder of Mattel Toy Company and the driving force behind the ultimate breasted female figure, the Barbie Doll, suffered from such chronic postmastectomy pain. She said that her pain never abated. Nevertheless she elected an ablation of her second breast twenty-two years after the first one, following a discovery of an in situ cancer in a routine check-up.[98]

Testimonies of women who underwent mastectomy and breast reconstruction illustrate the imperfections of this approach. One should add, however, that the great majority of these women are pleased with their decision to proceed with reconstruction. Breast cancer activist Rose Kushner claimed that her breast reconstruction played an important role in her successful recovery and fought for reimbursement of this surgery by health insurance. Her enthusiasm for this surgery was not dampened by the fact that her own breast implants got infected twice and had to be surgically replaced.[99] One of the first women who went public with narrative of prophylactic mastectomy for *BRCA* mutation explains that the consequences of this operation were more traumatic than she expected:

> One of the most difficult experiences to cope with was the lack of sensation in my breasts; it was something I was informed about, but was and is still a traumatic aspect of this surgery. Personally, it made the adjustment to the acceptance of the implants as part of my body difficult. . . . My recovery from the operation was a long, slow process. Pain and discomfort remained a feature of my life for a long time: a sensation of "cut glass" under the skin plus extreme tightness across the pectoral muscles. . . . I was physically exhausted and I felt apprehensive and vulnerable in a crowd. Emotionally the operation invoked an extreme sense of loss in terms of sexuality and femininity.[100]

Nevertheless she ended her story with the statement, "I have no regrets and I feel now I'm at a stage where I can truly celebrate my good fortune and feel happy about what I am and have." The prophylactic surgery, she stressed, "enabled me once again to feel in control of my life."[101]

Other women share similar convictions. Testimonies on breast cancer patho-blogs report satisfaction with the decision to undergo breast reconstruction, in spite of the fact that things often went wrong and that reconstruction surgery was often not a one-time event but rather a complex trajectory with numerous surgical episodes.

Carole underwent bilateral mastectomy in 1984 following a diagnosis of hyperplasia in lumpy breasts (that is, for a cancer risk). She had numerous complications: one year after the surgery she had to have her left breast implant repositioned, since it had shifted significantly to the left. A year later, because of further difficulties with the left implant, it was removed and replaced. In 1991, due to continuing difficulties with scar tissue capsular contraction and the hardening of the implants, she had surgery to remove and replace both implants. She is still not very pleased with her breasts, and, she explains that each surgery put her through the same mental and physical discomfort as the first surgery had. Nevertheless she does not regret her original decision: "I am happy to have taken away the fear of recurring lumpectomies and breast cancer . . . I am certain that mastectomy was the right decision for my continuing emotional well being."[102]

Laura had a succession of surgeries following breast reconstruction with implants: "First, my nipples got infected, causing huge holes to develop in each breast. After more than six months of healing the holes, I went to another surgeon to fix the mess. He did a reconstruction and put in different implants. After a few months, both implants started coming out through my skin." She changed doctors again and went to a third plastic surgeon: "I know people probably thought I was crazy trying to get a BEAUTIFUL look, but the truth is, I just had to have it fixed. Implants were making their way out through my skin." Her third surgery went well; she did lose one nipple, but felt that she could deal with that.[103]

Kim has a series of breast implants. Her first implant was purely saline: "hard as a rock! I hated it. It felt unnatural, looked unnatural, etc. That one was replaced with a combination saline/silicone implant. The core was silicone, and it had an outer saline shell. This one was softer, though still a bit firmer than I liked. It ruptured, so I again had to have surgery. Then I had chosen a silicone implant." She was still unhappy with the result and decided to have the silicone implant removed and to replace them with a DIEP flap procedure. She explains that the reason for all these surgeries is that her breasts are still not symmetrical, and she has to wear a small prosthesis on the reconstructed side.[104]

After the discovery of her breast cancer, Fabienne Rubert was advised to undergo a bilateral mastectomy because of family history of the disease. Her surgeon recommended an immediate reconstruction with saline implants, an option she and her husband accepted without giving it much thought. The surgery was a technical success, but for a long time Rubert had difficulty accepting her new breasts as part of herself. The reconstructed breasts, "two balls, hard and cold, laced with scars," were a permanent reminder of disease and loss.[105] Rubert points to the contrast between the real-life experience of the cancer patient—fragmented, incoherent, muddled—and the expectation, symbolically represented by the reconstruction of the removed breasts, that cancer patients will develop an optimistic attitude and will successfully erase all the visible signs of their encounter with disease. "We are expected to become 'meta-patients' capable of supporting with ease their treatments, but, above all able to alleviate the doctors' anguish of failure and death by presenting them a smooth, bland, comforting image of a patient that successfully transforms her suffering into an enhanced well-being."[106]

Prophylactic Surgery, Agency, and Risk

Prophylactic surgery may be compared to cosmetic surgery, not only because in breast cancer the two approaches are closely intertwined but also because both can be seen as ways by which people (in both cases, mainly women) attempt to regain control of their bodies and lives. Sociologist Kathy Davis, who studied cosmetic surgery, sees this approach as a narrative technique. Women are able to reclaim agency through a surgical modification of their appearance. Cosmetic surgery allows them to change the perception of their life as an uncontrollable downwards spiral, to attenuate a persisting feeling of failure, and to create new stories about themselves. The biographic narrative told about "before" and "after" cosmetic surgery, Davis explains, is often labile and shifts according to the context in which it is embedded. Women tend to hide and erase pain and suffering—psychological, but above all physical—from the cosmetic surgery stories. The disappearance of physical pain from such narratives may be also related to a response shift: a post hoc evaluation of what an acceptable pain and suffering is.[107] Downplaying of problems related to reconstructive breast surgeries may also reflect a sincere feeling of getting a control over one's life, coupled with a response shift that increases tolerance to problems linked with the surgery.

It is also possible that women who affirm (especially when answering a questionnaire) that they are truly happy with their prophylactic and reconstructive surgeries may tell only a part of the story.[108] A study of psychosocial effects of prophylactic mastectomy that compared answers to quantitative, close-ended questionnaires with those obtained thorough a qualitative, open-ended investigation found out that while in close-ended inquiry the great majority of women declared themselves to be very happy with their decision, in open-ended questionnaire over 70 percent provided a more negative evaluation. Negative comments were twice as common among women who underwent bilateral prophylactic ablation of the breasts as among those with contralateral prophylactic surgery.[109] Anthropologist Sandra Gifford made similar observation in the pre-*BRCA* era. She interviewed in depth "Alice," a young woman with lumpy breasts and suspicious calcifications. Alice was told that she had a 20 percent chance of developing breast cancer. She decided that she could not live with this level of risk and underwent a subcutaneous mastectomy. After the surgery she learned that her doctors had found in her breast "a tiny, tiny, the size of a pinhead, cell that was precancerous," and told her that her true cancer risk was in fact closer to 50 percent. The surgery left Alice with numerous undesirable effects, from heavy and unnatural feeling of the reconstructed breasts to a chronic pain, but she maintained nevertheless that she was very happy with her decision and could not imagine a life with her previous level of breast cancer risk. However, later in the conversation she told Gifford, close to tears: "but it is hard to get used to something that is not your own . . . My new breasts feel like stones on my chest, like big weight. But you know, the silicone was light, I held it. Why should it feel so heavy? When I lie down they feel like they're falling to the side but when I look at them they are not. Why do they feel like that?"[110]

Plastic and corrective surgery may have multiple meanings, exemplified in Lucy Grealy's *Autobiography of a Face*. Grealy, a talented poet and novelist, was diagnosed as a child with a tumor of face bones and underwent long and painful radiation treatment. The treatment was a success but it left her with long-term side effects of radiotherapy: facial deformation and necrosis of the bone. Grealy had elected to focus in her autobiography on the psychological pain of living with an unusual and "abnormal" look. *Autobiography of a Face* does not dwell on her physical distress, neither the functional difficulties that prompted her to seek surgical solutions in the first place nor the pain of reconstructive surgeries that failed to produce lasting results. Grealy, but also her friend and biographer Ann Patchett, speak very little about Grealy's swallowing problems, loss of teeth, difficulty in enjoying food, permanent physical discomfort, or repetitive bouts of pneumonia induced by inhalation of food particles.[111] Stories of women who underwent prophylactic removal of breasts and ovaries may reveal similar preference to bring to the foreground selected elements and mask others. Such stories tend to accentuate patients' agency and dwell less often on elements beyond their control.

The present-day Western biomedical discourse stresses the patients' "right to choose" and often downplays the role of other variables—from biological luck to medical division of labor and the organization of health services. Doctors who discuss prophylactic surgeries with *BRCA*-mutation carriers tend to stress unavoidable consequences of these operations, such as lack of feeling in reconstructed breasts or an early menopause induced by the removal of ovaries, but seldom speak about other problematic aspects of preventive treatments, such as postsurgical complications or chronic pain.[112] Such selective focus may reflect doctors' difficulty in dwelling on iatrogenic consequences of their interventions. It may also stem from a doctor's sincere conviction that a prophylactic surgery is the best available choice for mutation carriers and should therefore be encouraged for their own good. Henry Lynch complained in 2001 that prophylactic mastectomy is not used as frequently as it should be, because doctors and patients fail to properly understand its advantages: "Physicians often are reluctant to advocate new and particularly radical medical changes, such as bilateral prophylactic mastectomy, even though their patients may be inordinately at risk for the hereditary breast-ovarian cancer syndrome. . . . Women may find bilateral prophylactic mastectomy unacceptable. Indeed, they may not understand what the procedure entails, and/or the potential benefits of subsequent breast reconstruction. In short, they need to be educated."[113]

The publication of additional data on the efficacy of preventive surgery in reducing the cancer risk in mutation carriers strengthened Lynch's argument. Prophylactic surgery increasingly became an inescapable dilemma for a *BRCA*-positive woman.[114] Diffusion of genetic tests for *BRCA* mutations popularized the concept of hereditary forms of breast and ovarian tumors, extended the notion of susceptibility to malignancy to families, and increased the role played by genetic counselors in the management of such susceptibility. In clinical practice of the early twenty-first century the main effect of the introduction of these tests—and, as far as I know, one that was seldom discussed in numerous debates on ethical dimension of the new technology upon its introduction in the mid-1990s—was a massive comeback of prophylactic surgery for breast and ovarian tumors. As Masha Gessen put it: "There is maddening disconnect between the cutting edge science of oncogenetics and the barbaric state-of-art response to the discovery of a mutation: hack everything before it goes bad."[115]

Conclusion:
Uncertainty

The Wassermann Reaction: Screening for an Older "Dread Disease"

Preventive treatment of precancerous lesions is a twentieth-century innovation. Three developments favored the rise of this approach: (a) the transformation of cancer into a "pathologists' disease" in the 1910s and 1920s; (b) the introduction of mass screening for malignancies, which started in the 1940s with exfoliate cytology but expanded greatly in the 1970s and 1980s; and (c) the introduction, from the 1950s on, of population-based thinking to oncology and its consequence, the search for elements that increase cancer risk. This progression occurred in all the developed nations but took distinct forms and followed a different pace. In some cases, such as the diffusion of the Pap smear, divergent pathways—the intervention of a major cancer charity in the United States, an alliance between activists and politicians in the United Kingdom, development internal to the medical profession in France—produced a similar result: the generalization of screening for cervical cancer. In other cases, such as diagnosis and treatment of proliferative lesions of the breast, different local and national medical cultures generated divergent professional responses. Nevertheless, in spite of variability of practices, physicians who strived to diagnose and treat precancerous lesions faced a similar problem everywhere: the difficulty of correlating the presence of these lesions with the clinical disease of cancer.

The desire to transform precancer into a stable diagnostic category can be compared with earlier efforts to stabilize a diagnosis of another "dread disease," with deep social and cultural resonances: the history of the Wassermann reaction for the detection of syphilis. In the early twentieth century, syphilis was often perceived as a diagnostic puzzle. The proteiform manifestations of late syphilis were often confounded with other diseases: neurological disorders, bone and muscle ailments, malignant tumors, or cardiovascular pathologies. This difficulty, syphilis experts hoped, would disappear thanks to the development of a blood test—the Wassermann reaction—that detects the underlying cause of all the clinical manifestations of syphilis: an infection with the bacillus *Treponema pallidum*. Unfortunately, the blood test was problematic. First believed to display specific anti-*Treponema* antibodies, this test was redefined in the 1910s as revealing poorly understood "changes in syphilis blood" and the presence of a mysterious "Wassermann reagin." A strong aspiration to develop a diagnostic test for syphilis stimulated, however, a collective effort to adapt the Wassermann reaction to uses in the clinics. Scientists tinkered with this test until they obtained reproducible results. In the 1920s, experts viewed the link between positive Wassermann reactions and the infection by *Treponema pallidum* as a well-established scientific fact.[1]

Serologists and clinicians who employed the Wassermann test in the 1920s and 1930s did not fully understand its scientific basis. They were persuaded nevertheless that when performed by competent laboratory workers, the test rarely produced false positive results. Only people infected with *Treponema* tested positive. Accordingly, a positive result of "Wassermann serology" was seen as a sufficient reason to start treatment with antisyphilitic drugs and to expose patients to the toxicity of these compounds. At first, the Wassermann test was used only to confirm a suspicion of infection with *Treponema*. In the late 1930s increased confidence in the reliability of this test favored the introduction of mass screening for syphilis in large segments of the general population: people about to get married, pregnant women, newly recruited soldiers. The compilation of results of screening campaigns revealed unsuspected discrepancies between epidemiological and serological data. The Wassermann reaction was calibrated for high specificity (low tolerance of false positive results) and lower sensitivity (higher tolerance of false negative results) to avoid disastrous social consequences of an erroneous diagnosis of a shameful disease. Mass screening was therefore expected to underevaluate the prevalence of syphilis. Just the opposite was established: the percentage of positive results in tested populations was higher than the percentage expected on the basis of epidemiological data. The Wassermann reaction, the experts had found in the late 1940s, was considerably less specific than initially believed.[2] A positive Wassermann reaction, previously interpreted as a sure sign of an infection with *Treponema pallidum,* was transformed into an indication of a potential presence of a wide range of pathologies.[3]

The history of the Wassermann reaction illustrates conditions that favor the diffusion of diagnostic approaches grounded in an imperfect knowledge: Exis-

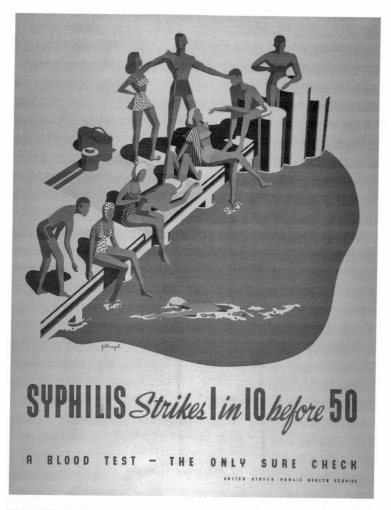

1945 U.S. Public Health Service poster promoting getting a blood test for syphilis. Wellcome Images.

tence of a highly visible and dreaded disease, doctors' desire to alleviate the burden of that disease and their wish to promote a cutting-edge medical technology, pressure from health authorities and the public, hope that an imperfect diagnostic tool will be improved with time, and difficulty in questioning well-established clinical practices. Cancer shares many traits with syphilis of the pre-penicillin era. It is also a poorly understood, frightening disease, associated with suffering and premature deaths of young and middle-aged people (malignant tumors are the highest cause of mortality of people under 70 in Western countries). Confronted with distressing and often-incurable pathology, doctors might have reacted like the advocates of the Wassermann reaction did. They promoted the stabilization of a partly understood diagnostic category—precancer—and of therapeutic and preventive practices linked with this category.

Tyranny and Tangle of Diagnosis

Diagnostic categories can be defined as *dispositifs,* a word that is literally translated as a "device." A *dispositif,* Michel Foucault proposed, is a network that links elements of a decidedly heterogeneous assembly: instruments and reagents; knowledge and practices; institutions, regulations, and laws; scientific statements and normative assessments; peoples, histories, and futures.[4] Such heterogeneous networks have a specific history and unique trajectory. Emergent diagnostic categories are often lists of constitutive traits: symptoms reported by patients, clinical findings, results of laboratory tests, and images produced by instruments.[5] When an additional element is added to such a list, a diagnostic category acquires new properties and a new shape, a process that frequently affects the classification of other pathological states as well. In a later stage of their trajectory, diagnostic categories are stabilized and integrated into routine clinical and administrative practices. The extent of their stabilization may, however, vary. Some diagnostic categories are rapidly transformed into "black boxed" entities, that is, they are not questioned for a long period of time. Others never reach a fully stabilized stage and continue to be seen by all the experts as open-ended, temporary units. Finally some diagnostic categories occupy an intermediary status—they are viewed as well-established by some specialists and questioned by others.

Stable diagnostic categories play a key role in management of sick bodies in the highly complicated world of modern, bureaucratized medicine.[6] They efficiently articulate heterogeneous components of medical enterprise, shape patients' subjective experiences, and standardize clinical practices and administrative decisions, tasks aptly captured by the historian Charles Rosenberg as the "tyranny of diagnosis."[7] Unstable, controversial diagnostic categories may have an opposite effect. They may increase tensions between the heterogeneous components of medical enterprise and produce a "tangle of diagnosis"—emotional, technical, ethical, and administrative dilemmas created by diagnostic uncertainty.[8] Doctors, patients, and health administrators share therefore a desire to untangle diagnoses and to produce stabilized classificatory categories. This desire may be especially strong facing a highly visible and emotional "dread disease." The stabilization of the diagnosis of precancerous lesions, like the consolidation and diffusion of the Wassermann test, reflected such an aspiration. And, in both

cases, the introduction of new diagnostic criteria was followed by the generalization of interventions grounded in these criteria: first, a treatment of syphilis by
Salvarsan (the trade name of arsphenamine) and akin compounds and, second,
a preventive surgery to reduce dangers of malignancy.[9]

Stabilizing Precancer

From the late nineteenth century on, cancer was defined as an abnormal proliferation of cells. Pathological phenomena observed in cancer patients were interpreted as a consequence of the presence of such deviant cells. Nevertheless, at first
diagnosis of cancer was made on the basis of clinical signs and macroanatomical
observations and only occasionally was confirmed under the microscope. The
growing reliance on cytological diagnosis of cancer led, however, to the inversion
of causal order. The pathologist's verdict became the main proof of the presence
of a malignant tumor, while clinical signs became increasingly interpreted as cor-
roborative rather than primary evidence.[10] Such an alteration of the causal order
was, however, problematic. In an advanced cancer, a disease with well-identified
manifestations and known trajectory, it is not too difficult to correlate microscopic observations with clinical evidence and data provided by medical imagery
and the laboratory. The linking of information provided by the pathology laboratory with events that take place in the body is more arduous in small, asymptomatic tumors. It is even more tricky when dealing with potentially precancerous lesions. Cytological diagnosis of premalignant lesions is more controversial
than the diagnosis of invasive tumors. Moreover, because such lesions point to a
danger of developing a malignancy in the future, their identification cannot be
consolidated through connecting them with other signs and symptoms. In spite
of this, cancer experts strived to stabilize the diagnostic category of precancer, because they were persuaded that an accurate recognition of precancerous conditions would lead to a cure or prevention of human malignancies. Three elements
facilitated such stabilization, which are outlined below.

A Unified Conceptual Framework

The linear view of cancer progression allowed the identification of borderline or
intermediary lesions as an early stage in the trajectory of malignant tumors. All
cancers, the specialist believed, should have a precancerous stage. Difficulties in
uncovering such a stage were accordingly attributed to technical problems: low
resolution power of diagnostic techniques, insufficient homogenization of cyto-

logical classifications, variability of local medical cultures, and paucity of reliable epidemiological data. The faith in the existence of an identifiable precancerous stage of each malignant tumor is aptly captured in the French word for cancer screening, *dépistage* (tracing). This word contains the implicit assumption that elements made visible by screening techniques reveal the presence of cancer or a lesion in process of becoming cancerous, in the same way that traces of an animal reveal the presence of that animal.[11] Traces can be distorted, imprecise, or faint and therefore difficult to read, but this does not invalidate the existence of a direct link between a traced animal and its imprints or between an early stage of the clinical disease cancer and precancerous lesions observed by pathologists.

The interpretation of all borderline morphological observations within the framework of cancer schemata favored the blurring of distinctions between correlations and causes. When pathologists observed a precancerous transformation of tissues in the immediate proximity of an invasive tumor, they viewed this as a proof that malignant lesions evolved from premalignant ones. Similarly, when epidemiologists observed a higher incidence of cancer in people previously diagnosed with premalignant lesions, they systematically interpreted it as evidence that these lesions became cancerous. Experts rarely evoked alternative explanations, such as the possibility that some malignant tumors lack a clearly identifiable precancerous stage, that invasive and noninvasive proliferative lesions can develop simultaneously and can represent two independent tissular reactions to the same stimulus or that noninvasive lesions are sometimes a local response to the presence of malignant cells.[12] The conceptual framework provided by cancer schemata gradually became an "incorrigible proposal."[13] Once all the ambivalent or intermediary lesions were defined as precancerous, it became very difficult to claim that they arise independently of cancerous lesions or that they develop later.

The Key Role of "Exemplary Tumors": Breast and Cervix

The diagnostic category of precancer became especially prominent in efforts of early detection of female malignancies: those of the breast and uterus. The visibility of these tumors may be related to a long tradition of medical interventions on women's bodies and to doctors' particular interest in female reproductive organs. It may be linked in parallel to the role of these tumors as exemplary malignancies. The emotionally laden image of terrifying, unpredictable "lived cancer" was constructed with memories, experiences, and fears drawn from a large variety of tumors, including those considered incurable, such as liver or pancreatic cancer, or those seen as too scary to be discussed in public, such as head and neck tumors.[14] By contrast, the rational image of "biomedical cancer," a disease open to an efficient medical intervention, was drawn to a large extent from studies of breast and cervical tumors. Breast cancer became a model for the development of radical surgery, the "local to regional to systemic" view of cancer progression in the body, the conviction that tumors spread mainly through the lymphatic system, and the rise of the "do not delay" paradigm. Cervical cancer became a model for the demonstration of a gradual progression from superficial to invasive epithelial lesions, the homogenization of staging of tumors, and the efficacy of mass screening campaigns.[15] In these malignancies, the diagnostic category of precancer was rapidly adopted by professionals. It was employed by oncologists, pathologists, radiologists, public health experts, and health administrators and incorporated into routine diagnostic procedures.

Circulation outside the Esoteric Circle of Experts

At the same time, the entity "precancer" was rapidly adopted by groups external to the medical profession: cancer charities, cancer activists, journalists, and politicians. Anthropologist Sarah Franklin uses the technical term *feeder layer* (a layer of irradiated cells that makes the growth of other, more delicate cells in the test tube possible) to describe the symbiotic reaction between media, public images, and new "future rich" technologies, such as cloning and stem cell therapies. This term can also be employed to explain the consolidation of diagnoses of precancerous states.[16] Selected diagnostic categories such as cystic mastitis, ductal carcinoma in situ (DCIS), lobular carcinoma in situ (LCIS), or cervical dysplasia, became inseparably linked with the early detection message and thrived on a feeder layer provided by public interventions of cancer experts, charities, patients, cancer activists, politicians, and the media.[17] The "unnatural history" of breast cancer is perhaps, partly at least, the history of an assisted growth on an especially dense feeder layer.[18]

A rich and sustaining environment can also favor the transformation of scientific terms into overdetermined and emotionally charged entities in themselves. Some scientific terms, the pioneer of social studies of science, Ludwik Fleck, proposed, became gradually disconnected from their original context: "Words which formerly were simple terms became slogans, sentences which once were simple statements become calls to battle . . . They no longer influence the mind through their logical meaning, but rather acquire a magical power and exert a mental influence simply by being used."[19] Precancer, initially a technical term employed by surgical pathologists, became an emotionally charged "slogan" through its wide circulation, prominence in the discourse of cancer experts and cancer charities, and key role in shaping clinical and public health practices.

Cancer as a "Productive Metaphor"

Susan Sontag's essay *Illness as Metaphor* was a reaction against theories of cancer personality that proposed that cancer developed in people unable to cope in a healthy way with the stress of life. Sontag contested the extensive use of the word "cancer" as a synonym of individual and collective self-destruction.[20] Cancer, she explained, is an ill-fated biological accident. It is deeply unjust to burden people who grapple with the dramatic consequences of this biological accident with an additional load of shame and guilt.[21] Sontag's study is focused on negative metaphoric connotations of cancer. One can propose that cancer was also a productive metaphor. The aspiration to "win the war against cancer" was a performative medical utopia. It mobilized professional and lay energies and became an important driving force in the making of twentieth-century medicine.

The terms *productive metaphor* and *performative medical utopia* point to the importance of ideology in promoting medical innovations. Striving to transform medicine into a science-grounded enterprise, historians of medicine proposed, influenced curricula of medical schools, the organization of hospitals, and the rise of medical specialties. It opened new spaces for technical and organizational developments and elaboration of better diagnoses and cures. Medicine first became scientific and then more efficient, not the other way around.[22] The history of cancer research, treatment, and activism illustrates the general principle that ideas and hopes are not less important than concrete technological achievements in furthering diagnostic and therapeutic change.[23] In the twentieth century, scientists made impressive advances in the understanding of the biology of malignant tumors, but these advances were not translated (yet) into an equally impressive reduction of cancer mortality or cancer-related suffering.[24] Nevertheless, an intensive collective effort to understand, prevent, and cure human malignancies stimulated major transformations of science, medicine, and society. It played a pivotal role in the organization of cancer diagnosis and care, the rise of cancer activism, and, more generally, in the development of "science rich" medical practices. Developments initially linked with prevention, detection, and cure of cancer, such as the rise of interdisciplinary teams, elaboration of international classifications, collaboration between doctors and disease-oriented charities or the blurring of boundaries between disease and disease risk—were extended in the second half of the century to numerous other domains of medical intervention.

Oncology was, from its very beginnings, a science-based specialty and a key site of development of collaborative approaches. In the interwar era, leading cancer centers promoted close cooperation among pathologists, surgeons, and radiotherapists. The wish to compare the efficacy of different treatments of cancer favored the homogenization of diagnoses and outcomes, while the use of expensive substances and instruments, such as radium and cobalt bombs or high voltage radiotherapy machines, promoted the centralization of cures. Cancer research, diagnosis, and treatment were at the forefront of the development of "big medicine," a multilevel, science-grounded endeavor.[25] In parallel, the "war against cancer" became an important model of a disease-oriented activism. One of the central targets of such cancer activism was the promotion of the early detection of malignant tumors. Doubts about the validity of cancer schemata, early, and "earlier than early" detection of malignancies, and the diagnostic category of precancer, could potentially have undermined key components of the twentieth-century biomedical enterprise.

The universal validity of cancer schemata was questioned by numerous specialists, but debates on this topic rarely left the esoteric milieu of oncologists.[26] Physicians' interventions and public policies continued to be dominated by the conviction that early detection of cancer was an attainable goal and an undivided blessing. The generalization of mass screening campaigns and a growing accent on the management of cancer risk further consolidated the confidence in the practical value of early detection, as did the rise of a new identity—"cancer survivor." Many cancer patients who remained symptom free believed that they had saved themselves by rapidly recognizing the danger of malignancy and acting upon it, or, alternatively, that they owed their life to skillful physicians who promptly made a correct diagnosis and provided an appropriate therapy. A fortunate outcome—long-term survival—became a proof that they or their doctors had the right attitude, a message some patients are eager to diffuse. By contrast, people who believe that the advent of their illness and its outcome reflects mainly random events (bad or good biological luck) seldom join the survivors' community. "Cancer survivors" and then "cancer pre-vivors" (people diagnosed with a hereditary predisposition to cancer) became new additions to the feeder layer that sustained the diagnosis of precancerous conditions and cancer risk and interventions destined to eliminate such risk.

Doctors' Might and Doctors' Responsibility

In 1899 Polish philosopher of medicine Edmund Biernacki published an investigation into the theoretical foundations of medical thought. His study, *The Essence and the Limits of Medical Knowledge*, pointed to the existence of a gap between advances in the understanding of human diseases and therapeutic progress. The impressive accumulation of physiological, biochemical and bacteriological knowledge had not been converted into efficient means of curing disease.[27] Circa 1900, the number of truly efficient therapies was indeed very small. Physicians, Biernacki pointed out, learned how to accurately recognize tuberculosis, typhoid fever, diabetes, syphilis, or uremia but were unable to help patients diagnosed with these conditions. Proud of their newly acquired scientific knowledge and their ability to make differential diagnoses, doctors were reluctant to recognize the extent of their impotence. The confusion between medical science and medical practice and maintaining the illusion that a better understanding of pathophysiological mechanisms is sufficient to produce a cure, was, Biernacki argued, a major obstacle for the development of an efficient, therapy-oriented medical practice.

In hindsight, Biernacki's view of the future of therapy was excessively pessimistic. In the second half of the twentieth century, physicians learned how to treat nearly all the diseases listed by him as incurable. Nevertheless, an impressive therapeutic progress did not eliminate the central problem discussed in Biernacki's book: the difficulty of aligning medical science and medical practice and conducting high level clinical research without forgetting doctors' duty to avoid unnecessary harm. Eighty years after the publication of Biernacki's book, another physician and philosopher of medicine, Lester King, examined the theoretical foundations of medical thinking. The medicine studied by King was, however, very different from the powerless profession observed by Biernacki. Thanks to the development of new diagnostic approaches, powerful drugs, and innovative surgical techniques, doctors acquired the capacity to modify physiological functions and transform human bodies.[28] The capacity of intervention of modern medicine heightened public expectations and favored the development of medical activism. It also increased doctors' capacity to hurt their patients. A manifold increase in medicine's technical efficacy, King argued, does not free doctors from their traditional obligation to carefully evaluate how good the evidence is, how sound the reasoning, what hangs on their decision, and what the alternatives are.[29]

Powerless physicians, Biernacki proposed, need to be aware of the limits of their art. Powerful physicians, King claimed, need to develop critical skills that will enable them to evaluate the consequences of their interventions and guard them against misuse of their newly acquired might. Such a misuse may arise from doctors' sincere wish to help suffering patients, an aspiration to advance their professional interests, or, frequently, a combination of both. It may also be influenced by actions undertaken by other social groups. Multiple stakeholders in the increasingly complicated arena of present-time biomedicine—health providers and regulatory bodies, legislators and judges, politicians, administrators and the pharmaceutical industry, consumer organizations, patients' associations, and health activists—also need to develop their ability to critically appraise medical interventions. Such an ability may be especially important when evaluating medical interventions that aim to reduce embodied health risks, that is, technologies that manipulate and modify healthy bodies.[30] The growing popularity of these interventions can be related to an unease generated by the gap between a rapidly growing capacity to investigate changes in the body and a much slower capacity to correlate these changes with prevention and treatment of diseases.[31] A focus on management of embodied health risks may reduce such unease. It may also promote interventions that do more harm than good.

In medicine, the term *risk* describes a danger for two very different groups: the oft-debated risk for the patient (or, when dealing with healthy people, the health care user or consumer) and the less frequently discussed risk for health professionals.[32] People diagnosed with predisposition of developing malignant tumors face multiple risks: the cancer itself, life with a permanent fear of the "ticking bombs" in their bodies, agonizing choices, lasting medical surveillance, and overtreatment.[33] Doctors who treat such people face consequences of erroneous medical decisions: risk of juridical pursuits (especially in litigious societies), damage to their reputation and professional status, and loss of self-esteem and self-confidence. Finally health administration and politicians who deal with the susceptibility to cancer on a population level are at risk of being blamed for inadequate allocation of resources and poor management of a public health problem.[34] A preventive excision of dangerous parts of the patient's body may be an efficient way to remove these multiple risks. One should bear in mind, however, that in a war against cancer, like in a real war, preventive strikes are frequently driven by a problematic mixture of desire to be in control and of fear and that in both the replacement of a reaction to an already existing harm with prevention of the risk of such harm may lead to making suspicion rather than evidence the new threshold for action.[35] Or, the consequences of a deterrent action grounded in a suspicion rather than in evidence may sometimes be worse than the event one seeks to avert. In Pierre Denoix's words: "One should not attempt to open a cupboard if one does not know how to deal with the skeleton that may be discovered there. One should be careful not to replace a healthy individual found in a cupboard with a skeleton."[36]

In Praise of Complexity

Science schematizes. Sociologists and historians of science reveal the role of purification and elimination of superfluous elements in the production of entities that can be successfully studied and manipulated in the laboratory. As Lorraine Daston and Peter Galison put it: "Working objects can be atlas images, type specimens or laboratory processes—any manageable, communal representatives of the sector of nature under investigation. No science can do without such standardized working objects, for unrefined natural objects are too quirkily particular to cooperate in generalization and comparisons."[37] And few scientific disciplines, Fleck had already noted in 1927, can compete with the irreducible quirkiness of pathology.[38] Hence the importance of simplifications and schematic representations in medicine. But such schemata may occasionally take on a life of their own. Paul Edwards's description of the attractiveness of computer simulation can be applied to diagnostic categories that, like the much more recent computer simulations "are by nature partial, internally consistent but externally incomplete . . . [each] has an unique ontological and epistemological structure, simpler than the world it represents . . . [they] are thus intellectually useful and emotionally appealing for the same reason: they create words without irrelevant or unwanted complexity."[39]

Simplified understanding of disease may sustain faith in the progress of science and encourage clinical research and public health interventions. It may also facilitate management across disciplinary boundaries and alignment of heterogeneous practices. The schematization of complex pathological situations may be therefore an indispensable stage in the elaboration of efficient clinical interventions. It may be important, however, not to lose sight of the original complexity of pathological phenomena. Simple models, French philosopher of science Gaston Bachelard argued, cannot be employed correctly without an accurate understanding of the process of simplification from which they are derived and without keeping in mind that they are inescapably a historical product of a refinement procedure.[40] However, the knotty, convoluted origins of scientific and medical concepts often became invisible with the generalization of their use. When undetermined traces become stable signs, Hans Jörg Rheinberger proposed, they erase their historicity, original complexity, and uncertainty and "create through their action the origin of their non-origin . . . the 'after' becomes the constitutive of the 'before.' "[41] The transformation of the initially problematical and convoluted diagnostic category of precancer into a simplified, overdetermined, and emotionally charged "slogan" made the original complexities of construction of boundaries between the normal and the pathological during a pre-refinement stage invisible.

The diagnostic category of precancer efficiently articulated doctors' and patients' preoccupations. It was linked with the tradition of surgical management of gynecological problems and became rapidly embedded in increasingly dense networks of scientific, clinical, institutional, and political practices.[42] The success of this category was not without a price: a systematic overlooking of uncertainties concerning relationships between candidate precancerous lesions and the disease of cancer. Parts of the impressive edifice of early detection and screening for cancer were constructed on imperfectly stabilized foundations.

Leaps of faith, open-ended classifications, loosely defined boundary objects, and heterogeneous arrangements are constitutive traits of modern science and medicine.[43] Not every heterogeneous alignment is, however, equally compelling and viable. The prevention of cervical cancer is an example of the efficient alignment of heterogeneous and sometimes imperfect data. Pathologists were unable to define exactly what a precancerous lesion of the cervix was but the technical ability to remove all suspicious lesions with a relatively low cost to patients and to the community led to a transformation of a loosely defined entity, cervical dysplasia, into an indication for a preventive intervention. In cervical cancer, a precise correlation of morphological data with clinical outcomes no longer mattered, because eliminating the lesions simultaneously eliminated any uncertainty about their future.

The history of breast cancer was different. A century of difficulties of correlating diagnoses of proliferative lesions of the breast, such as cystic mastitis, DCIS, LCIS, or atypia, with reliable prediction of their future fate illustrate the persistence of obstacles to a dependable linking of cytological observations with the natural history of a malignant tumor. Current dilemmas of screening for other malignancies, diagnosis of precancerous lesions, detection of hereditary predisposition to cancer, and prophylactic surgery, may reflect the "lumpiness" of today's oncological practice—persisting zones of uncertainty, opacity, and ignorance hidden under a smooth surface of impressive technological achievements.

Introduction

1. The disease of cancer is usually defined as the presence of major disturbances of physiological functions that, if left untreated, usually lead to the patient's death. An early stage in the natural history of this disease includes the period—which may be very long for slow-growing tumors—that precedes the production of such major disturbances.

2. "Ensemble prenons le cancer de vitesse" (together we'll be faster than cancer) is the slogan of the Curie Institute, one of the main French centers for treating cancer. Note that the Curie Foundation (Fondation Curie) began in 1920. In 1965 it changed its name to the Curie Institute (Institut Curie).

3. Georges Canguilhem, *The Normal and the Pathological*, trans. Carolyn R. Fawcett (1964; New York: Zone Books, 1989).

4. Soraya de Chadarevian and Harmke Kamminga, eds., *Molecularization of Biology and Medicine* (Amsterdam: Harwood Academic Publishers, 1998); Alberto Cambrosio, Peter Keating, Thomas Schlich, and George Weisz, "Regulatory objectivity and the generation and management of evidence in medicine," *Social Science and Medicine* 63 (2006): 189–99.

5. R. L. Carter, Introduction, in *Precancerous States*, ed. R. L. Carter (Oxford: Oxford University Press, 1984), xvi.

6. Elliott Foucar, "Predictive genetics and predictive morphology have certain similarities," *British Medical Journal* 323 (2001): 514.

7. The term *embodied risk* was proposed in the 1990s by sociologists and anthropologists of medicine; e.g., Deborah Lupton, "Taming uncertainty: Risk discourse and diagnostic testing," in *The Imperative of Health: Public Health and the Regulated Body*, ed. Deborah Lupton (London: Sage, 1995), 77–105; Anne M. Kavanagh and Dorothy H. Broom, "Embodied risk: My body, myself?" *Social Science and Medicine* 46 (1998): 437–44; Margaret Lock, "Breast cancer: Reading the omens," *Anthropology Today* 14 (1998): 7–16. Robert Aronowitz's book *Unnatural History: Breast Cancer and American Society* (Cambridge: Cambridge University Press, 2007) studies the history of embodied risk for breast malignancies.

8. Professional reactions and public debates currently focus on "genetic risk," but practical considerations may favor a joint management of morphological and genetic risks. This is the usual practice in U.S. "breast health centers."

9. Charles Rosenberg, "The tyranny of diagnosis: Specific entities and individual experience," *The Milbank Quarterly* 80 (2002): 237–60. According to the Merriam-Webster dictionary, the word *diagnosis*, from Greek *dia* (by) and *gnosis* (knowledge), has a second, more general meaning: the investigation or analysis of the cause or nature of a condition. The latter meaning reflects the role of medicine as an exemplary profession that sets standards for expertise in other domains. Andrew Abbott, *The System of Professions: An Essay on the Division of Expert Labor* (Chicago: University of Chicago Press, 1988).

10. Mary Douglas, *The World of Good: Towards the Anthropology of Consumption* (New York: Basic Books, 1978).

11. One way to make a disease "real" (that is, somatic) is to find a drug that cures it. The approval by the FDA for a drug for fibromyalgia was a step toward an official recognition of fibromyalgia as a valid diagnostic category. Alex Berenson, "Drug approved. Is disease real?" *New York Times,* Jan. 14, 2008. Another, more frequent pattern of emergence of new diagnostic categories is the mutual adaptation of diagnostic tests and definition of the disease.

12. Charles E. Rosenberg, "Managed fear: Contemplating sickness in an era of bureaucracy and chronic disease," American Osler Society, 2008. A shorter version of this text was published in 2009 in *Lancet* 373: 802–3.

13. I propose the expression "fear by numbers" as an extension of Jeremy Greene's description of the preventive use of drugs, or "prescription by numbers." Jeremy A. Greene, *Prescribing by Numbers: Drugs and the Definition of Disease* (Baltimore: Johns Hopkins University Press, 2007).

14. Paul Rabinow speaks about "biosociality," Ian Hacking about "making up people," and Nicolas Rose about "vital politics," for him a state in which selfhood is presented and conceptualized as an increasingly somatic entity. Paul Rabinow, "Artificiality and enlightenment: From sociobiology to biosociality," in *Essays on the Anthropology of Reason*, ed. Paul Rabinow (Princeton: Princeton University Press, 1996), 99–103; Ian Hacking, "Making up people," in *Historical Ontology*, ed. Ian Hacking (Cambridge, MA: Harvard University Press, 2002), 99–114; Carlos Novas and Nicolas Rose, "Genetic risk and the birth of the somatic individual," *Economy and Society* 29 (2000): 485–513. The rise of the category of "pre-vivor"—people diagnosed with hereditary susceptibility to cancer—who produce networks of activism and mutual support is a telling example of this new type of somatic identity. See, e.g., www.pre-vivor.org/pre-vivors_and_survivors/cancer_pre-vivors.html (accessed Sept. 15, 2008).

15. Nicholas Rose, *The Politics of Life Itself: Biomedicine, Power and Subjectivity in the Twenty-First Century* (Princeton: Princeton University Press, 2007).

16. Some lesions classified as premalignant, such as an atypical mole or an adenoid polyp in the intestine, can be observed with the naked eye, but their definitive diagnosis as a premalignant structure is nearly always made in the pathology labora-

tory. One possible exception is the diagnosis of a rare hereditary condition, familial adenomatous polyposis (discussed in detail in chapter 7). Doctors who observe the presence of multiple polyps in the intestine can define the carrier of these polyps as being at very high risk of developing a colon cancer on the basis of this macroscopic finding alone.

17. Polish philosopher Leon Chwistek was probably the first to point out differences between "scientific reality" and "commonsensical reality." Leon Chwistek, *Wielosc rzeczywistosci* (Crakow: Jaslo, 1921; reproduced in L. Chwistek, *Pisma filozoficzne i logiczne*, Warsaw: PWN, 1961), 30–105. English translation by Hannah Rosnerowa, in *Aesthetics in Twentieth Century Poland*, ed. Jean G. Harzell and Alina Wierzbianska (Lewisburg: Bucknell University Press, 1973), 66–97.

18. He was paraphrasing Gertrude Stein's "a rose is a rose is a rose." Stein first used this expression in a poem (written in 1913 and published in 1922); she then employed this expression in other works.

19. The standard work on this subject is Ian Hacking's *Representing and Intervening: Introductory Topics in the Philosophy of Natural Science* (Cambridge: Cambridge University Press, 1983). The role of methods used by scientists in the production of "scientific facts" was discussed earlier in Ludwik Fleck's *Genesis and Development of a Scientific Fact*, trans. Fred Bradley and Thaddeus J. Trenn (Chicago: Chicago University Press, 1979, first published in German in 1935).

20. Images from this exhibition can be seen at www.albany.edu/museum/www museum/schneider/index.html (accessed Sept. 3, 2008)

21. Berenike Pasweer, "Knowledge of shadows: The introduction of X-ray images in medicine," *Sociology of Health and Illness* 11 (1989): 360–81.

22. Nicolas Rasmussen, *Picture Control: The Electron Microscope and the Transformation of Biology in America, 1940–1960* (Palo Alto, CA: Stanford University Press, 1997).

23. Hans Jörg Rheinberger, "Preparations," in *Iconoclash*, ed. Bruno Latour and Peter Weibel (Cambridge, MA: MIT Press, 2002), 143–45.

24. "Epistemic things" were described by Hans Jörg Rheinberger in *Toward a History of Epistemic Things: Synthesizing Proteins in the Test Tube* (Palo Alto, CA: Stanford University Press, 1997). The term *quasi-objects* was coined by Michel Serres and applied by Bruno Latour in his book *Nous N'avons Jamais Eté Modernes* (Paris: La Decouverte, 1991), 71–84. Quasi-objects (as I understand them) are less exclusively dependent on specific forms of laboratory life than are "epistemic things." They can exist outside experimental systems and can become part of the layperson's universe.

25. The lay interpenetration of biomedical knowledge adds an additional level of complexity. People tend to interpret signs sent by their bodies using by a mixture of medical knowledge, information derived from other sources, and personal views. See, e.g., Jessica Gregg, *Virtually Virgins, Sexual Strategies and Cervical Cancer in Recife, Brazil* (Palo Alto, CA: Stanford University Press, 2003).

26. On the history of cancer, see J. Lelland Rather, *The Genesis of Cancer: A Study in the History of Ideas* (Baltimore: Johns Hopkins University Press, 1978); Sigismund Peller, *Cancer Research since 1900: An Evaluation* (New York: Philosophical Library,

1979); Pierre Darmon, *Les Cellules Folles: L'homme Face au Cancer, de l'Antiquité à Nos Jours* (Paris: Plon, 1993); David Cantor, "Cancer," in *Companion Encyclopedia of the History of Medicine*, ed. William Bynum and Roy Porter (London: Routledge, 1993), 1:537–61; Ilana Löwy, "Cancer; The century of the transformed cell," in *Science in the Twentieth Century*, ed. John Krige and Dominique Pestre (Amsterdam: Harwood Academic Publishers, 1997), 461–78.

27. There is a rapidly expanding literature on the rise of risk society and its consequences in medicine, e.g., Ulrich Beck, *The Risk Society: Towards a New Modernity*, trans. Mark Ritter (London: Sage, 1992), Nicolas Rose, "The politics of life itself," *Theory, Culture and Society* 18 (2001): 1–30; Robert A. Aronowitz "Situating health risks: An opportunity for disease prevention policy," in *History and Health Policy in the United States: Putting the Past Back In*, ed. Charles Rosenberg, Rosemary Stevens, and Lawton R. Burns (New Brunswick, NJ: Rutgers University Press, 2006) 153–65. On the history of risk factors and the development of probabilistic evaluations of health risks, see Robert Aronowitz, *Making Sense of Illness: Science, Society and Diseases* (Cambridge: Cambridge University Press, 1998); William G. Rothstein, *Public Health and the Risk Factor: A History of an Uneven Medical Revolution* (Rochester, NY: University of Rochester Press, 2003); Greene, *Prescribing by Numbers*. This study draws on concepts developed by researchers in this area, while focusing on the management of embodied risk, that is, changes in the body seen as fraught with danger.

28. Ornella Moscucci, "Gender and cancer in Britain, 1860–1910: The emergence of cancer as a public health concern," *American Journal of Public Health* 95 (2005): 1312–21.

29. Organization d'Hygiène de la Société des Nations, *Bibliographie Technique* (Geneva: World Health Organization, 1946), 40–47.

30. Ella Shohat, "Lasers for ladies: End discourse and the inscription of science," in *The Visible Woman: Imaging Technologies, Gender and Science*, ed. Paula Treichler, Lisa Cartwright, and Constance Penlzy (New York: New York University Press, 1998), 240–70, on p. 259.

31. Ornella Moscucci, *The Science of Woman: Gynecology and Gender in England, 1800–1929* (Cambridge: Cambridge University Press, 1990); Mary Jacobus, Evelyn Fox-Keller, and Sally Shuttleworth, *Body/Politics: Women and the Discourse of Science* (London: Routledge, 1990); Charles Rosenberg, "The female animal: Medical and biological views of women," in *No Other Gods: On Science and American Social Thought*, ed. Charles Rosenberg (1976; Baltimore: Johns Hopkins University Press, 1997), 54–70.

32. Judith Walkowitz, *Prostitution in Victorian Society: Women, Class and the State* (Cambridge: Cambridge University Press, 1980); Barbara Ehrenreich and Deirdre English, *For Her Own Good: 150 Years of Experts' Advice to Women* (New York: Anchor Books, 1978); Moscucci, *The Science of Woman*.

33. Ellen Leopold, *A Darker Ribbon: Breast Cancer, Women, and Their Doctors in the Twentieth Century* (Boston: Beacon Press, 1999); Baron Lerner, *The Breast Cancer Wars: Hope, Fear, and the Pursuit of a Cure in Twentieth-Century America* (Oxford: Oxford University Press, 2000), 222–40.

34. Erin O'Connor, *Raw Material: Producing Pathology in Victorian Culture* (Durham: Duke University Press, 2000), 78–99.

35. Barbara Katz Rothman, *The Book of Life: A Personal and Ethical Guide to Race, Normality and the Implications of Human Genome Project* (Boston: Beacon Press, 1998), 154–58.

36. Testimonies of people with head and neck cancers, such as Lucy Grealy's *Autobiography of a Face* (Boston: Houghton Mifflin, 1994) or John Diamond's, *C: Because Cowards get Cancer Too* (London: Vermillion, 1998), are seldom mentioned in the context of the "war against cancer."

37. Sander Gilman, *Making the Body Beautiful: A Cultural History of Aesthetic Surgery* (Princeton, NJ: Princeton University Press, 1999); Kathy Davis, *Reshaping the Female Body: The Dilemma of Cosmetic Surgery* (New York: Routledge, 1995); Kathy Davis, *Dubious Equalities and Embodied Differences: Cultural Studies on Cosmetic Surgery* (Lanham, MD: Rowman & Littlefield, 2003).

38. Edward P. Gelmann, "Complexities of prostate cancer risk," *The New England Journal of Medicine* 358 (2008): 961–63.

39. C. Warlick, B. J. Trock, P. Landis, J. I. Epstein, and H. B. Carter, "Delayed versus immediate surgical intervention and prostate cancer outcome," *Journal of the National Cancer Institute* 98 (2006): 355–57; Laurence Klotz, "Low-risk prostate cancer can and should often be managed with active surveillance and selective delayed intervention," *Nature Clinical Practice Urology* 5 (2008): 2–3. European doctors are usually more favorable toward watchful observation of already present prostate malignancies. Jerome Groopman, "The prostate paradox: Prostate cancer," *The New Yorker*, May 29, 2000.

40. Howard J. Burstein, K. Polyak, J. S. Wong, S. C. Lester, and C. M. Kaelin, "Ductal carcinoma in situ of the breast," *New England Journal of Medicine* 350 (2004): 1430–41.

41. For example, women diagnosed with *BRCA* mutation legitimize their willingness to undergo prophylactic ablation of ovaries by mentioning their responsibility as mothers. Nina Hallowel, Ian Jacobs, Martin Richards, James Mackay, and Martin Gore, "Surveillance or surgery? A description of the factors that influence high risk premenopausal women's decisions about prophylactic oophorectomy," *Journal of Medical Genetics* 38 (2001): 683–91.

42. The expression "good to think with" is borrowed from Claude Lévi-Strauss, who proposed that "ce qui est bon à manger doit être bon à penser." Claude Lévi-Strauss, *La Pensée Sauvage* (Paris: Mouton, 1962; English version, *The Savage Mind*, trans. John Weightman and Doreen Weightman [Chicago: Chicago University Press, 1966]).

43. The choice of case studies mirrors the availability and accessibility of archival materials. For the same reason, the studied cases mainly illustrate medical practices in leading teaching and research hospitals.

44. Rosenberg, "Managed fear."

45. Louise B. Russell, *Educated Guesses: Making Policy about Medical Screening Tests* (Berkeley and Los Angeles: University of California Press, 1994), 1–2.

46. Progress of chemotherapy and other cancer treatments led to a partial "chronicization" of some forms of this disease: people with disseminated breast or prostate cancer may live many years while undergoing cycles of treatment. In contrast, advanced cancer continues to be seen as model of "awareness of dying" and of unavoidable downhill trajectory, culminating in death.

47. It is reasonable to believe that all malignant tumors have a "precancerous" stage, but this does not necessary mean that it is always possible to identify such a stage or that the elimination of a precancerous lesions will each time be more efficient than a later intervention.

48. This difficulty will probably disappear when scientists are able to follow individual malignant cells in the body and study these cells in real time.

Chapter One · Biopsy

1. This is true for solid tumors. The diagnosis of hematological malignancies is more complicated. See, e.g., Peter Keating and Alberto Cambrosio, *Biomedical Platforms: Realigning the Normal and the Pathological in Late-Twentieth-Century Medicine* (Cambridge, MA: MIT Press, 2003).

2. Soraya de Chadarevian and Harmke Kamminga, eds., *Molecularization of Biology and Medicine* (Amsterdam: Harwood Academic Publishers, 1998); Keating and Cambrosio, *Biomedical Platforms.*

3. Ornella Moscucci, "Gender and cancer in Britain, 1860–1910: The emergence of cancer as a public health concern," *American Journal of Public Health* 95 (2005): 1312–21.

4. Joyce Hemley, ed., *Description of Fanny Burney's operation for cancer of the breast performed by Larrey,* leaflet (London: The Wellcome Library, 1975; extract from *Journals and Letters of Fanny Burney, Madame D'Arblay,* Oxford: Oxford University Press, 1974, 4:596–707). James S. Olson, *Bathsheba's Breast: Women, Cancer, and History* (Baltimore: Johns Hopkins University Press, 2002). Burney was operated on in 1811; she died in 1840 at the age of 88.

5. Ornella Moscucci, *The Science of Women: Gynecology and Gender in England, 1800–1929* (Cambridge: Cambridge University Press, 1990).

6. On Crile's surgical approach, see Gert H. Brieger, "From conservative to radical surgery in late nineteenth century America," in *Medical Theory, Surgical Knowledge: Studies in the History of Surgery,* ed. Christopher Lawrence (London: Routledge, 1992), 216–31. In the 1950s Crile's son, surgeon George Barney Crile, became a champion of the conservative surgery for breast cancer. Barron Lerner, *The Breast Cancer Wars: Fear, Hope and the Pursuit of Cure in Twentieth-Century America* (New York: Oxford University Press, 2001), 61–68.

7. Peter English, *Shock, Physiological Surgery and George Washington Crile* (Westport, CT: Greenwood Press, 1980).

8. William S. Halsted, "The results of operations for the cure of cancer of the breast from June, 1889 to January, 1894," *Annals of Surgery* 20, no. 5 (1894): 497–555; William S. Halsted, "The results of radical operation for the cure of carcinoma of the breast," *Annals of Surgery* 46 (1907): 1–18; Daniel De Moulin, *A Short History of Breast*

Cancer (Dordrecht: Kluwer, 1989), 82–86; John L. Cameron, "William Stewart Halsted: Our surgical heritage," *Annals of Surgery* 225 (1997): 445–58.

9. Dean Lewis, "Surgical principles in cancer of the breast," *Annals of Surgery* 102 (1935): 252–53, on p. 253.

10. Physicians, one may assume, do not like to dwell on suffering produced by their activities, especially if it can be presented as minor, short-term, or derivative. The neglect of such suffering is a constant trait of cancer diagnosis and treatment. The invisibility of distress produced by skin grafts made during radical mastectomy may be compared to invisibility of pain produced by routine complications of radiotherapy (e.g., skin burns) and surgical interventions presented as minor, such as biopsies.

11. Such descriptions were for example always present in reports from the pathological laboratory of the London Hospital in the years 1909–39. Pathological Institute, Surgical Department, Director's Book, the Archives of the Royal London Hospital, London, England (Archives of London Hospital).

12. For a classical description of training of the eye to recognize typical visual patterns, see Ludwik Fleck, *Genesis and Development of a Scientific Fact*, trans. Fred Bradley and Thaddeus J. Trenn (Chicago: University of Chicago Press, 1979; first published in German in 1935).

13. Loraine Daston and Peter Galison, "The image of objectivity," *Representations* 40 (1992): 81–128, on p. 83.

14. Lelland J. Rather, *The Genesis of Cancer: A Study in the History of Ideas* (Baltimore: Johns Hopkins University Press, 1978); David Cantor, "Cancer," in *Companion Encyclopedia to the History of Medicine*, ed. William F. Bynum and Roy Porter (London, Routledge, 1993), 1:537–61; Ilana Löwy, "Cancer—The century of the transformed cell," in *Science in the Twentieth Century*, ed. John Krige and Dominique Pestre (Amsterdam: Harwood Academic Press, 1997), 461–78.

15. The slow integration of cytology into understanding of clinical cancer may be compared to the equally slow incorporation of new bacteriological knowledge into routine diagnosis and treatment of transmissible diseases in late 19th century. See, e.g., Michael Worboys, *Spreading Germs: Disease Theories and Medical Practice in Britain, 1865–1900* (Cambridge: Cambridge University Press, 2000); Jean-Paul Gaudillière and Ilana Löwy, eds., *Heredity and Infection: The History of Disease Transmission* (London and New York: Routledge, 2001).

16. L. Stephen Jacyna, "The laboratory and the clinics: The impact of pathology on surgical diagnosis in the Glasgow Western Infirmary, 1875–1910," *Bulletin of the History of Medicine* 62 (1988): 384–406.

17. Jacyna, "The laboratory and the clinics."

18. Series GC/152, box 1, notes of William Sampson Handley (1862–1962) from 1894, Wellcome Library, Archives and Manuscripts Department, London, England (Wellcome Archives).

19. William S. Halsted, "The results of operations for the cure of cancer," 497–555.

20. Forty percent of women who underwent Halsted's mastectomy were still alive five years after the initial diagnosis, compared with 22% of the patients in the un-

treated group. Ernest M. Dalland, "Untreated cancer of the breast," *Surgery, Gynecology and Obstetrics* 44 (1927): 264–68. The untreated group often included many women diagnosed with "inoperable," that is, very advanced cancer. The curative efficacy of radical mastectomy was thus probably even smaller.

21. Some surgeons, such as Gordon Taylor, claimed that up to 90% of their "early" breast cancer cases were still alive five years after mastectomy. R. S. Handley, "Gordon Taylor, breast cancer and the Middlesex Hospital," *Annals of the Royal College of Surgeons of England* 49 (1971): 151–64.

22. W. Sampson Handley, "The dissemination of mammary carcinoma," *The Lancet* 1 (1905): 909–13.

23. W. Sampson Handley, *Cancer of the Breast and its Operative Treatment* (London: John Murray, 1906), 1–2.

24. The majority of historians believe today that Halstead's radical surgery was unnecessarily mutilating and was not more efficient than more conservative operations. On the history of breast cancer surgery and of early detection campaigns, see Cordelia Shaw Bland, "The Halsted mastectomy: Present illness and past history," *Western Journal of Medicine* 134 (1981): 549–55; Jane Austoker, " 'The treatment of choice': Breast cancer surgery 1860–1895," *Society of the Social History of Medicine Bulletin* 37 (Dec. 1985): 100–107; Lerner, *The Breast Cancer Wars;* Robert Aronowitz, "Do not delay: Breast cancer and time 1900–1970," *The Milbank Quarterly* 79 (2001): 355–86. For a more positive evaluation of the efficacy of Halsted's mastectomy, see Olsen, *Bathsheba's Breast.*

25. American Medical Association, Prevention of cancer series, leaflet no. 1 (undated); Aronowitz, "Do not delay."

26. Joseph Colt Bloodgood, *What Every One Should Know about Cancer* (American Medical Association [AMA] leaflet, undated). *Time* magazine claimed that Bloodgood motto was "get an early diagnosis, no matter if you must scare the wits out of the people." *Time,* "Bloodgood v. fear," Jan. 2, 1933. Bloodgood (1867–1935) was a clinical professor of surgery at the Johns Hopkins University. He first made important contributions to surgical pathology of bone tumors and then became a national leader in the movement to educate the public about cancer prevention, treatment, and research.

27. R. Ledouc-Lebard, *La Lutte Contre le Cancer* (Paris: Masson & Cia, 1906), 87.

28. Bloodgood, *What Every One Should Know about Cancer.* Aronowitz rightly points out to the absence of quantitative data on the efficacy of the "do not delay" campaigns (in terms of reduction of cancer mortality or shift to diagnosis of less advanced tumors); Aronowitz, "Do not delay." Data in medical articles seem to indicate, however, an increase in the number of women who consulted physicians for small, localized lumps in their breasts, at least among those seen in major cancer treating centers.

29. See, for example, Alfred Velpeau, *Traité des Maladies de Sein et de la Région Mammaire* (Paris: Mason, 1858); Samuel W. Gross, *A Practical Treatise of Tumors of the Mammary Gland. Embracing their Histology, Pathology, Diagnosis and Treatment* (New York: Appleton and Co, 1880); A. Marmaduke Shield, *A Clinical Treatise on Dis-*

eases of the Breast (London: Macmillan, 1898); W. Sampson Handley, *Cancer of the Breast and Its Operative Treatment* (London: John Murray, 1906).

30. Edred M. Corner, "Discussion of the diagnosis and treatment of cancer of the breast," *British Medical Journal* ii (Oct. 31, 1908): 970–81.

31. Joseph Colt Bloodgood, "Control of Cancer," Prevention of Cancer Series, AMA leaflet no. 7 (text of a speech delivered by Bloodgood, June 17, 1913).

32. Corner, "Discussion of the diagnosis and treatment of cancer of the breast."

33. James Ewing, "Precancerous diseases and precancerous lesions, especially in the breast," *Fourth Report of the Collin P. Huntington Fund for Cancer Research and the Memorial Hospital, 1913–14* (New York: William Wood and Company, 1913–14), 4:1–32.

34. Rather, *The Genesis of Cancer.*

35. William De Morgan, "On the origin of cancer," *The Lancet* 2 (1871): 6–7, 41–42, 80–81, 118–19, 154–56, 165–66. Charles Moore, "Antecedents of cancer: Discussions in scientific medicine," *British Medical Journal* 1 (1865): 165–66. Quoted by Moscucci, "Gender and cancer in Britain, 1860–1910."

36. The "local to general" model was first explicitly elaborated for breast cancer. Handley, "The dissemination of mammary carcinoma."

37. Charles Creighton, *Cancers and Other Tumors of the Breast* (London: Williams & Norgale, 1902), 156–62, 275–93.

38. Shield, *A Clinical Treatise on the Diseases of the Breast,* 34.

39. Ewing, "Precancerous diseases and precancerous lesions"; William L. Rodman, *Diseases of the Breast with Special Reference to Cancer* (Philadelphia: P. Blackinson & Sons, 1908).

40. J. B. Lockwood, "Early microscopic diagnosis of tumors," *British Medical Journal* 2, no. 5 (1905), quoted by William Seaman Bainbridge, "Biopsy and cancer: A review," *Medical Record* (New York) 92, no. 17 (Apr. 28, 1917): 705–15.

41. J. Collins Warren, "The surgeon and the pathologist: A plea for reciprocity as illustrated by the consideration of classification and treatment of benign tumors of the breast," a talk at the 56th annual session of AMA, Portland, Oregon, July 11–14, 1905.

42. Rodman, *Diseases of the Breast,* 235.

43. Joseph Colt Bloodgood, "The relation of surgical pathology to surgical diagnosis," *Detroit Medical Journal* 3 (1903): 337–52, on p. 338. After the demise of radical mastectomy, the "quotability" of this sentence likening radical surgery to lynching was enhanced by its parallel between brutal treatment of Blacks and women.

44. J. Clark Stewart, "What is the proper surgical treatment of suspicious tumors of the involuting breast," *JAMA* 53 (1904): 365–69, on p. 366. An "involuting" breast is one that underwent some degenerative changes, usually a breast of a woman past her reproductive years.

45. Georges Herbert Fink, *Cancer and Precancerous Changes* (London: H.K. Lewis, 1903). This is the first time I found the term *precancerous* in a title of a publication.

46. Fink, *Cancer and Precancerous Changes,* 93–95.

47. Stewart, "What is the proper surgical treatment of suspicious tumors," 366–67.

48. William Jepson, "A comment on Clark Stewart's, 'What is the proper surgical treatment of suspicious tumors of the involuting breast,'" *JAMA* 53 (1904): 368.

49. MR 16/56, surgical register, female, 1907. Service of M. Harrison Cripps. Patients' records, St Bartholomew's Hospital, London, series MR /16. Archives of St Bartholomew's Hospital (Archives of St Bart's) Patient records allow the examination of "real life" practices on a hospital ward. One should remember, however, that this is an imperfect source: data are seldom complete, and records may vary greatly among institutions and individual practitioners. On uses of case studies by historians of medicine, see, e.g., Gunter B. Risse and John H. Warner, "Reconstructing clinical activities," *Social History of Medicine*, 5 (1992): 183–205; Brian Hurwitz, "Form and representation in clinical case reports," *Literature and Medicine* 25 (2006): 216–40.

50. Ibid. The treatment for benign tumors of the breast at St Bart's was often partial mastectomy.

51. John M. T. Finney, "Joseph Colt Bloodgood 1867–1935," *Annals of Surgery* 105 (1937): 150–51.

52. Bloodgood, *Control of Cancer*.

53. Harold J. Stiles, "The diagnosis and treatment of malignant disease of the breast," in "Discussion on the diagnosis and treatment of cancer of the breast," *British Medical Journal* 1 (1908): 970–81, on p. 973.

54. Bloodgood, *Control of Cancer*.

55. Handley, *Cancer of the Breast and Its Operative Treatment*, 191.

56. The evolution of biopsy techniques was summed up by J. Arthur B. McGraw and Frank W. Hartman, "Present status of biopsy," *JAMA* 101 (1933): 1205–9.

57. Bloodgood, *Control of Cancer*.

58. T. S. Cullen, "A rapid method of making permanent sections from frozen sections by the use of formalin," *Johns Hopkins Hospital Bulletin* 6 (1895): 67; Louis B. Wilson, "A method for the rapid preparation of frozen tissues for the microscope," *JAMA* 45 (1905): 1737; Anthony A. Gall and Philip T. Cagle, "The 100-year anniversary of the description of the frozen section procedure," *JAMA* 294 (2005): 3135–36.

59. James Wright, "The 1917 New York biopsy controversy: A question of surgical incision and the promotion of metastasis," *Bulletin of the History of Medicine* 62 (1988): 546–62.

60. W. P. Cunningham, "The peril of biopsy," *Medical Record* (New York), Feb. 24, 1917, 336 (letter); James Ewing, "Incising tumors for diagnostic purposes, *Medical Record*, Mar. 3, 1917, 376 (letter); "Biopsy" (editorial), *Medical Record*, Mar. 3, 1917, 371.

61. Samuel R. Haythor, "Advantages and disadvantages of the frozen section method for the diagnosis of malignancy" (Pittsburgh: *Reports of the William H. Singer Memorial Research Laboratory*, 1931); McGraw and Hartman, "Present status of biopsy"; James Wright, "The development of the frozen section technique, the evolution of surgical biopsy and the origins of surgical pathology," *Bulletin of the History of Medicine* 59 (1985): 295–326; Wright, "The 1917 New York biopsy controversy." Some surgeons claimed, nevertheless, that they made diagnostic biopsies of breast tumors several days before radical surgeries with no ill results for the patients. See, for ex-

ample, Kenneth W. Monsarrat, "Discussion on the diagnosis and treatment of cancer of the breast, *British Medical Journal* 1 (1908): 970–81, on pp. 976–77.

62. Stiles, "The diagnosis and treatment of malignant disease of the breast"; Wright, "The development of the frozen section technique."

63. Joseph Colt Bloodgood, "Borderline breast tumors: Encapsulated and non encapsulated cystic adenomata observed from 1890 to 1931," *American Journal of Cancer* 16 (1932): 103–76, on p. 104. It is not sure to what extent the Johns Hopkins data represented a general trend. They may overrepresent both women's readiness to consult physicians rapidly for breast lumps and doctors' willingness to make careful investigations to avoid unnecessary mutilation.

64. Joseph Colt Bloodgood, "When cancer becomes a microscopic disease, there must be a tissue diagnosis in the operating room," *JAMA* 88 (1927): 1022–23; Joseph Colt Bloodgood, "Biopsy in the treatment of malignancy," *Journal of Clinical Laboratory Medicine* 16 (1931): 632–703; Joseph Colt Bloodgood, "Biopsy in breast lesions in relation to diagnosis, treatment and prognosis," *Annals of Surgery* 102 (1935): 239–49; McGraw and Hartman, "Present status of biopsy"; Wright, "The development of the frozen section technique."

65. William Seaman Bainbridge, "Biopsy and cancer: A review," *Medical Record* (New York) 92 (Apr. 28, 1917): 705–15.

66. Bloodgood, "Borderline breast tumors," 141–43.

67. Committee for the treatment of malignant diseases of the American College of Surgeons (R. B. Greenough, chairman), "Organization of a service for diagnosis and treatment of cancer," *Surgery, Gynecology and Obstetrics* 51 (1930): 570–74, on p. 572. The College of Surgeons officially recognized at that time that surgeons cannot provide a diagnosis of malignancy solely on the basis of their impressions during an operation. The American College of Surgeons established its first "standardization commission" in 1912. Murray E. Brennan, Rosemarie E. Clive, and David P. Winchester, "The COC: Its roots and destiny," *American College of Surgeons Bulletin* 79 (1994): 14–21.

68. File, breast cancer 1914–1915, second surgical division, Archives of New York Hospital, Weill Cornell Medical Library, Ithaca, New York (Archives of New York Hospital).

69. Surgery dept files, for 1920, ward II, carcinoma, Archives of New York Hospital

70. Mixed benign tumors, 1925–1928, General hospital, first division, Archives of New York Hospital.

71. Ibid.

72. Breast carcinoma, 1930–32, Archives of New York Hospital.

73. Ibid. Not all the lymph nodes were excised, only those "selected for their hardness."

74. On national variations in medical practice, see, e.g., Ilana Löwy and George Weisz, "French hormones: Progestins and therapeutic variation in France," *Social Sciences and Medicine* 60 (2005): 2609–22.

75. Surgery block notebooks (Cahiers de chirurgie), 1923–1939, Archives of the

Department of Medical Files, Musée Curie Historical Resources Center, Curie Institute, Paris (Archives of the Curie Institute).

76. See, for example, Jean Louis Roux Berger, "Cinquante et une observations des récidives post-opératoires de cancer du sein," *Bulletin et Memoires de la Société de Chirurgie de Paris*, meeting of May 31, 1922.

77. Soraya Boudia, *Marie Curie et son Laboratoire* (Paris: Archives d'Histoire Contemporaine, 2001); Patrice Pinell, *Naissance d'un Fléau* (Paris: Anne Marie Metaillé, 1992; English version, *The Fight against Cancer: France 1890–1940*, trans. David Maddell [London: Routledge, 2002]).

78. Surgery block notebooks, 1919–1939, Archives of the Curie Institute.

79. File, breast-radiotherapy, 1919–1939. Archives of the Curie Institute. All the translations from French are mine, if not indicated otherwise.

80. Ibid.

81. Ibid.

82. Ibid. Adherence to skin is often a sign of malignancy.

83. File breast-radiotherapy, 1919–1939. Archives of Curie Institute. The case does not appear in surgical files of the Curie Foundation, probably because the person in question underwent surgery elsewhere. The foundation's surgeons, Jean Louis Roux Berger and André Tailhefer, performed some of the breast operations at the Hôtel-Dieu Hospital, Paris.

84. For example, about half of people treated with x-rays for breast cancer at the Curie Foundation did not undergo a biopsy. One should add, however, that the great majority of these individuals had advanced tumors or a recurrence of cancer.

85. Notes: Cervical cancer, 1930s, box, gynecological cancers, Archives of the Curie Institute.

86. See, for example, case nos. 15 and 25 of 1919; case nos. 137, 147, and 175 of 1920; case no. 366 of 1923; and case no. 474 of 1924.

87. File, breast-radiotherapy, 1919–1939, Archives of the Curie Institute.

88. Notebooks, cervical cancer, 1919–1939, box gynecological cancers, Archives of the Curie Institute.

89. Memorandum no. 716 of Sept. 16, 1926, British Ministry of Health, London: Whitehall.

90. Janet E. Lane-Claypon, *Report on the Late Results of Operation for Cancer of the Breast, Reports on Public Health and Medical Subjects*, Ministry of Health, publication no. 51 (London: His Majesty's Stationery Office [HMSO], 1928). Lane-Claypon's work is extensively discussed in chapter 2.

91. Bloodgood, "Borderline breast tumors," 108.

92. Bloodgood, "Biopsy in breast lesions," 248.

Chapter Two · Classifications

1. The performative role of classifications in producing knowledge, practices, and identities was discussed by many philosophers, historians, and sociologists, e.g., Michel Foucault, *Sécurité, Territoire, Population, Cours de College de France, 1977–1978*

(Paris: Gallimard 2005; English version, *Security, Territory, Population,* trans. Graham Burchell [Basingstoke: Palgrave, McMillan, 2007]); Ian Hacking, *The Taming of Chance* (Cambridge: Cambridge University Press, 1990); Alain Desrosières, *La Politique des Grands Nombres: Histoire de la Raison Statistique* (Paris: Editions La Découverte, 1993; English version, *The Politics of Large Numbers,* trans. Camille Naish [Cambridge MA: Harvard University Press, 1998]); Theodore M. Porter, *Trust in Numbers: The Pursuit of Objectivity in Science and Public Life* (Princeton: Princeton University Press, 1995); Paul Rabinow, *Essays on the Anthropology of Reason* (Princeton: Princeton University Press, 1996); Ian Hacking, *Historical Ontology* (Cambridge, MA: Harvard University Press, 2002).

2. Barron Lerner, *The Breast Cancer Wars: Fear, Hope and the Pursuit of Cure in Twentieth-Century America* (New York: Oxford University Press, 2001), 197–202.

3. Ellis McDonald and William C. Hueper, "Cancer and the laboratory," *Journal of Laboratory and Clinical Medicine* 16 (1931): 713–33.

4. Pierre Masson, *Diagnostic de Laboratoire: Tumeurs—Diagnostic Histologique* (Paris: A. Maloine & Fils, 1923), 301.

5. James Ewing, *Neoplastic Diseases: A Treatise on Tumors* (London: W. B. Saunders Company, 1922), 541. Some French authors viewed attempts to correlate histological diagnoses with outcomes as a hopeless task. See, e.g., Pierre Hermert, "La radiotherapie dans le traitement du cancer du sein," *Paris Médical* 26 (1936): 233–46.

6. Janet E. Lane-Claypon, *Report on the Late Results of Operation for Cancer of the Breast,* Reports on Public Health and Medical Subjects, Ministry of Health, publication no. 51 (London: His Majesty's Stationery Office [HMSO], 1928). An alternative explanation may be that some of these patients did not have cancer, or had a "pseudodisease"—a lesion that does not induce clinical symptoms in the patient's lifetime.

7. Cohnheim is mainly known for his studies on inflammation; his work on cancer was part of the effort to differentiate inflammatory "tumefaction" from "tumors," an excessive proliferation of tissue that is not a result of an inflammatory process. Lelland J. Rather, *The Genesis of Cancer: A Study in the History of Ideas* (Baltimore: Johns Hopkins University Press, 1978).

8. The Bellevue Hospital Nomenclature of Diseases and Conditions, one of the first general classifications of human pathologies, was elaborated by doctors from the Bellevue Hospital in New York City and then adopted by numerous hospitals in the United States.

9. Robert J. Carlisle, Warren Coleman, Thomas A. Smith, and Edmund L. Dow, *The Bellevue Hospital Nomenclature of Diseases and Conditions, with Rules for the Recording and Filing of Histories.* Adapted by the Board of Trustees in 1903 and conformed to the international classification in 1911 (1911; reprinted, New York: Clarence S. Nathan, 1922), 95–99.

10. Committee on Clinical Records, *The Revised Bellevue Hospital Nomenclature of Diseases and Conditions* (New York: Paul B. Hoeber Institute, 1929).

11. Goustave Roussy, *Le Cancer* (Paris: Armand Collin, 1929).

12. Roussy, *Le Cancer,* 67.

13. Ibid., 71–72.

14. Ibid., 776.

15. Ibid., 783. Goustave Roussy, "Les principes de la lutte contre le cancer," *Revue d'Hygiène* 7 (July 1931): 503–9, on pp. 507–8. "Cancer can be cured, if treated early" was the slogan of Institut de Cancer de la Faculté de Médecine de Paris, headed by Roussy.

16. Ernest M. Dalland, "Untreated cancer of the breast," *Surgery, Gynecology and Obstetrics* 44 (1927): 264–68.

17. "L'effroyante enigme qui dépuis les temps les plus reculés est restée aussi tenebreuse." Robert Le Bret, "La recherche sur le cancer," *La Lutte Contre le Cancer* 1 (1923): 15–25, on p. 19; James Ewing, "Precancerous diseases and precancerous lesions, especially in the breast," *Fourth Report of the Collin P. Huntington Fund for Cancer Research and the Memorial Hospital, 1913–14,* 4:1–32.

18. Warren Winkelstein, "Vignettes of the history of epidemiology: Three firsts by Janet Elisabeth Lane-Claypon," *American Journal of Epidemiology* 160 (2004): 97–101; Ellen Leopold and Warren Winkelstein, "Unsung heroines: Unveiling history, Janet Elisabeth Lane-Claypon," *Breast Cancer Action Newsletter* 81 (May–June 2004).

19. Nigel Paneth, Ezra Susser, and Mervyn Susser, "Origins and early development of case control study. Part 2: The case control study from Lane-Claypon to 1950," *Sozial und Präventivmedizin* 47 (2002): 359–65.

20. Janet E. Lane-Claypon, *Report on the Late Results.*

21. Ibid., 120.

22. Robert Aronowitz, *Unnatural History: Breast Cancer and the American Society* (Cambridge and New York: Cambridge University Press, 2007).

23. Lane-Claypon, *Report on the Late Results,* ii.

24. Ibid.

25. Lane-Claypon only analyzed the fate of operable breast tumors. She did not include data on survival of women diagnosed with distant metastases.

26. Lane-Claypon, *Report on the Late Results,* 90–94; Janet E. Lane-Claypon "Evaluation of statistics relating to effectiveness of treatment," in *Report of the International Conference on Cancer,* London, July 10–17, 1927 (Bristol: John Wright and Sons, 1928), 181–88.

27. Lane-Claypon, *Report on the Late Results,* vi.

28. Lane-Claypon's results were summed up and presented in issues of *La Lutte Contre le Cancer,* e.g., 4 (July–Sept. 1926): 7–14; 5 (Oct.–Dec. 1927): 74–76.

29. Janet E. Lane-Claypon, *Cancer of the Uterus: A Statistical Inquiry into the Results of Treatment, Being the Analysis of the Existing Literature,* Reports on Public Health and Medical Subjects, Ministry of Health, publication no. 40 (London: HMSO, 1927), 58–59. Cervical cancer has a much lower rate of late recurrence than breast cancer and women who survived five years after their diagnosis were usually classified as cured.

30. Janet E. Lane-Claypon, *A Report on the Treatment of Cancer of the Uterus at the Samaritan Free Hospital,* Reports on Public Health and Medical Subjects, Ministry of Health, publication no. 47 (London: HMSO, 1927).

31. On the controversy between radiological and surgical treatment of cervical cancer, see Ornella Moscucci, " 'The ineffable freemasonry of sex': Feminist surgeons and the establishment of radiotherapy in early twentieth-century Britain," *Bulletin of the History of Medicine* 81 (2007): 139–63.

32. Henri Rubens Duval and Antoine Lacassagne, *Classification Pratique des Cancers Derivés des Epithelium Cutanés et Cutaneo-muceux* (Paris: Octave Doin, 1922), 6.

33. Note of Regaud, with the title "erreurs à rectifier dans les listes du Dr. Lacassagne" joined to the typed notes: cervical cancer, 1930s, box, gynecological cancers, Archives of the Department of Medical Files, Musée Curie Historical Research Center, Curie Institute, Paris (Archives of the Curie Institute).

34. "Rapport de la Commission du Cancer de la Societé des Nations sur le Traitement Radiotherapique du Col d'Uterus," *La Lutte Contre le Cancer*, 27 (Jan.–Mar. 1930): 507–36. On controversies in treatment of cervical cancer, see, e.g., Antoine Lacassagne, "Importance respective des causes du succès ou de l'échec en radiotherapie des epitheliomes du col utérin," manuscript from a conference organized by the British Empire Cancer Campaign, London, July 17–20, 1927, Archives of the Curie Institute.

35. Gerry B. Hill, "Editorial: Counting cancers," *Canadian Medical Association Journal* 29 (1983): 1262–63.

36. Clinical Research subcommittee meeting of Nov. 1, 1934. Minutes of the meeting of Clinical Research subcommittee of BECC, 1934–37. British Empire Cancer Campaign (BECC), series SA/CRC: clinics, pathology, research, box 34, Wellcome Library, Archives and Manuscripts Department, London, England (Wellcome Archives).

37. Minutes of the meeting of Clinical Research subcommittee of BECC, Feb. 25, 1935. BECC archive, box 34, Wellcome Archives.

38. Minutes of the meeting of Clinical Research subcommittee of BECC, July 19, 1938, and Mar. 27, 1939, BECC archive, box 34, Wellcome Archives.

39. Stebbing to Scarff, May 3, 1946. BECC archive, box 38, file A.30: Consultant Panel in Morbid Histology, 1946–70, Wellcome Archives.

40. Ibid.

41. Benedetto Terracini and Roberto Zanettini, "A short history of pathology registries, with an emphasis on cancer registries," *Sozial und Präventivmedizin* 48 (2003): 3–10.

42. Jean François Picard, "Poussé scientifique ou demande des médecins? La recherche médicale en France de l'Institut National d'Hygiène à l'INSERM," *Sciences Sociales et Santé* 10 (1992): 47–106.

43. Marie Ménoret, "The genesis of the notion of stages in oncology: The French Permanent Cancer Survey, 1943–1952," *Social History of Medicine* 15 (2002): 291–302.

44. "Nomenclature des cancers," *Receuil de Travaux d'INH* 3 (1946), L'Institut National d'Hygiène, Paris; Ménoret, "The genesis of the notion of stages in oncology."

45. Ménoret, "The genesis of the notion of stages in oncology." Cushman Haagensen from Columbia University proposed an alternative clinical classification of breast tumors, the "Columbia clinical classification." Haagensen's classification in-

cluded indications on the pathophysiology of the tumor (presence of edema, of ulceration, adherence to chest wall). "Old-fashioned" clinical signs, Haagensen argued, have an important prognostic value, lost in the tumor, nodes, metastases (TNM) classification. Cushman Haagensen and Edith Cooley, "The clinical classification of mammary carcinoma according to stage advancement," in *Symposium on the Prognosis of Malignant Tumors of the Breast,* ed. P. Denoix and C. Roquette (Basel: S. Krager, 1963), 195–98.

46. WHO's Expert Committee on Health Statistics, "Statistical code for human tumors," Document number WHO/HS/CANC/24.1 (Geneva: World Health Organization, 1956).

47. *Manual of Tumor Nomenclature and Coding* (Atlanta: American Cancer Society, 1951).

48. Simone Laborde, in name of the working group on cervical cancer "Cancer du col d'utérus, defintion du stade o," *Bulletin de l'Institut National d'Hygiène* 7 (1952): 549–54. The French Cancer Survey set up a special commission, active between 1952 and 1959, to discuss the definition of premalignant states. Ménoret, "The genesis of the notion of stages in oncology," 299–300.

49. Georges Gricouroff, "Le problème du cancer du col d'utérus a stade zéro," *La Presse Médicale* 34 (1952): 743–44. Gricouroff's argument was reproduced in the report of the Institut National d'Hygiène commission on classification of cervical cancer. Groupe de travail sur le cancer du col, "Cancer du col d'utérus: Definition du stage 'o,' " L'Institut National d'Hygiène, Paris.

50. Gerald A. Galvin and Richard W. TeLinde, "The present day status of noninvasive cervical carcinoma," *American Journal of Obstetrics and Gynecology,* 57 (1949): 15–36.

51. Eliot Foucar, "Carcinoma in situ of the breast: Have pathologists run amok?" *Lancet* 347 (1996): 707–8; David L. Page, William D. Dupont, Roy A. Jensen, and Jean F. Simpson, "Editorial: When and to what end do pathologists agree," *Journal of the National Cancer Institute* 90 (1998): 88–89.

52. On the central role of insurance companies in the rise of the health risk concept, see William G. Rothstein, *Public Health and the Risk Factor: A History of an Uneven Medical Revolution* (Rochester, NY: University of Rochester Press, 2003).

53. J. Paterson MacLaren, *Medical Insurance Examination: Modern Methods and Rating of Lives* (New York: William Wood and Company, 1943).

54. Ibid., 531.

Chapter Three · Borderline Lesions

1. Dermatologists also promoted surgical elimination of suspicious skin lesions. Surgical removal of suspected skin lesions such as moles ("beauty spots") usually is not seen as a prophylactic surgery for cancer.

2. Ornella Moscucci, "Gender and cancer in Britain, 1860–1910: The emergence of cancer as public health concern," *American Journal of Public Health* 95 (2005): 1312–21.

3. Erin O'Connor, *Raw Material: Producing Pathology in Victorian Culture* (Durham: Duke University Press, 2000), 60–61.

4. Ornella Moscucci, "The 'ineffable freemasonry of sex': Feminist surgeons and the establishment of radiotherapy in early twentieth-century Britain," *Bulletin of the History of Medicine* 81 (2007): 139–63.

5. Moscucci, "Gender and cancer in Britain, 1860–1910."

6. Howard C. Taylor, "Controversial points in the treatment of carcinoma of the cervix," *Cancer* 5 (1952): 435–44.

7. Erich Burghart, "Radicality in gynecological cancer surgery: A historical perspective," *Gynecologic Oncology* 70 (1998): 172–75. In the 1960s and 1970s, German and Austrian gynecologists gradually accepted the principle that an early cervical carcinoma usually could be safely treated by local elimination.

8. Alvin M, Cotlar, Joseph J. Dubose, and D. Michael Rose, "History of surgery for breast cancer: Radical to sublime," *Current Surgery* 60 (2003): 329–37.

9. James Ewing, "The prevention of cancer," in *Cancer Control: Proceedings of the ASCC Conference, Lake Moonok, NY, Sept. 20–24, 1926* (Chicago: The Surgical Publishing Company, 1927), 165–74, on p. 174.

10. For a summary, see Cushman Haagensen, *Carcinoma of the Breast* (New York: American Cancer Society, 1950); Victor Riddel, "Carcinoma of the breast: A review of treatment," *Annals of the Royal College of Surgeons* 14 (1954): 215–46.

11. James Ewing, "Precancerous diseases and precancerous lesions, especially in the breast," in *Fourth Report of the Collins P. Huntington Fund for Cancer Research and the Memorial Hospital* (New York: William Wood and Company, 1913–14), 4:1–31.

12. Archives of the British Empire Cancer Campaign (BECC), series SA/CRC: Clinics, pathology, research, box 51, file E.3/9: Papers of William Sampson Handley (1872–1962), Wellcome Library, Archives and Manuscripts Department, London, England (Wellcome Archives). Handley, a surgeon at Middlesex Hospital, was active in the BECC before World War II.

13. Claudius Regaud, "Revue critique de quelques travaux sur le cancer: Statistiques, pathogenese, étiologie et prophylactique," *Paris Médical,* 18 (1928): 237–54; Claudius Regaud, "Sur l'existence ou l'absence des phenomènes d'irritation cellulaire et d'inflamation et sur l'importance relative des facteurs locaux et des facteurs géneraux dans la preparation des tissus à la cancerisation," *Bulletin de l'Academie de Médicine* (Paris) 110 (1934): 170–73.

14. Captain E. J. C. Chapman, secretary to the BECC, *The Truth about Cancer* (London: John Murray, 1930), 55–66.

15. Margaret E. A. Bleck, "What did popular women's magazines from 1929 to 1949 say about breast cancer?" *Cancer Nursing* 18 (1995): 270–77.

16. W. Sampson Handley, "The prevention of cancer," *The Lancet* 1 (1936): 987–91. In the 1930s, the view that cancer was the result of mutation was limited to a handful of specialists. The systematic linking of radioactivity to mutations and cancer took place only in the aftermath of the Second World War and was linked with the development, testing, and use of atomic bombs.

17. Bloodgood made this statement in a public talk in Paris on anticancer measures in the United States. Joseph Colt Bloodgood, "La lutte contre le cancer aux Etats Unis," *La Lutte Contre le Cancer* 10 (Apr.–June 1932): 74–80.

18. Ewing, "The prevention of cancer."

19. Alfred Louis Velpau, *Traité des Maladies de Sein* (Paris: Masson, 1856).

20. Pierre Reclus, "Maladies cystiques de la mamelle," *Bulletin de la Societé d'Anatomie de Paris* 68 (1883): 424–28; Charles Monod and Felix Jayle, *Cancer du Sein* (Paris: Rueff et Cie Editeurs, 1894).

21. Charles F. Geschichter, "The early literature on chronic cystic mastitis," *Bulletin of the Institute of History of Medicine* 2 (1934): 249–56, on p. 251.

22. The characterization of breasts of women aged 40 to 50 as "senile" is a telling comment on the perception of women's aging in early twentieth century.

23. Joseph Colt Bloodgood, "Senile parenchymatous hypertrophy of the female breast," *Surgery, Gynecology and Obstetrics* 3 (1906): 721–30.

24. Ewing, "Precancerous diseases and precancerous lesions," 2.

25. Ibid., 19.

26. Ibid., 25; James Ewing, *Neoplastic Diseases: A Treatise on Tumors* (London, W. B. Saunders Company, 1922), 493; James Ewing, "Classification of mammary cancer," *Proceedings of the Round Table Conference on Cancer, Memorial Hospital, New York, New York, Annals of Surgery* 162 (1935): 249–52.

27. M. C. Tod and E. K. Dawson, "The diagnosis and treatment of doubtful mammary tumors," *The Lancet* 2 (1934): 1041–45, on p. 1041. Tod and Dawson described French surgeons as "overanxious" and insufficiently committed to their patient's long-term well-being and criticized their view that mastectomy for Reclus's disease was an unnecessary mutilation.

28. Simple mastectomy, at first called "plastic resection of the breast," was developed in 1905 by Warren and improved by Gibson. Ewing, "Precancerous diseases and precancerous lesions," 24–25.

29. Sir G. Lenthal Cheatle, "Cancer of the breast. Treatment of the proemial breast," *British Medical Journal* 1 (1922): 869–71, quotation on p. 870. Cheatle's typical patient was a woman 40 to 45 years old, with swollen, painful, and lumpy breasts; she was treated with subcutaneous, nipple-sparing mastectomy.

30. Sir Lenthal Cheatle and Max Cutter, *Tumours of the Breast: Their Pathology, Symptoms, Diagnosis and Treatment* (London: Edward Arnold, & Co., 1931), 120–34, esp. 132. Cheatle worked in King's College, London, and Cutter in Michael Reese Hospital, Chicago.

31. Arthur Purdy Stout, *Human Cancer* (London: Henry Kimpton, 1932), 317–19.

32. William H. Sternberg, "The pathology of breast cancer," in *Breast Cancer*, ed. Albert Segaloff (St. Louis, MO: The C.V. Mosby Company, 1958).

33. William C. White, *Cancer of the Breast* (New York and London: Harper and Brothers, 1930), 39.

34. Barbara Maria Stafford, "Picturing ambiguity," in *Good Looking, Essays on the Virtue of Images*, ed. Barbara Maria Stafford (Cambridge, MA: MIT Press, 1996), 146–67, on p. 147.

35. Guido de Manjo and Isabelle Joris, *Cells, Tissues and Disease: Principles of General Pathology* (Oxford: Blackwell, 1996), 727–77, reproduction on p. 753.

36. Ellis Macdonald and William C. Hueper, "Cancer and the laboratory," *Journal of Laboratory and Clinical Medicine* 16 (1931): 713–33; Ewing, *Neoplastic Diseases*, 541;

Pierre Hermert, "La radiotherapie dans le traitement de cancer du sein," *Paris Médical*, 26 (1936): 233–46; Pierre Masson, *Diagnostic de Laboratoire: Tumeurs—Diagnostic Histologique* (Paris: A. Maloine & Fils, 1923), 301.

37. The choice of these institutions reflects the availability of suitable material. Pathology diagnoses in New York Hospital files are usually very concise. The pathologists communicated their conclusions but did not provide description of slides that led them to these conclusions. The Arthur Purdy Stout Society files do not contain verbal descriptions of slides, probably because participants in the society meetings looked collectively at the preparations.

38. Autobiography (unpublished manuscript) of Professor Hubert Maitland Turnbull (1875–1955), Fellow of the Royal Society, pathologist at London Hospital, Archives of the Royal London Hospital, London, England (Archives of London Hospital). On the history of cytology and the key role of German pathologists in the development of this specialty, see Cay-Rüdiger Prüll, "Pathology and surgery in London and Berlin, 1800–1930: Pathological theory and surgical practice," in *Pathology in the 19th and 20th Centuries*, ed. Cay-Rüdiger Prüll (Sheffield: European Association for the History of Medicine, 1998), 71–99.

39. Hubert Maitland Turnbull, "Teaching notes in Morbid Anatomy," Notes from lectures, 1925 and 1928, revised (partly) in 1943, Turnbull's papers, Archives of the London Hospital.

40. Turnbull, "Teaching notes in Morbid Anatomy."

41. Turnbull, "Teaching notes in Morbid Anatomy."

42. Card indexes of pathology books, surgery materials, biopsies, and body liquids, 1906–54, Archives of London Hospital.

43. Registers of all surgical cases at the London Hospital for 1909 and for 1919, Archives of London Hospital. The number of cases was relatively small, five to ten per year. Pathology notebooks of St Bartholomew's Hospital for 1900–35 reveal a similar pattern, with breast amputations peaking in the 1910s. Pathology registers, St Bartholomew's Hospital, codes PA 8/1-PA8/18, Archives of St Bartholomew's Hospital (Archives of St Bart's). In both hospitals, pathology notebooks do not distinguish simple mastectomy from radical surgery.

44. Pathological Institute, Surgical Department, Director's Book, Archives of London Hospital. I sampled the voluminous pathology books for every ten years, starting in 1909.

45. Pathological Institute, Surgical Department, Director's Book, Archives of London Hospital, notes from 1909. The level of detail in Turnbull's descriptions seems to be exceptional.

46. Pathological Institute, Surgical Department, Director's Book, Archives of London Hospital, notes from 1919.

47. Pathological Institute, Surgical Department, Director's Book, Archives of London Hospital, notes from 1929.

48. Pathological Institute, Surgical Department, Director's Book, Archives of London Hospital, notes from 1939.

49. Gricouroff was appointed in 1927 and remained the Institute's main pathologist

until late 1950s. Extracts of pathology reports, activity reports, Archives of the Department of Medical Files, Musée Curie Historical Resources Center, Curie Institute, Paris (Archives of the Curie Institute). All the extracts of pathology reports are from 1931–35.

50. Notebooks, cervical cancer, 1919–39. Notebook 1931–1935, without case numbers, box, gynecological cancers, Archives of the Curie Institute.

51. Records of patients, classified by pathology, breast, section 86, Archives of Addenbrooke's Hospital, Cambridge, England (Archives of Addenbrooke's Hospital).

52. J. Collins Warren, "The surgeon and the pathologist," *JAMA* 2 (1905): 149–65.

53. Joseph Colt Bloodgood, "Senile parenchymous hyperthrophy of female breast," *Surgery, Gynecology and Obstetrics* 3 (1906): 721–30.

54. Joseph Colt Bloodgood, "Borderline breast tumors," *American Journal of Cancer* 16 (1932): 103–76.

55. Ewing, *Neoplastic Diseases*, 541. Italics mine, IL. The obvious parallel is with "complete" mastectomy.

56. Robert B. Greenough, "Early diagnosis of cancer of the breast," in *Proceedings of the Round Table Conference on Cancer, Memorial Hospital, New York, New York, Annals of Surgery* 162 (1935): 233–38.

57. M. C. Tod and E. K. Dawson, "The diagnosis and treatment of doubtful mammary tumors," *The Lancet* 2 (1934), 1041–45.

58. Tod and Dawson, "The diagnosis and treatment of doubtful mammary tumors," 1045.

59. R. J. Behan, *Cancer, With Specific Reference to Cancer of the Breast* (St. Louis, MO: The C.V. Mosby Company, 1938), 330–31.

60. Joseph Colt Bloodgood, "Biopsy in breast lesions, in relation to diagnosis, treatment and prognosis," *Proceedings of the Round Table Conference on Cancer, Memorial Hospital, New York, New York, Annals of Surgery* 162 (1935): 239–49, on p. 248.

61. All the data were collected from Annual Reports of the Harvard University Cancer Commission, Department of Rare Books, Countway Library, Harvard Medical School.

62. File, breast cancer cases, 1914–1915, First Surgical Division, Archives of New York Hospital, Weill Cornell Medical Library, Ithaca, New York (Archives of New York Hospital).

63. Records of cystoma patients, 1918–1923, Archives of New York Hospital.

64. Mixed benign tumors, 1923–1925, Archives of the New York Hospital; general hospital, second division, section on breast, Archives of New York Hospital.

65. Mixed benign tumors, 1925–1928, Archives of the New York Hospital; general hospital, first division, Archives of New York Hospital.

66. Mixed benign tumors, 1925–1929, Archives of the New York Hospital; general hospital, second division, Archives of New York Hospital.

67. Breast carcinoma, 1928, Archives of New York Hospital.

68. File, breast cancer cases, 1930–1932, Archives of New York Hospital.

69. Maurice Lenz's papers, box 15, file 5: breast cancer, Columbia University Health Sciences Library, Archives and Special Collections, Columbia University, New York, New York (Columbia University Health Services Library).

70. Lenz's papers, Box 15, file 5: breast cancer. Columbia University Health Sciences Library. In this case, too, Lenz noted that the decision to perform a radical surgery gave the patient "the benefit of doubt."

71. Janet Lane-Claypon, *A Further Report on Cancer of the Breast, With Special Reference to Its Associated Antecedent Conditions* (London: His Majesty Stationary Office, 1926), 175–85. Six of the participating hospitals were in London—The Cancer Hospital, University College Hospital, St Bartholomew's Hospital, London Hospital, Elisabeth Garrett Anderson Hospital, and Samaritan Hospital—and three were in Glasgow: Western Infirmary, Royal Infirmary, and Victoria Infirmary. Lane-Claypon relied on pathologists' diagnoses. She lumped together data provided by nine pathology laboratories that might have had very different criteria for, e.g., classifying a breast lesion as "cystic mastitis."

72. Lane-Claypon, *A Further Report on Cancer of the Breast*, 175–77. Lane-Claypon's data seem to indicate that, when in doubt, doctors often elected radical mastectomy, while when the diagnosis of cystic mastitis was confirmed, practices varied greatly.

73. Lane-Claypon observed also an opposite diagnostic error. Seven women in her sample underwent radical mastectomy for cancer; the pathologist's verdict was that they only had cystic mastitis. Lane-Claypon, *A Further Report on Cancer of the Breast*, 177.

74. Lane-Claypon, *A Further Report on Cancer of the Breast*, 178–85.

75. Ibid., 177–78, 185–89.

76. Records of patients, classified by pathology: breast: section 86, 1937, Archives of Addenbrooke's Hospital.

77. Ibid. Paget's disease of the nipple is a proliferative lesion that has invasive and pre-invasive variants.

78. Breast, section 86, 1937, Archives of Addenbrooke's Hospital.

79. Breast, section 86, 1942, Archives of Addenbrooke's Hospital. The emphasis in the last sentence is in the text. To judge from notes in the records, simple mastectomy for proliferative condition of the breast was not seen as a problematic operation, while radical mastectomy needed to be justified.

80. Breast, section 86, 1942, Archives of Addenbrooke's Hospital, Cambridge. It is not clear why the patient was discharged without further surgery. It is possible that she refused such surgery, or, alternatively, that she underwent mastectomy later or elsewhere.

81. Breast, section 86, 1947, Archives of Addenbrooke's Hospital.

82. Ibid. The case seems to be typical. Several other simple mastectomies for cystic mastitis were performed around that time, all in women in their forties and fifties.

83. Breast, section 86, 1947 and records of patients, classified by pathology, Archives of Addenbrooke's Hospital. Letters to the patients' physicians are a post–World War II innovation, probably related to the development of the National Health Service.

84. Ibid. Italics mine, IL.

85. Ibid. Italics mine, IL.

86. Cancer patient files, Archives of the Curie Institute. French medical tradition—

from Claude Bernard on—stressed the importance of physiological considerations in clinical decisions.

87. Cancer patient files, Archives of the Curie Institute. The Curie Institute files include correspondence between medical experts involved in the case and patients and their family members.

88. This complication was developed by a woman treated in August 1938. Case no. 8, series: benign breast tumors treated by radiation, file: breast-radiotherapy, 1919–1939, Archives of the Curie Institute.

89. Ibid.

90. Howard C. Taylor, "A case of 'chronic mastitis' treated by irradiation of the ovary, *Bulletin of the Memorial Hospital for the Treatment of Cancer and Allied Diseases* (New York: William Wood and Company, 1930), 59–60. One may assume that in this case doctors did not hesitate to shut off ovarian function, because the patient, deprived of her uterus, was already sterile, and irradiation just made her hysterectomy "complete." Taylor did not mention the well-established practice of treating patients with advanced breast cancer by surgical or radiological castration. Michael J. Clarke, "Ovarian ablation in breast cancer, 1896 to 1998," *British Medical Journal* 17 (1998): 1246–48.

91. W. Sampson Handley, "The prevention of cancer," *The Lancet* 1 (1936): 987–91. Handley explained that to settle the question of the preventive effect of x-rays, one should take a thousand 40-year-old women, treat one breast of each woman with low level x-ray radiation, follow up these women for twenty years, and compare the number of malignancies in irradiated and nonirradiated breasts. Alas, he added, such experiment is not possible. Ibid., 989.

92. Bloodgood, "Senile parenchymatous hypertrophy of the female breast."

93. Joseph Colt Bloodgood, "The pathology of chronic cystic mastitis of the female breast," *Archives of Surgery* 3 (1921): 446–542.

94. Joseph Cold Bloodgood, "Borderline breast tumors: Encapsulated and non encapsulated cystic adenomata observed from 1890 to 1931," *American Journal of Cancer* 16 (1932): 103–76.

95. Joseph Colt Bloodgood, "Comments on an article of Charles F. Geschichter, 'The early literature on chronic cystic mastitis,'" *Bulletin of the Institute of History of Medicine* 2 (1934): 256–57.

96. Bloodgood, "Comments on an article of Charles F. Geschichter."

97. He explicitly mentions Cheatle and Cutler's influential 1931 textbook, *Tumours of the Breast.*

Chapter Four · In Situ Cancers

1. John Williams, *Cancer of the Uterus; Being the Harveian Lectures for 1886* (London: H. K. Lewis, 1888), 12; see also plate I, p. 119. William added that such lesions remain superficial for a long time; he believed that they could be cured by a local treatment. Ibid., 108.

2. The history of this lesion is summed up in Walter Schiller, "Early diagnosis of carcinoma of the cervix" *Surgery, Gynecology and Obstetrics* 56 (1933): 212–22.

3. Surgery department files, for 1920, ward II: carcinoma, Archives of New York Hospital, Weill Cornell Medical Library, Ithaca, New York (Archives of New York Hospital).

4. Notebooks "Cervical cancer, 1919–1939, box, gynecological cancers, Archives of the Department of Medical Files, Musée Curie Historical Resources Center, Curie Institute, Paris (Archives of the Curie Institute). On the rarity of observation of proliferative lesions of the cervix before the generalization of Pap smears, see Walter E. O'Donnell, Emerson Day, and Louis Venet, *Early Detection and Diagnosis of Cancer* (Saint Louis, MO: The C.V. Mosby Company, 1962), 154–155.

5. Schiller, "Early diagnosis of carcinoma of the cervix."

6. Ibid., 214.

7. Walter Schiller, "Clinical behaviour of early carcinoma of the cervix," *Surgery, Gynecology and Obstetrics* 66 (1938): 129–39. Italics mine, IL.

8. Schiller, "Early diagnosis of carcinoma of the cervix," 218.

9. E. Novak, "The pathological diagnosis of early cervical and corporeal cancer," *American Journal of Obstetrics and Gynecology* 8 (1929): 2–24; K. Martzloff, "Leucoplasia in cervix uteri," *American Journal of Obstetrics and Gynecology* 24 (1932): 57–67.

10. Charles Summers Stevenson and Elmer Scipiade, "Non invasive potential 'carcinoma' of the cervix," *Surgery, Gynecology and Obstetrics* 66 (1938): 822–35; Randolph H. Hoge, "Carcinoma in situ of the cervix: A survey of its treatment in the United States and Canada," *American Journal of Obstetrics and Gynecology* 61 supplement 5 (1950): 618–27, on pp. 621–624. Before the generalization of Pap smear, superficial lesions of the cervix were usually diagnosed in women with clinical symptoms (bleeding, vaginal discharge, pain). It is not to be excluded that in some cases presumed premalignant lesions were in fact misdiagnosed invasive malignancies.

11. O'Donnell, Day, and Venet, *Early Detection and Diagnosis of Cancer,* 154.

12. Chandler Smith, "Carcinoma in situ," *Human Pathology* 9 (1978): 373–74.

13. Howard C. Taylor, "Controversial points in the treatment of carcinoma of the cervix," *Cancer* 5 (1952): 435–41, on p. 435. The Cancer Campaign Committee (the precursor of the Committee on Cancer, or COC) was appointed in 1913 by the Board of Regents of the American College of Surgeons to analyze records of patients with cancer of the uterus to promote standardized surgical practices. Murray F. Brenna, Rosemary E. Clive, and David P. Winchester, "The COC: Its roots and destiny," *American College of Surgeon's Bulletin* 79 (1994): 14–21.

14. Adele Clarke, *Disciplining Reproduction: Modernity, American Life Sciences and the Problem of Sex* (Berkeley and Los Angeles: University of California Press, 1998).

15. George N. Papanicolaou, "The sexual cycle in the human female as revealed by vaginal smears," *American Journal of Anatomy* 52 (1933): 519–27.

16. George N. Papanicolaou, "New cancer diagnosis," *Proceedings of the Third Race Betterment Conference, January 2–6, 1928,* Battle Creek, Michigan, 528–34. Charles

Stockard, the head of the department of anatomy at the Cornell Medical Center where Papanicolaou was employed, had a long-standing interest in eugenics and might have suggested to Papanicolaou to present his finding at a "race betterment" conference.

17. George N. Papanicolaou and Herbert F. Traut, "The diagnostic value of vaginal smears in carcinoma of the uterus," *American Journal of Obstetrics and Gynecology* 42 (1941): 193–206; George N. Papanicolaou and Herbert F. Traut, *Diagnosis of Uterine Cancer by Vaginal Smear* (New York: The Commonwealth Fund, 1943).

18. George N. Papanicolaou and V. F. Marshall, "Urine sediments as a diagnostic procedure in cancers of the bladder," *Science* 101 (1945): 145–49; George N. Papanicolaou, "A survey of the actualities and the potentialities of exfoliate cytology in cancer diagnosis," *Annals of Internal Medicine* 31 (1949): 661–66. These attempts were made in collaboration with Dr. McLellan from the Memorial Hospital, New York, New York, Papanicolaou's papers, Archives of New York Hospital.

19. Daniel McSweeney and Donald G. McKay, "Uterine cancer: Its early detection by simple screening methods," *New England Journal of Medicine* 238 (1948): 867–70.

20. G. A. Galvin and R. W. TeLinde, "The present day status of non-invasive cervical carcinoma," *American Journal of Obstetrics and Gynecology* 57 (1949): 15–36.

21. Taylor, "Controversial points in the treatment of carcinoma of the cervix."

22. Galvin and TeLinde, "The present day status of non-invasive cervical carcinoma."

23. Randolph H. Hoge, "Carcinoma in situ of the cervix: A survey of its treatment in the United States and Canada," *Obstetrics and Gynecology* supplement 5 (1950): 621–28.

24. Bayard Carter, Kenneth Cuyler, Walter L. Thomas, Robert Creadick, and Robert Alter, "The methods of management of carcinoma in situ of the cervix," *American Journal of Obstetrics and Gynecology* 64 (1952): 833–45. The results were first presented at the 75th annual meeting of the American Gynecological Society in Hot Springs, Virginia, May 12–14, 1952.

25. George Weisz, *Divide and Conquer* (Oxford University Press, 2005).

26. Georges Gricouroff, "Le problème du cancer du col d'utérus a stade zéro," *La Presse Médicale* 34 (1952): 743–44.

27. Antoine Lacassagne, "A propos du cancer du col utérin: Que penser du stade 0?" *Actes du 57e Congrès Français de Chirurgie,* Paris, 1955, 122–24.

28. Olaf Petersen, *Precancerous Changes of the Cervical Epithelium* (Copenhagen: Danish Science Press, 1955), 11.

29. Petersen, *Precancerous Changes of the Cervical Epithelium;* P. C. Meyer, "Diagnosis of pre-invasive carcinoma of the uterine cervix, *Journal of Clinical Pathology* 18 (1965): 414–23. The majority of the women in this trial were relatively young (ages 25 to 45).

30. This is a surprisingly high percentage of invasive tumors, compared with more recent data on the fate of noninvasive cervical lesions. The high incidence of malignancies may reflect the fact that the great majority of women enrolled in Petersen's study were recruited because they consulted physicians for gynecological

complaints and had symptoms such as bleeding or pain. By contrast, women diagnosed with proliferative changes in the cervix following a positive Pap smear are nearly always symptom free.

31. Petersen, *Precancerous Changes of the Cervical Epithelium*, 77–79.

32. Ibid., 91–92.

33. Ibid., 102.

34. Ibid., 129–31.

35. Frantz Bushke to Maurice Lenz, Feb. 13, 1959, Maurice Lenz Papers, box 1, folder 12, Columbia University Health Sciences Library, Archives and Special Collections, Columbia University, New York, New York (Columbia University Health Services Library).

36. O'Donnell, Day, and Venet, *Early Detection and Diagnosis of Cancer*, 154–55.

37. Leopold G. Koss, Fred Stewart, Frank Foote, et al., "Some histological aspects of behavior of epidermoid carcinoma in situ and related lesions of uterine cervix. A long term prospective study," *Cancer* 12 (1963): 1160–1211, on p. 1204.

38. Koss, Stewart, Foote, et al., "Some histological aspects of behavior," 1188.

39. Ralph Richard, "The natural history of cervical intraperithelial dysplasia," *Clinical Obstetrics and Gynecology* 10 (1967): 748.

40. C. Gad, "The management and the natural history of severe dysplasia and carcinoma in situ of the uterine cervix," *British Journal of Obstetrics and Gynecology* 83 (1976): 554–59.

41. Gerald A. Galvin, Howard W. Jones, and Richard W. TeLinde, "Clinical relationship of carcinoma in situ and invasive carcinoma of the cervix," *Journal of the American Medical Association* 149 (1952): 744–48.

42. On differences between U.S. and French gynecologists, see, for example, Lynn Payer, *Medicine and Culture: Varieties of Treatment in the United States, England, West Germany and France* (New York: Henry Holt, 1988).

43. Sue Fisher, *In the Patient's Best Interest: Women and the Politics of Medical Decisions* (New Brunswick, NJ: Rutgers University Press, 1986). French gynecologists were more conservative, while UK specialists held an intermediary position.

44. O'Donnell, Day, and Venet, *Early Detection and Diagnosis of Cancer*, 166. Cervical biopsies were not seen as problematic interventions. By contrast the same authors were more reluctant to recommend systematic removal of suspect polyps during colonoscopy, fearing complications such as bleeding, perforation of colon, or scarring. Ibid., 218.

45. Erich Burghart, "Radicality in gynecologic cancer surgery: A historical perspective," *Gynecologic Oncology* 70 (1998): 172–75.

46. Koss, Stewart, Foote, et al., "Some histological aspects of behavior."

47. H. W. Jones, and R. E. Buller, "The treatment of cervical intraepithelial neoplasia by cone biopsy," *American Journal of Obstetrics and Gynecology* 137 (1980): 882–86; J. L. Benedet, G. H Anderson, M. L. Simpson, and D. Shaw, "Colposcopy, conization and hysterectomy practices, A current perspective, *Obstetrics and Gynecology* 60 (1982): 539–45.

48. See, for example, series of angry testimonies of the "castrated women" who belatedly discovered the complications of premature menopause and then wrote in the 1970s to Boston Women's Health Book Collective. Letters, 1975–1979, series 99M147, folder 3, box 99-M147, menopause questionnaires, Boston Women's Health Book Collective Archives, 1976.

49. Charles Geschichter, *Diseases of the Breast* (Philadelphia: J. B. Lippincott, 1945), 280.

50. In 2008 "cystic changes of the breast" are not seen as a condition that increases the risk of breast tumors. See, for example, www.thedoctorsdoctor.com/diseases/proliferative_breast_disease.htm, accessed Feb. 5, 2008.

51. Edith K. Dawson, "Malignant tumors of the breast," in *Cancer,* ed. Ronald W. Raven (London, Butterworth & Co, 1959), 2:269–97, esp. 274 and 277.

52. Pathological Institute, Surgical Department, Director's Book, Archives of the Royal London Hospital, London, England (Archives of London Hospital). The pathology laboratory book became gradually thicker, up to nearly 1,500 pages in 1959. In 1969, for the first time, the pathology laboratory reports were collected in nine bound books. I sampled the reports for every ten years.

53. Records of patients, classified by pathology: breast, section 86, Archives of Addenbrooke's Hospital, Cambridge, England (Archives of Addenbrooke's Hospital). In 1942 A. M. Barett replaced Dr. C. H. Whittle as the hospital's pathologist. From the late 1940s on, Addenbrooke's hospital records were no longer classified according to pathologies, making a search for diagnoses of malignant tumors difficult.

54. The irritation theory is, however, alive and well in lay representation of cervical cancer. In 2008, many women still believe that the risk of this malignancy is increased by the trauma of childbirth and by high frequency of sexual relations (rather than having multiple sexual partners), events linked with "harm" to the cervix. Natalie Armstrong and Elisabeth Murphy, "Weaving meaning? An exploration of the interplay between lay and professional understanding of cervical cancer risk," *Social Sciences and Medicine* 67 (2008): 1074–82.

55. Antoine Lacassagne, *Certain Biological Problems Relating to Cancer, Hormones, and Radiation* (Philadelphia: International Cancer Research Foundation, 1936); Antoine Lacassagne, *Les Cancers Produits par les Substances Chimiques Endogènes* (Paris: Hermann, 1950); Alexander Haddow, ed., *Advances in Cancer Research* (New York: Academic Press, 1953).

56. Manuel Garcia, "The etiology of cancer: A review," *Bulletin of the American Association for the Control of Cancer* 20 (1938): 3–5; Carrington Williams, "The etiology of malignant tumors," *Bulletin of the American Association for the Control of Cancer* 20 (1938): 2–6.

57. O'Donnell, Day, and Venet, *Early Detection and Diagnosis of Cancer,* 23.

58. Albert C. Broders, "Carcinoma in situ contrasted with benign penetrating epithelium," *JAMA* 99 (1932): 1670–74.

59. Frank W. Foote and Fred W. Stewart, "Lobular carcinoma in situ: A rare form of mammary carcinoma," *American Journal of Surgical Pathology* 19 (1941): 74–99;

Frank W. Foote and Fred W. Stewart, "Comparative studies of cancerous versus non-cancerous breasts," *Annals of Surgery* 121 (1945): 6–53.

60. Ilana Löwy, "Cancer—the century of the transformed cell," in *Science in the Twentieth Century,* ed. John Krige and Dominique Pestre (Amsterdam: Harwood Academic Press, 1997), 461–77.

61. Sir Lenthal Cheatle and Max Cutter, *Tumours of the Breast: Their Pathology, Symptoms, Diagnosis and Treatment* (London: Edward Arnold and Co., 1931), 162.

62. Robert B. Greenough, "Early diagnosis of cancer of the breast," *Proceedings of the Round Table Conference on Cancer, Memorial Hospital, New York, New York, Annals of Surgery* 162 (1935): 233–38, on p. 233.

63. Records of patients, classified by pathology, breast, section 86, 1942, Archives of Addenbrooke's Hospital. Italics mine, IL.

64. Ibid. It is possible that in these two cases the fact that the patient underwent a radical mastectomy favored an ulterior classification of her tumor as true malignancy.

65. Albert Broders, "Carcinoma in situ contrasted with benign penetrating epithelium," *JAMA* 99 (1932): 1670–74. Italics mine, IL. Schiller employed a similar rhetoric technique in his descriptions of in situ carcinoma of the cervix. Walter Schiller, "Early diagnosis of carcinoma of the cervix," *Surgery, Gynecology and Obstetrics* 56 (1933): 212–22.

66. Foote and Stewart, "Lobular carcinoma in situ," Italics mine, IL.

67. Foote and Stewart, "Comparative studies," Italics mine, IL.

68. Georges Gricouroff, "Différenciation pratique et dogmatique entre lesions benignes et lesions malignes," *Acta Union Internationale Contre le Cancer* 10 (1954): 125–36; Georges Gricouroff, "Essai de définition de la prolifération cellulaire maligne," *Bulletin du Cancer* 42 (1955): 97–111. Italics mine, IL. Gricouroff's views may reflect purely personal preferences but perhaps also the interest of some French surgeons for physiological explanations, in the tradition of Claude Bernard.

69. William H. Sternberg, "The pathology of beast cancer," in *Breast Cancer,* ed. Albert Segaloff (St. Louis, MO: The C.V. Mosby Company, 1958), 46–52.

70. Fred Waldorf Stewart, *Tumors of the Breast: Atlas of Tumor Pathology,* section 9, fasicle 34 (Washington, DC: Armed Forces Institute of Pathology, 1950).

71. Robert V. Hutter, "What is a premalignant lesion," in *Early Breast Cancer: Detection and Treatment,* ed. H. Stephen Gallagher (New York: John Wiley and Sons, 1975), 165–69, on p. 165.

72. Stewart, *Tumors of the Breast.*

73. John R. Benfield, Aaron G. Gingerhut, and Nancy E. Warner, "Lobular carcinoma of the breast, 1969," *Archives of Surgery* 99 (1969): 129–31.

74. Edward F. Lewinson, "Lobular carcinoma in situ of the breast: The feminine mystique," *Military Medicine* 129 (1964): 115–23. The title is an allusion to Betty Friedan's book, published a year earlier. Betty Friedan, *The Feminine Mystique* (New York: Norton, 1963).

75. Lewinson, "Lobular carcinoma in situ of the breast."

76. Robert W. McDivitt, Robert V. P. Hutter, Frank W. Foote, and Fred W. Stewart,

"In situ lobular carcinoma: A prospective follow-up study indicating cumulative patients' risks," *JAMA* 201 (1967): 96–100, on pp. 99–100.

77. Papers of the Arthur Purdy Stout Society of surgical pathologists, box 1, papers 1957–1986, folder 6. Undated, probably 1970s. Columbia University Health Sciences Library.

78. Ibid.

79. Nancy E. Warner, "Lobular carcinoma of the breast," *Cancer* 23 (1969): 840–46.

80. Lewinson, "Lobular carcinoma in situ of the breast."

81. Virginia L. Ernster, "The epidemiology of benign breast disease," *Epidemiological Reviews* 3 (1981):184–202.

82. Barron Lerner, *The Breast Cancer Wars: Hope, Fear and the Pursuit of a Cure in Twentieth-Century America* (New York: Oxford University Press, 2001), 223–41.

83. John E. Martin, Charles H. Hayden, William E. Powers, William W. Shingleton, Reuven K. Snyderman, and Herbert B. Taylor, "The management of premalignant or histologically dubious lesions: A panel discussion," in *Early Breast Cancer: Detection and Treatment*, ed. H. Stephen Gallagher (New York: John Wiley and Sons, 1975), 171–77.

84. From the 1940s on, experts who noted that childless women or those who deferred childbirth have higher incidence of breast cancer linked these observation with influence of female sex hormones on breast cells. I. T. Nathanson, "The relations of hormones to diseases of the breast," in *Endocrinology of Malignant Diseases*, ed. G. H. Twombley and G. T. Pack (Oxford: Oxford University Press, 1947), 119–37. Some doctors viewed higher frequency of breast cancer in childless women and those who delayed birth as an indication that nature punishes women who reject their traditional role. Cancer advocate Rose Kushner accepted the evidence about the protective effect of early childbirth but not the proposed solution—to put women back in the nursery. Scientists, she proposed, should find a way to hormonally manipulate women to artificially mimic the protection accorded by pregnancy. Rose Kushner, draft of a text, "Career before carriages," Mar. 1, 1983. Kushner's papers, MC 453, box 3, folder 46, Arthur and Elizabeth Schlesinger Library on the History of Women in America, Radcliffe Institute of Advanced Study, Harvard University (Schlesinger Library).

85. Nicholas L. Petrakis, Virginia L. Ernster, Eileen B. King, and Susan T. Sacks, "Epithelial dysplasia in nipple aspirates of breast fluid: Association with family history and other breast cancer risk factors," *Journal of the National Cancer Institute* 68 (1982): 9–12; William D. Dupont and David L. Page, "Risk factors for breast cancer in women with proliferative breast disease," *New England Journal of Medicine* 312 (1985): 146–51; David L. Page, "The clinical significance of atypical hyperplasia, multicentricity and bilaterality," in *Breast Cancer: Controversies in Management*, ed. Leslie Wise and Huston Johnson (Armonk, NY: Futura Publishing, 1994), 203–214. D. L. Page, R. Wande Zwaag, L. W. Rogers, L. T. Williams, W. E. Walker, and W. H. Farmann, "Relation between component parts of fibrocystic disease complex and breast cancer," *Journal of the National Cancer Institute* 61 (1978): 1055–63.

86. John E. Martin, Charles H. Hayden, William E. Powers, William W. Shingle-

ton, Reuven K. Snyderman, and Herbert B Taylor, "The management of premalignant or histologically dubious lesions: A panel discussion," in *Early Breast Cancer: Detection and Treatment,* 171–77, on p. 175. Italics mine, IL.

87. Martin et al., "The management of premalignant or histologically dubious lesions."

88. P. P. Rosen, D. W. Braun, B. Lynghom, J. A. Urban, and D. W. Kinne, "Lobular carcinoma in situ of the breast: preliminary report of treatment by ipsilateral mastectomy and contralateral breast biopsy," *Cancer* 47 (1981): 813–15.

89. J. P. Sloane, "Precancerous changes of the breast," in *Precancerous States,* ed. R. L. Carter (Oxford: Oxford University Press, 1984), 93–128, on p. 125.

90. Haagensen was, on the one hand, an enthusiastic advocate of radical and even ultraradical surgery for "operable" cases of breast cancer. On the other hand, he was reluctant to extend this approach to all proliferative breast lesions. In the early 1980s, the percentage of conservative treatments for breast cancer doubled in the United States, but in spite of the growing popularity of this approach, the majority of American women treated for breast cancer at that time underwent a mastectomy (70% of all those diagnosed with breast cancer and 85% of women over 65). Anne Butler Nattinger, Raymond G. Hoffman, Alicia Howel Peltz, and James S. Goodwin, "Effect of Nancy Reagan's mastectomy on choice of surgery for breast cancer by US women," *JAMA* 279 (1998): 762–66.

91. Benfield, Fingerhut, and Warner, "Lobular carcinoma of the breast," 129.

92. Cushman D. Haagensen, Nathan Lane, Raffaele Lattes, and Carol Bodian, "Lobular neoplasia (so called lobular carcinoma in situ) of the breast," *Cancer* 42 (1978): 737–69.

93. Paul H. O'Brien, "The management of lobular carcinoma in situ of the breast," in *Breast Cancer: Controversies in Management,* ed. Leslie Wise and Huston Johnson (Armonk, NY: Futura Publishing, 1994), 217–21.

94. J. A. Anderson, "Lobular carcinoma of the breast. An approach to rational treatment," *Cancer* 39 (1977): 2597–2602.

95. Susan M. Love, Rebecca Sue Gelman, and William Se, "Fibrocystic disease of the breast—A nondisease," *New England Journal of Medicine* 307 (1982): 1010–14.

96. Papers of the Arthur Purdy Stout Society of Surgical Pathologists, box 1, papers 1957–1986, folder 8, papers of the meeting of Mar. 28, 1976. Stenciled form, unsigned, on "benign lesions of the breast" and a letter from C. D. Haagensen to Dr. Hartmann, Jan. 24, 1976, on the classification of breast lesions, Columbia University Health Sciences Library.

97. Paolo Bruzzi, Luigi Doliotti, Carlo Naldoni, et al., "Cohort study of association of risk of breast cancer with cyst type in women with gross cystic disease of the breast," *British Medical Journal* 314 (1997): 935–41; Elisabeth Tan-Chiu, Ji Ping Wang, Joseph P. Costantino, et al., "Effects of tamoxifen on benign breast disease in women at high risk of breast cancer," *Journal of the National Cancer Institute* 95 (2003): 302–7; David M. Page, "Cancer risk assessment in benign breast biopsies," *Human Pathology* 17 (1986): 871–73.

98. Richard R. Monson, Stella Yen, and Brian MacMahon, "Chronic mastitis and

carcinoma of the breast," *The Lancet* 1 (1976): 224–26. Other reports did not find, however, an excess of cancer in chronic mastitis patients. The discrepancies in results were attributed to divergent diagnoses of "cystic mastitis." Robert P. Huttern "What is a premalignant lesion," in *Early Breast Cancer: Detection and Treatment*, ed. H. Stephen Gallagher (New York: John Wiley and Sons, 1975), 165–81, on p. 167.

99. D. L. Page and W. D. Dupont, "Histopathological risk factors for breast cancer in women with benign breast disease," *Seminars in Surgical Oncology* 4 (1988): 213–17; Grazia Arpino, Rodolfo Laurica, and Richard M. Elledge, "Premalignant and in situ breast disease: Biology and clinical implications," *Annals of Internal Medicine* 143 (2005): 446–57, on p. 447.

100. J. Andersen, M. Blichert-Toft, and U. Dyreborg, "In situ carcinoma of the breast. Types, growth pattern, diagnosis and treatment," *European Journal of Surgical Oncology* 13 (1987): 105–7; I. S. Fentima, "The treatment of in situ breast cancer," *Acta Oncologica* 28 (1989): 923–26. An aggressive surgical approach to treatment of ductal carcinoma in situ (DCIS) affected also the therapy of Paget's disease of the nipple. Oncologists distinguished between a malignant Paget disease, similar to an invasive breast cancer, and a nonmalignant Paget's disease, akin to DCIS. This distinction remained, however, theoretical. In practice, experts recommended mastectomy for all the patients diagnosed with Paget's disease regardless of its invasiveness. H. Freund, M. Maydovnik, N. Lauer, and A. L. Durst, "Paget's disease of the breast," *Journal of Surgical Oncology* 9 (1977): 93–98.

101. However, women diagnosed with DCIS were found to have a better quality of life than women diagnosed with localized invasive carcinoma, especially in regard to general health, sex life, and social life. This difference was attributed to the fact that women with DCIS did not receive systemic chemotherapy, a treatment known to produce a long-term effect on patients' quality of life. Y. R. B. M. van Gestel, A. C. Voogd, A. J. J. M. Vingerhoets, et al., "A comparison of quality of life, disease impact and risk perception in women with invasive breast cancer and ductal carcinoma in situ," *European Journal of Cancer* 43 (2007): 549–56.

102. Frantz Uyttenbroeck, *Aspects Chirurgicaux en Cancérologie Gynécologique et Mammaire* (Paris: Masson, 1983), 323–25. The author, a professor of gynecology and obstetrics at the University of Antwerp, was one of the leading European experts on gynecological cancers.

103. Christopher I. Li, Kathleen E. Malone, B. S. Saltzman, and Janet R. Daling, "Risk of invasive breast carcinoma among women diagnosed with ductal carcinoma in situ and lobular carcinoma in situ, 1988–2001," *Cancer* 106 (2006): 2104–12.

104. Specialists estimated in 2004 that 30% of U.S. women with DCIS were overtreated, while 33% were undertreated. N. N. Baxtern, B. A. Virnig, S. B. Durham, and T. M. Tuttle, "Trends in the treatment of ductal carcinoma in situ of the breast," *Journal of the National Cancer Institute* 96 (2004): 443–48. Recent studies confirmed the persistence of important disparities in treatment of DCIS. E. Rakowitch, J. P. Pignol, C. Chartier, et al., "The management of ductal carcinoma in situ of the breast: A screened population-based analysis," *Breast Cancer Research and Treat-*

ment 101 (2007): 335–47; W. E. Sumner, L. G. Koniaris, S. E. Snell, et al., "Results of 23,810 cases of ductal carcinoma in situ," *Annals of Surgical Oncology* 14 (2007): 1638–43.

105. Li, Malone, Saltzman, and Daling, "Risk of invasive breast carcinoma."

106. Ibid. One may argue, however, that women with DCIS are more "breast cancer prone" than women in the general population.

107. Chandler Smith, "Carcinoma in situ," *Human Pathology* 9 (1978): 374–74.

108. A. Bernard Ackerman, "Carcinoma in situ," *Human Pathology* 10 (1979): 127–28.

109. David L. Page, "Cancer risk assessment in benign breast biopsies," *Human Pathology* 17 (1986): 871–73.

110. Arkady M. Rivlin, "Terminology of premalignant lesion in light of the multistep theory of carcinogenesis," *Human Pathology* 15 (1984): 806–7.

111. Elliot Foucar, "Carcinoma in situ of the breast: Have pathologists run amok?" *The Lancet* 347 (1996): 707–8; S. W. Duffy, L. Tabar, B. Vitak, N. E. Day, R. A. Smith, H. H. Chen, and M. F. Yen, "The relative contribution of screen-detected in situ and invasive breast carcinomas in reducing mortality from the disease," *European Journal of Cancer* 39 (2003): 1755–60.

112. David L. Page, "Breast lesions, pathology and cancer risk," *The Breast Journal* 10 supplement 1 (2004): S3–S4; Edwin R. Fisher, "Pathobiological considerations relation to the treatment of ductal carcinoma in situ of the breast," *CA: Cancer Journal for Clinicians* 47 (1996): 52–64; David P. Winchester, Jan M. Jeske, and Robert A. Goldschmidt, "The diagnosis and management of ductal carcinoma in situ of the breast," *CA: Cancer Journal for Clinicians* 50 (2000):184–200; A. Ringberg, H. Nordgreen, S. Thorstensson, et al., "Histopathological risk factors for ipsilateral breast events after breast conserving treatment for ductal carcinoma in situ of the breast)—Results from the Swedish randomized trial," *European Journal of Cancer* 43 (2007): 291–98; Monica Morrow and Martin J. O'Sulllivan, "The dilemma of DCIS," *The Breast* 16 supplement 2 (2007): S59–S62.

113. A 2004 review reported that "after 10 years of follow up, 14 to 60 percent of the women who underwent diagnostic biopsy alone received a diagnosis of invasive cancer in the affected breast." H. J. Burstein, K. Polyack, J. S. Wong, S. C. Lester, and C. M. Kaelin, "Ductal carcinoma in situ of the breast," *New England Journal of Medicine* 350 (2004): 1430–41.

114. Michael D. Lagions and Melvin J. Silverstein, "Ductal carcinoma in situ: Through a glass, darkly," *Annals of Surgical Oncology* 15 (2008): 16–17. The detection of localized prostate cancer leads to similar dilemmas. Ian Thompson and Lucia M. Scott, "Diagnosing prostate cancer: Through a glass, darkly," *Journal of Urology* 175 (2006):1598–99.

115. Rainer was not persuaded: "I did my research, found a more conservative surgeon and weighed my odds." Yvonne Rainer, "MURDER and murder. Screenplay; *Performing Arts Journal* 55 (1997): 76–117, on pp. 102–3. For discussion of Rainer's view of cancer and cancer risk, see Kathleen Woodward, "Statistic panic," *Differences: A Journal of Feminist Cultural Studies* 11 (1999): 177–203.

116. Li, Malone, Saltzman, and Daling, "Risk of invasive breast carcinoma." In par-

allel, women diagnosed with DCIS occasionally develop cancer in the contralateral breast. Shaheenah Dawood, Kristine Broglio, Ana M. Gonzales-Angulo, et al., "Development of new cancer in patients with DCIS. The M.D. Anderson experience," *Annals of Surgical Oncology* 15 (2008): 244–49.

117. M. Nielsen, J. L. Thomsen, S. Primdahl, U. Dyreborg, and J. A. Andersen, "Breast cancer and atypia among young and middle aged women: A study of 110 medico-legal autopsies," *British Journal of Cancer* 56 (1987): 814–19; M. E. Sander, P. A. Schuyler, W. D. Dupont, and D. L. Page, "The natural history of low grade ductal carcinoma in situ of the breast in women treated by biopsy only revealed over 30 years of long-term follow up," *Cancer* 103 (2005): 2481–84; Richard J. Santen, "Benign breast disorders," *New England Journal of Medicine* 353 (2006): 275–85; Grazia Arpino, Rodolfo Laurica, and Richard M. Elledge, "Premalignant and in situ breast disease: Biology and clinical implications," *Annals of Internal Medicine* 143 (2005): 446–57.

118. A recent publication proposes that women diagnosed with lobular carcinoma in situ (LCIS) face the same increase in risk of breast malignancy as obese women do (those with a body mass index over 30). The latter are, however, less often presented as living with a ticking bomb in their breast. Jennifer Chun, Mahmoud El-tamer, Kathie-Ann Joseph, Beth Ann Ditkoff, and Freya Schnabel, "Predictors of breast cancer development in high risk populations," *The American Journal of Surgery* 192 (2006): 474–77.

119. Maurice M. Black and Reinhard E. Zachrau, "The use and abuse of therapeutic modalities in breast cancer," *Preventive Medicine* 19 (1990): 723–29. The observation that cancer in the contralateral breast was not detected at an earlier stage than the first one was (and, occasionally, was detected at a more advanced stage), in spite of the fact that women who had cancer are usually submitted to intensive medical surveillance, may be an additional indication of limits of efficacy of such surveillance.

120. "Forum: When primary cancer of the breast is treated, should the second breast be prophylactically removed?" *Modern Medicine* 34 (1966): 242–60. Bilateral mastectomies for DCIS and LCIS and preventive mastectomies for women with family history of breast cancer follow a similar logic.

121. John R. Benfield, Aaron G. Fingerhut, and Nancy E. Warner, "Lobular carcinoma of the breast—1969," *Archives of Surgery* 99 (1969): 129–31; A. Ringbert, B. Palmer, and F. Linell, "The contralateral breast at reconstructive surgery after breast cancer operation—a histopathological study," *Breast Cancer Research and Treatment* 2 (1982): 151–61; C. E. Alpers and S. R. Wellings, "The prevalence of carcinoma in situ in normal and cancer associated breasts," *Human Pathology* 16 (1985): 796–807.

122. Robert S. Pollack, *Treatment of Breast Tumors* (Philadelphia: Lea & Feibiger, 1958), 83–84; Walter L. Mersheimer, "The problem of second primary breast cancer," *CA: A Cancer Journal for Clinicians* (Jan.–Feb. 1966): 33–35; Henry Patrick Leis, "Prophylactic removal of the second breast," *Hospital Medicine* (Jan. 1968): 45–49.

123. George T. Pack, "Editorial: Argument for bilateral mastectomy," *Surgery* 29 (1952): 929–31, quotation pp. 930–31. The song "Pack the Knife" (to the tune of Bertolt Brecht's and Kurt Weill's "Mack the Knife") is mentioned by Lerner, *The*

Breast Cancer Wars, 73. Lerner provides a detailed analysis of the surgical activism in post–World War II United States.

124. Henry Patrick Leis, "Selective, elective, prophylactic contralateral mastectomy," *Cancer* 28 (1971): 956–62, on p. 958.

125. Leis, "Selective, elective, prophylactic contralateral mastectomy." In 1971, "one stage breast surgery" was still the rule in the United States, and women diagnosed with a suspicious lump in their breast agreed to an operation without knowing what its outcome would be.

126. Karl Bader, Edmund Pelletiere, and John W. Courtin, "Definitive surgical therapy for the premalignant of equivocal breast lesion," *Plastic and Reconstructive Surgery* 46 (1970): 120–24.

127. Richard M. Goldwyn, "Subcutaneous mastectomy," *New England Journal of Medicine* 297 (1977): 503–5. Prophylactic subcutaneous mastectomy became much less popular in the 1990s, because this approach does not eliminate all the breast tissue.

128. Goldwyn, "Subcutaneous mastectomy," 504. The argument that delayed reconstruction protects the surgeon against malpractice claims is an interesting twist on the more frequent suggestion that a delay in breast reconstruction helps the patient to mourn the loss of body integrity and to accept an imperfect, "alien feeling" breast.

129. See, for example, Saul Hoffman and Peter I. Pressman, "Prophylactic mastectomy," *The Mount Sinai Journal of Medicine* 49 (1982): 102–9.

130. John J. Mulvihill, Andrew W. Safyer, and Jane K. Bening, "Prevention in familial breast cancer," *Preventive Medicine* 11 (1982): 500–511.

131. Mulvihill, Safyer, and Bening, "Prevention in familial breast cancer," 507–8. In the 1980s, fibrocystic disease of the breast was removed from the list of risk factors for breast cancer; accordingly it was no longer seen as an indication for preventive mastectomy.

132. John Bostwick, "Editorial: Preventive mastectomy," *Annals of Surgery and Oncology* 1 (1994): 455–56.

133. Ibid., 456.

134. Leslie L. Montgomery, Katherine N. Tran, Melissa C. Heelan, et al., "Issues of regret in women with contralateral prophylactic mastectomies," *Annals of Surgical Oncology* 6 (1999): 546–52. Thirty-two percent of women reported that their decision reflected the combination of more than one reason. Younger women (under 50) and those with "good prognosis" tumors received recommendations to undergo a prophylactic mastectomy more frequently.

135. Kushner's papers, MC 453, box 2, folder 28: materials on the book *Alternatives*, Schlesinger Library.

136. Rose Kushner, "Prophylactic mastectomies," manuscript for a talk given on Jan. 14, 1984. Kushner's papers, MC 453, box 3, folder 53, Schlesinger Library.

137. Jeremy Weir Alderson, "An indecent proposal," *Mother Jones*, May 1985, 52–56. Boston Women's Health Book Collective Archives 99-M147, box 4, Schlesinger Library.

138. Sandra M. Gifford, "The meaning of lumps: A case study of the ambiguities of risk," in *Anthropology and Epidemiology: Interdisciplinary Approaches to the Study of Health and Disease,* ed. Craig R. Janes, Ron Stall and Sandra Gillford (Dordrecht: Reidel, 1986), 213–46.

139. Hoffman and Pressman, "Prophylactic mastectomy."

140. Ibid.

141. Gifford, "The meaning of lumps," on p. 236.

Chapter Five · The Origins of Screening

1. Chapter 6 discusses screening for men's tumors, such as prostate cancer, introduced in the 1990s. In the case of prostate cancer, however, screening detects a "true" (that is, invasive) cancer, not a precancerous condition. The therapeutic dilemmas of screening for prostate malignancies stem from the fact that some invasive cancers evolve very slowly and do not put the patient's life or health at risk.

2. *Cancer, Be Quick! Cancer Control Is a Race against Time* (Boston: Massachusetts Department of Public Health, 1928).

3. James Ewing, "The prevention of cancer," in *Cancer Control: Proceedings of the ASCC Conference, Lake Moonok, New York, Sept. 20–24, 1926* (Chicago: The Surgical Publishing Company, 1927), 165–74, on p. 174. Sir Lenthal Cheatle similarly argued that when breast cancer manifests itself, it is too often beyond the reach of a surgical cure. Sir G. Lenthal Cheatle, "Cancer of the breast, Treatment of the proemial breast," *British Medical Journal* 1 (1922): 869–71, on p. 869.

4. James T. Patterson, *The Dread Disease: Cancer and the Modern American Culture* (Cambridge, MA: Harvard University Press, 1987).

5. Editorial, "Quelques principes géneraux deduits de l'état actual de la thérapeutique anitcancereuse," *La Lutte Contre le Cancer* 1 (1923): 114–19. Some of the Ligue's posters used, however, a stronger formulation "dépistée à temps toute tumeur est guérissable" (if detected in time, every tumor can be cured). Goustave Roussy's version of this slogan, "Le cancer est guérissable si traité à temps (cancer is curable if caught at the right time)," did not speak about "early" diagnosis (tôt), but about a "right time" (à temps), another ambivalent term. Goustave Roussy, "Les principes de la lutte contre le cancer," *Revue d'Hygiène* (July 7, 1931): 503–9.

6. Jean Firket, *Notions d'Anatomo-pathologie Humaine* (Paris: Masson & Cie, 1943), 44–47.

7. Joseph Colt Bloodgood, "Discussion of Charles Gaschicter's paper, 'The early literature on chronic cystic mastitis,' " *Bulletin of the Institute of History of Medicine* 2 (1934): 256–57; Groupe de travail sur la classification internationale des cancers d'utérus de Institut National d'Hygiène (president, Antoine Lacassagne), "Cancer du col d'utérus, definition du stade '0,' " *Bulletin de l'INH* 7 (1952): 549–54.

8. Amadé Baumgarten, *Les Maladies de la Mammelle* (Paris: Libraire J.B. Ballière & Fils, 1908), 275.

9. Robert B. Greenough, "Early diagnosis of cancer of the breast," in *Proceedings of the Round Table Conference on Cancer, Memorial Hospital, New York, New York, An-*

nals of Surgery 162 (1935): 233–38, on pp. 233, 238. "Early diagnosis" is in quotation marks in the text. In the 1930s Greenough headed the Committee on Treatment of Malignant Diseases of the American College of Surgeons.

10. Patterson, *The Dread Disease*.

11. Notes of William Sampson Handley (1862–1962) from 1894, series GC/152, box 1, Wellcome Library, Archives and Manuscripts Department, London, England (Wellcome Archives).

12. Sherwin B. Nulland, *William Steward Halsted, Surgical Scholar,* introductory pamphlet to William Steward Halsted, Surgical Papers (Birmingham: The Classics of Surgery Library, 1984).

13. R. Ledoux-Lebard, *La Lutte Contre le Cancer* (Paris: Masson, 1906), 85–90.

14. Gustave Roussy, "Autour du problème du cancer" *La Lutte Contre le Cancer* 6 (Jan.–Mar. 1929): 160–69.

15. Paterson, *The Dread Disease,* 56–87.

16. G. Jeannay, "Comment éviter et comment reconnaître le cancer de la langue," *La Lutte Contre le Cancer* 12 (July–Sept. 1934): 224–26.

17. Barbara Clow, "Who is afraid of Susan Sontag? Of the myth and metaphors of cancer reconsidered," *Social History of Medicine* 14 (2001): 293–312; Patterson, *The Dread Disease*.

18. R. Cale, J. P. Pilleron, and P. Schlinger, "Therapeutiques à visé conservatrice des épitheliomes mammaires," *Bulletin du Cancer* 69 (1973): 217–34.

19. Clow, "Who is afraid of Susan Sontag?" 301.

20. Poster included in *La Lutte Contre le Cancer* 7 (Apr.–June 1929). This poster was signed by Professor T. Maire and the dean of science faculty of Toulouse University, Paul Sabatier.

21. For example, R. Le Bret, "Autour du problème de cancer," *La Lutte Contre le Cancer* 6 (Jan.–Mar., 1929): 160–69; Professor Forge, "Le cancer du sein peut être guéri s'il est traité dès son débout," *La Lutte Contre le Cancer* 9 (July–Sept. 1931): 14–17; Robert Le Bret, "Lorsqu'on le soigne à ses debouts, le cancer est très souvent guérissable," *La Lutte Contre le Cancer* 12 (July–Sept. 1934): 211–14; and for discussion, Patrice Pinell, *Naissance d'un Fléau* (Paris: Anne Marie Metaillé, 1992) English version, *The Fight against Cancer: France 1890–1940,* trans. David Maddell [London: Routledge, 2002]). In the United States, surgeons not radiotherapists played a central role in the development of oncology.

22. French activists noticed this difference, e.g., Germaine Lavignac, "La lutte anti-cancereuse aux Etats Unis," *La Lutte Contre le Cancer* 5 (Jan.–Mar. 1928): 139–50.

23. Undated British Empire Cancer Campaign (BECC) internal document, probably early to mid-1920s; Memorandum on cancer, prepared by Departmental Committee on Cancer, appointed by the Minister of Health, and chaired by Sir George Numann, published July 1923, box 90, BECC papers, Collection SA/CRC, Wellcome Library, Archives and Manuscripts Department, London, England (Wellcome Archives).

24. Malcolm Donaldson, "A plea for periodical examination to reduce the mortality from cancer," *The Practitioner,* 129 (Aug. 1932), 209–15, box 92, BECC papers,

Wellcome Archives; undated BECC internal document, probably late 1930s, folder, "Propaganda 1936–1939," box 90, BECC papers, Wellcome Archives.

25. *Advice for Medical Lecturers Who Speak to Lay Public,* leaflet, 1936, box 90, BECC papers, Wellcome Archives.

26. Lesley J. Reagan, "Engendering the dread disease: Women, men and cancer," *American Journal of Public Health* 87 (1997): 1779–87.

27. From Maurice B. Judd, "Art aids the doctor," *Hygiea* 17 (Feb. 1939), reproduced in Reagan, "Engendering the dread disease."

28. Kirsten Elizabeth Gardner, *Early Detection: Women, Cancer, and Awareness Campaigns in the Twentieth-Century United States* (Chapel Hill: University of North Carolina Press, 2006), 53–92.

29. Gardner, *Early Detection,* 60n17; Reagan, "Engendering the dread disease," 1781.

30. Lester Breslow, "The prevention of cancer," in *Cancer,* ed. Ronald W. Raven (London: Butterworth & Co, 1959), 6:464–93, on p. 469. The link between cigarette smoking and lung cancer was demonstrated in the 1950s, but at that time smoking was not seen as a major public health problem. Allan Brandt, *The Cigarette Century: The Rise, Fall and Deadly Persistence of the Product That Defined America* (New York: Basis Books, 2007); Virginia Berridge, *Marketing Health: Smoking and the Discourse of Public Health in Britain 1945–2000* (Oxford: Oxford University Press, 2007).

31. Le Bret, "Autour du problème de cancer."

32. Emerson Day, "Value of simple procedures in cancer examination," in *Cancer,* ed. Ronald W. Raven (London: Butterworth & Co, 1959), 3:445–57, on pp. 448–51; Breslow, "The prevention of cancer," 485–86. Day was the director of the division of preventive medicine of Sloan Kettering Institute for Cancer Research, New York.

33. George N. Papanicolaou and Herbert F. Traut, "The diagnostic value of vaginal spears in carcinoma of the uterus," *American Journal of Obstetrics and Gynecology* 42 (1941): 193–206, on pp. 193–94.

34. J. E. Ayre, "A simple officine test for cancer diagnosis," *Journal of the Canadian Medical Association* 51 (1944): 17–22; L. H. Lombard, M. Middletown, S. Warren, and O. Gates, "The use of vaginal smears as a screening test," *New England Journal of Medicine* 238 (1948): 867–71; Heinz Grunze and Arthur I. Spriggs, *History of Clinical Cytology* (Darmstadt: Verlag Ernst Giebler, 1980), 88–90.

35. Charlotte A. Jones, Theodore Neustaaedeter, and Locke L. MacKenzie, "The value of vaginal smears in the diagnosis of early malignancy," *American Journal of Obstetrics and Gynecology* 49 (1945): 159–68.

36. Claudius Regaud, "L'organisation et les conditions d'efficacité de la lutte contre le cancer d'utérus," *Archives de l'Institut du Radium* 2 (1930): 81–94.

37. Walter Schiller, "Early diagnosis of carcinoma of the cervix," *Surgery, Gynecology and Obstetrics* 56 (1933): 212–22, on p. 222.

38. Walter Schiller, "Clinical behavior of early carcinoma of the cervix," *Surgery, Gynecology and Obstetrics* 66 (1938): 129–40.

39. "Advancement of science," *Time,* Jan. 11, 1937.

40. E. Forgue, "Pour le diagnostique acceleré de cancer du col utérin," *La Lutte*

Contre le Cancer 13 (July–Sept. 1935): 138–46; Annual report of the Curie Foundation for 1932. Minutes from the meeting of the Foundation's administration council of May 4, 1934, Archives of the Curie Institute.

41. Bayard Carter, Kenneth Cuyler, Walter L. Thomas, Robert Creadick, and Robert Alter, "The methods of management of carcinoma in situ of the cervix," *American Journal of Obstetrics and Gynecology* 64 (1952): 833–45.

42. Ibid., 834–36.

43. John E. Dunn, "The relationships between carcinoma in situ and invasive cervical carcinoma: A consideration of the contribution to the problem to be made from general population data," *Cancer* 6 (1953): 873–86.

44. Georges Gricouroff, "Différenciation pratique et dogmatique entre lesions benignes et lesions malignes," *Acta Union Internationale Contre le Cancer* 10 (1954): 125–36, on p. 134.

45. Leopold G. Koss, Fred Stewart, Frank Foote, et al., "Some histological aspects of behavior of epidermoid carcinoma in situ and related lesions of uterine cervix. A long term prospective study," *Cancer* 12 (1963): 1160–1211.

46. Koss, Stewart, Foote, et al., "Some histological aspects of behavior"; R. Morocard, "Anatomie pathologique des epitheliomas intraepithéliaux du col utérin: Essai de définir le stade 0," *Journal de Chirurgie* 71 (1955): 737–41; C. Gad, "The management and the natural history of severe dysplasia and carcinoma in situ of the uterine cervix," *British Journal of Obstetrics and Gynecology* 83 (1976): 554–59.

47. J. L. Benedet, G. H Anderson, M. L. Simpson, and D. Shaw, "Colposcopy, conization and hysterectomy practices: A current perspective, *Obstetrics and Gynecology* 60 (1982): 539–45.

48. Daniel McSweeney and Donald G. McKay, "Uterine cancer: Its early detection by simple screening methods," *New England Journal of Medicine,* 238 (1948): 867–70.

49. Howard C. Taylor, "Controversial points in the treatment of carcinoma of the cervix," *Cancer* 5 (1952): 435–41, on p. 437.

50. Adele E. Clarke and Monica J. Casper, "From simple technology to complex arena: Classification of Pap Smears, 1917–1990," *Medical Anthropology Quarterly* 10 (1996): 601–23.

51. Edward E. Sieler, "Microdiagnosis of carcinoma in situ of the uterine cervix," *Cancer* 9 (1956): 463–69.

52. Ibid., 469.

53. A. D. Govan, M. R. Haiens, F. A. Langley, C. W. Taylor, and A. S. Woodcock, "The histology and cytology of changes in the epithelium of the cervix uteri," *Journal of Clinical Pathology* 22 (1969): 383–95.

54. P. C. Meyer, "Diagnosis of preinvasive carcinoma of the uterine cervix," *Journal of Clinical Pathology* 18 (1965): 414–23.

55. Peter Keating and Alberto Cambrosio, *Biomedical Platforms: Realigning the Normal and the Pathological in Twentieth Century Medicine* (Cambridge, MA: MIT Press, 2003).

56. See, for example, a letter from Edward Rimley to Charles Cameron, medical and scientific director of American Cancer Society (ACS), from July 6, 1955, on the

importance of endorsing Pap smears by the ACS, Mary Lasker Papers, Box 98, Columbia University Health Sciences Library, Archives and Special Collections, Columbia University, New York, New York (Columbia University Health Services Library); letter of Eugene Pendergrass, chairman of the committee on professional and public education of ACS, to Mary Lasker, Oct. 10, 1956, on the importance of including Pap smears in doctors' annual checkups, Mary Lasker Papers, box 99, Columbia University Health Sciences Library.

57. Eftychia Vayena, "Cancer detectors: An international history of the Pap test and cervical cancer screening, 1928–1970," PhD thesis, University of Minnesota, 1999. Vayena's unpublished thesis is a detailed study of ACS's role in the implementation of Pap smear in the United States.

58. H. Gilbert Welch, "Editorial: Right and wrong reasons to be screened," *Annals of Internal Medicine* 140 (2004): 754–55.

59. Monica J. Casper and Adele E. Clarke, "Making Pap smear into the 'right tool' for the job: Cervical cancer screening in the USA, circa 1940–1995," *Social Studies of Science* 28 (1998); 255–90.

60. Leopold G. Koss, "Precancerous lesions," in *Persons at High Risk of Cancer: An Approach to Cancer Etiology and Control,* ed. Joseph F. Fraumeni (New York: Academic Press, 1975), 85–101, on p. 87; Leopold Koss, "Dysplasia: A real concept or a misnomer," *Obstetrics and Gynecology* 51 (1978): 374–79.

61. Casper and Clarke, "Making Pap smear into the 'right tool' for the job."

62. Petersen, *Precancerous Changes of the Cervical Epithelium,* 27–28.

63. M. Gronroos, P. Hautera, O. Jarvi, S. Kangas, L. Rauramo, "Cytology and colposcopy in mass screening for cervical cancer," *Acta Cytologica* 11 (1967): 37–38; Leopold G. Koss, "The Papanicolau test for cervical cancer detection: A triumph and a tragedy," *JAMA* 261 (1989): 737–43.

64. Quoted by Per Kolstad, "Carcinoma of the cervix, stage 0: Diagnosis and treatment," *American Journal of Obstetrics and Gynecology* 96 (1966): 1098–1111, on p. 1109.

65. J. Curtial, "Sur le dépistage précoce des cancers," *La Lutte Contre le Cancer* 30 (Jan.–Mar., 1952): 7–11.

66. Papers of the Arthur Purdy Stout Society of surgical pathologists, 1957–1986, box 1, folder 6, undated, probably 1970s, Columbia University Health Sciences Library.

67. H. W. Jones and R. E. Butler, "The treatment of cervical intraepithelial neoplasia by cone biopsy," *American Journal of Obstetrics and Gynecology* 137 (1980): 882–86; Benedet, Anderson, Simpson, and Shaw, "Colposcopy, conization and hysterectomy practices; Kolstad, "Carcinoma of the cervix, stage 0: Diagnosis and treatment."

68. A. I. Springgs, "Precancerous states of the cervix uteri," in *Precancerous States,* ed. R. L. Carter (Oxford: Oxford University Press, 1984), 317–53; M. C. Anderson, C. L. Brown, C. H. Buckley, et al., "Current views on cervical intraepithelial neoplasia," *Journal of Clinical Pathology* 44 (1991): 969–78; S. Payne, N. M. Kernohan, and F. Walker, "Proliferation in the normal cervix and in preinvasive cervical lesions," *Journal of Clinical Pathology* 49 (1996): 667–71; Koss, "Dysplasia," 79; Koss, "The Papanicolaou test for cervical cancer detection.

69. Guido de Manjo and Isabelle Joris, *Cells Tissues and Disease: Principles of General Pathology* (Oxford: Blackwell, 1996), 867–83, on p. 875, italics in the text.

70. D. Salomon, D. Davey, R. Kurman, et al., "The 2001 Bethesda system: Terminology for reporting results of cervical cytology," *JAMA* 287 (2002): 2114–19; T. C. Wright, J. T. Cox, L. S .Massad, et al., "Consensus guidelines for the management of women with cervical cytological abnormalities," *JAMA* 287 (2002): 2120–29.

71. Malcolm Donaldson, "Education of the public concerning cancer," Medical Officer, Sept. 9, 1950, box 90, BECC papers, series SA/CRC, Wellcome Archives. ACS was especially active in promoting diagnosis of precancerous conditions. Such conditions were found in a high number of people who consulted ACS's sponsored cancer detection clinics.

72. Series SA/MWF, Documents of the Medical Women Federation, file F.13/3, Wellcome Archives.

73. Preliminary debates on cervical cancer screening, House of Lords, vol. 269, no. 120, Nov. 2, 1965, Documents of the Medical Women Federation, file F.13/3, Wellcome Archives.

74. Julian Snow, the parliamentary secretary to the Minister of Health, to Joyce Butler, MP, the president of Women's Campaign, July 12, 1967, Documents of the Medical Women Federation, file F.13/3, Wellcome Archives.

75. Press conference of Minister of Health, Kenneth Robinson, on cervical cytology, Oct. 21, 1966. Documents of the Medical Women Federation, file F.13/4, Wellcome Archives.

76. Women's National Cancer Control Campaign (previously National Cervical Cancer Prevention Campaign), Report on activities, 1968, Documents of the Medical Women Federation, file F.13/5, Wellcome Archives.

77. Talk, by John Wakefield, Head of Dept. of Social Research, Christie Hospital, and Holt Radium Institute, and chairman of the committee on public education of International Union Against Cancer, Mar. 27, 1968, Documents of the Medical Women Federation, file F.13/5, Wellcome Archives.

78. Report from mobile unit in Hackney, summer 1969, Documents of the Medical Women Federation, file F.13/6, Wellcome Archives.

79. Vicky Singleton, "Actor networks and ambivalence: General Practitioners in the UK cervical screening program," *Social Studies of Science* 23 (1993): 227–64; Vicky Singleton, "Stabilizing instabilities: The role of the laboratory in the United Kingdom cervical screening program," in *Differences in Medicine: Unraveling Practices, Techniques and Bodies,* ed. Marc Berg and Anne Marie Mol (Durham: Duke University Press, 1998), 86–103.

80. Series SA/MWF, Documents of the Medical Women Federation, file F.13/10, Wellcome Archives; documents from the Meeting of the "Film Working Party of the Women's National Cancer Control Campaign," Dec. 13, 1967.

81. David Cantor, "Uncertain enthusiasm: The American Cancer Society, public education and the problem of the movie, 1921–1960," *Bulletin of the History of Medicine* 81 (2007): 39–69.

82. Louise B. Russell, *Is Prevention Worse Than Cure?* (Washington DC: The Brookings Institution, 1986).

83. Editorial, "Diagnostic problems in cervical cancer," *British Medical Journal* 1 (1974): 471; Editorial, "Cancer of the cervix: Death by incompetence," *The Lancet* 326 (1985): 363–64; Angela R. Raffle, B. Alden, and E. D. Mackenzie, "Detection rates for abnormal cervical screens: What we are screening for?" *The Lancet* 345 (1995): 1469–73.

84. Julian Peto, Clare Gilham, Olivia Fletcher, and Fiona E. Matthews, "The cervical cancer epidemic that screening has prevented in the UK," *The Lancet* 364 (2004): 249–56.

85. Ruth Etzioni and David B. Thomas, "Modeling the effect of screening for cervical cancer on the population," *The Lancet* 364 (2004): 224–26. See also debate on the article by Peto et al. in *The Lancet* 364 (2004): 1483–85. The reduction of incidence of cervical cancer, critics of Peto and his colleagues propose, started well before the generalization of the Pap smear. The incidence of another malignancy induced by an infectious agent, stomach cancer (this malignancy is associated with the infection by the bacterium *Helicobacter pylori*) declined precipitously in the majority of Western countries, without medical intervention.

86. D. R. Brunet, in the name of the working group on cervical cancer screening, "Rapport au sujet de l'organization d'une campagne de dépistage du cancer du col de l'uterus en France," Ministre de la Santé, Direction Generale de la Santé, Commission du Cancer de Conseil Permanent d'Hygiène, Nov. 24, 1976, folder: Commission du Cancer, Archives of the Institut National de la Santé et de la Recherche Médicale (INSERM Archives).

87. R. Laumonier and C. Marsan, "Rapport sur la formation, les activities et les responsabilités des cytotechniciens," Ministre de la Santé, Direction Generale de la Santé, Commission du Cancer de Conseil Permanent d'Hygiène, June 1976, folder: Commission du Cancer, INSERM Archives.

88. A. Sicard, "L'introduction des frottis cervico-vaginaux en France," *Bulletin de l'Academie de Médicine* 180 (1996): 1109–13; A. Garnier, C. Exbrayat, M. Bolla, et al., "Une campagne de dépistage de cancer du col avec des frottis vaginaux," *Bulletin de Cancer* 84 (1997): 791–95.

89. In France medical gynecology is a feminine specialty oriented toward routine surveillance of women's reproductive health. Medical gynecologists are concentrated in the cities. Women living outside important cities, and those from more modest socioeconomic strata, are usually followed by their GPs.

90. Nora Liberetto, master's thesis, Paris, Ecole des Hautes Etudes en Science Sociale, 2005.

91. G. Dubois, "Cytologic screening for cervix cancer: Each year or each 3 years," *European Journal of Obstetrics, Gynecology and Reproductive Medicine* 65 (1996): 57–59.

92. Institut National du Cancer, "Bilan Plan Cancer 2003–2006: Dépistage: Des avantages quantitatives et qualitatives," Paris: 2006. Institute de Cancer experts found the number of people receiving Pap smears in France unacceptably low (according to this document, only 7% of American women do not have regular cervical smears);

however, the incidence of cervical cancer in France is not higher than in other Western European countries or than in the United States.

93. This problem was evoked in debates on the introduction of the 1999 Breast and Cervical Cancer Prevention and Treatment Act, "Breast and cervical cancer federally funded screening programs." Hearings before the subcommittee on health and environment of the committee on commerce, House of Representatives, 106 sess., on H.R. 1070, July 21, 1999 (Washington, DC: U.S. Government Printing Office, 1999).

94. B. E. Sirovich and H. G. Welch, "The frequency of Pap smear screening in the United States," *Journal of General Internal Medicine* 19 (2004): 243–50.

95. G. F. Sawaya, J. McConnell, S. L. Kulasingam, et al., "Risk of cervical cancer associations with extending the interval between cancer screenings," *New England Journal of Medicine* 349 (2003): 1501–9.

96. Andran A. Renshaw, "Editorial: Increased cervical cancer risk screening intervals: A risky investment," *Diagnostic Cytology* 30 (2004): 137–38. Renshaw's claim is that an increased frequency of screening is always beneficial to the individual health care user.

97. F. Gagnon, "Contribution to the study of etiology and prevention of cancer of the cervix of the uterus," *American Journal of Obstetrics and Gynecology* 60 (1950): 516–22; Johannes Clemmesen, "On the etiology of some human cancers," *Journal of the National Cancer Institute*, 12 (1951): 1–22.

98. This claim was illustrated by data on incidence of cervical cancers in Los Angeles County: the number of cases per year and per 100,000 women was 8.8% for White women, 16.1% for Black, 17.4% for U.S.-born Mexican Americans, and 31.4% for Mexico-born Mexican Americans. Brian E. Henderson, "Sexual factors and pregnancy," in *Persons at High Risk of Cancer: An Approach to Cancer Etiology and Control*, 267–83, table p. 275. Frederick Hoffman had noted already that cancer of the uterus was twice as frequent among Black women as among Whites, but he explained this difference by a presumed "racial susceptibility" of the Black, not by differences in sexual behavior. Frederick L. Hoffman, "Cancer in the North American Negro," *American Journal of Surgery and Gynecology*, 22 (1908–9): 229–63.

99. M. Durst, L. Gissmann L. H. Ikenberg, and H. zur Hausen, "A papillomavirus DNA from a cervical carcinoma and its prevalence in cancer biopsy samples from different geographic regions," *Proceedings of the National Academy of Science* 80 (1983): 3812–15; P. J. Baird, "Serological evidence for the association of papillomavirus and cervical neoplasia," *The Lancet* 322 (1983): 17–18. Premalignant transformations were related mainly to infection with two HPV strains, HPV-16 and HPV-18. R. Reid, "Genital warts and cervical cancer. II: Is human papillomavirus infection the trigger to cervical carcinogenesis?" *Gynecologic Oncology* 15 (1983): 239–52.

100. The difficulty in homogenizing readings of Pap smears continues to be a cause for concern for experts. See, for example, S. Ruba, M. Schoolland, S. Allpress, and G. Sterrett, "Adenocarcinoma in situ of the uterine cervix: Screening and diagnostic errors in Papanicolaou smears," *Cancer* 102 (2004): 280–87.

101. Mark Schiffman, "Human Papilloma virus and cervical cancer," *The Lancet* 370 (2007): 890–907; Carolyn D. Runowicz, "Molecular screening of cervical cancer: Time to give up Pap tests?" *New England Journal of Medicine* 357 (2007): 1650–52.

102. James S. McCormick, "Cervical smears: A questionable practice?" *The Lancet* 334 (1989): 207–9; Linda McKie, "The art of surveillance of reasonable prevention? The case of cervical cancer screening," *Sociology of Health and Illness* 17 (1995): 441–57.

103. Jeremy Groopman, "Contagion: Papilloma virus," *The New Yorker*, Sept. 13, 1999.

104. Editorial, "Outcome of pregnancy after a cone biopsy," *British Medical Journal* i (1980): 1393–94; McCormick, "Cervical smears." On a—rare—discussion of pain and suffering following "routine" biopsies, see Vered Levy-Barzilai, "Hey doc— It hurts," *Haaretz*, Apr. 14, 2006.

105. Ruba, Schoolland, Alpress, and Sterrett, "Adenocarcinoma in situ of the uterine cervix." Aggressive attitudes of some U.S. doctors toward the prevention of gynecological cancers were studied by Sue Fisher. Sue Fisher, *In the Patient's Best Interest: Women and the Politics of Medical Decisions* (New Brunswick, NJ: Rutgers University Press, 1986).

106. Patricia A. Kaufert, "Screening the body: The Pap smear and the mammogram," in *Living and Working with the New Medical Technologies*, ed. Margaret Lock, Allan Young, and Alberto Cambrosio (Cambridge: Cambridge University Press, 2000), 165–83.

107. McKie, "The art of surveillance or reasonable prevention."

108. Annette Forss, Carol Tishelman, Catarina Widmark, and Lisbeth Sachs, "Women's experiences of cervical cellular changes: An unintentional transition from health to liminality?" *Sociology of Health and Illness* 26 (2004): 306–25.

109. Gilbert Welch, *Should I Be Tested for Cancer: Maybe Not, And Here's Why* (Berkeley and Los Angeles: University of California Press, 2004).

110. On trauma of local treatment for cervical dysplasia, see Nicky Britten, "Personal view: Colposcopy," *British Medical Journal* 1 (1988): 296.

111. Naomi Pfeffer, "If you think you have a lump they'll screen you: Informed consent and health promotion," *Journal of Medical Ethics* 30 (2004): 227–30.

112. Forss, Tishelman, Widmark, and Sachs, "Women's experiences of cervical cellular changes."

113. In French the word *screening* (criblage) is reserved for the testing of pharmaceutically active substances and for a selection of a few active compounds among many studied.

114. Nicolas Rose, "Genetic risk and the birth of the somatic individual," *Economy and Society* 29 (2000): 485–513; Nicolas Rose, "The politics of life itself," *Theory, Culture and Society* 18 (2001): 1–30.

115. Deborah Lupton, "Taming uncertainty: Risk discourse and diagnostic testing," in D. Lupton, *The Imperative of Health: Public Health and the Regulated Body* (London: Sage, 1995), 77–105; Kaufman, "Screening the body."

Chapter Six · The Generalization of Screening

1. Kirsten E. Gardner, *Early Detection: Women, Cancer and Awareness Campaigns in the Twentieth Century United States* (Chapel Hill: University of North Carolina Press, 2006), 217.

2. Leopold G. Koss, "From koilocytosis to molecular biology: The impact of cytology on concepts of early human cancer," *Modern Pathology* 2 (1989): 526–35. However, it should be noted that other tumors, such as head and neck malignancies, do not progress in a regular and predictable way. Pierre Denoix and G. Violet, "Données sur la durée d'evolution de certains cancers," *Bulletin de l'Institut National d'Hygiène* 3 (Oct.–Dec. 1948): 523–25.

3. Ian MacDonald, "Biological predetermism in human cancer," *Surgery, Gynecology and Obstetrics* 92 (1951): 443–52; Neil McKinnon, "The present status of the treatment and the diagnosis of cancer of the breast," *Canadian Medical Association Journal* 78 (1958): 781–85.

4. Bushke to Lentz, Aug. 19, 1957. Lenz's papers, box 1, folder 12. Columbia University Health Sciences Library, Archives and Special Collections, Columbia University (Columbia University Health Sciences Library).

5. Barron Lerner, *The Breast Cancer Wars: Hope Fear and the Pursuit of Cure in Twentieth Century America* (New York: Oxford University Press, 2001), 92–114.

6. Lester Breslow, "The prevention of cancer," in *Cancer,* ed. Ronald W. Raven (London: Butterworth & Co, 1959), 6:464–93, on p. 479. French experts made the same point in 1952. Groupe de travail sur le cancer du col, "Cancer du col d'utérus: Definition du stade '0,'" *Bulletin de l'Institut National d'Hygiène* 7 (1952): 549–54.

7. Robert Sutherland, *Cancer: The Significance of Delay* (London: Butterworth & Co, 1960).

8. Ibid., viii; 8–9, 47.

9. Ibid., 13, 14. Such evaluation is possible only in "accessible" cancers.

10. Ibid., 147–50.

11. Ibid., 195, 202.

12. Not all oncologists accepted a parallel between breast and cervical cancers. By the early twentieth century, some specialists argued that these two malignancies were very different and that one should not extrapolate from one to the other. This was, however, a minority opinion. Ornella Moscucci, "The 'ineffable freemasonry of sex': Feminist surgeons and the establishment of radiotherapy in early twentieth century Britain," *Bulletin of the History of Medicine* 81 (2007): 139–63.

13. William R. Hendee, "History and status of X-ray mammography," *Health Physics* 69 (1995): 636–48.

14. Early history of mammography in the United States was studied by Robert Aronowitz. R. Aronowitz, *Unnatural History: Breast Cancer and American Society* (New York: Cambridge University Press, 2007).

15. Sam Shapiro, Philip Strax, and Louis Vernet, "Evaluation of periodic breast cancer screening with mammography: Methodology and early observations," *JAMA* 196 (1966): 731–38. On reevaluation of the Canadian trial, see C. K. Baines, "The Canadian National Breast Cancer Screening Study: A perspective on criticism," *Annals of Internal Medicine* 120 (1994): 326–34.

16. Some activists protested nevertheless against what they saw as systematic confusion between prevention and early detection. See, for example, Maryann Napoli, "Early breast cancer detection reconsidered" *Medical Self-Care* (Summer 1983): 19–

22, series 99M147, box 3, documents of the Raising Sun Alliance, Boston Women Health Book Collective Archives.

17. "Use of mammography, United States, 1990," *CDC- Morbidity and Mortality Weekly Reports* 39 (1990): 621–30.

18. Funds for screening were obtained thanks to the vote of the Breast and Cervical Cancer Mortality Prevention Action of 1990. D. S. May, M. R. Nadel, R. M. Henson, and D. S. Miller, "The National Breast and Cervical Early Detection Program: Report on the first 4 years of mammography provided to medically undeserved women," *American Journal of Roentgenology* 170 (1998): 97–104. The Centers for Disease Control and Prevention program pays for detection but not for treatment of detected cancer: states and municipalities organize such treatment programs for uninsured women, with variable efficacy.

19. Cut from *New York Post* of Jan. 19, 1976, Barbara Seaman papers, 82-M33–84-M82, box 2, folder 107, Arthur and Elizabeth Schlesinger Library on the History of Women in America, Radcliffe Institute of Advanced Study, Harvard University (Schlesinger Library).

20. Curtis Merlin and Charles R. Smart, "Breast cancer detection guidelines for women aged 40 to 49: Rationale for American Cancer Society reaffirmation of recommendations," *CA: Cancer Journal for Clinicians* 44 (1994), 248–55; Charles Smart, R. E. Hendrick, J. H. Routledge, and R. A. Smith, "Benefits of mammography screening in women aged 40 to 49 years: Current evidence from clinical trials," *Cancer* 75 (1995): 1619–26.

21. The vigor of such protests reflected, among other things, the rise of breast cancer activism in the 1980s and 1990s and the growing public visibility of this disease. On breast cancer activism, see, e.g., Sharon Batt, *Patient No More: The Politics of Breast Cancer* (Charlottetown, PEI, Canada: Gynergy Books, 1994); Roberta Altman, *Waking Up / Fighting Back: The Politics of Breast Cancer* (Boston: Little Brown, 1996); Maureen Hogan Casamayou, *The Politics of Breast Cancer* (Washington DC: Georgetown University Press, 2001), and for a more critical view of such activism, see Samantha King, *Pink Ribbons, Inc., Breast Cancer and the Politics of Philanthropy* (Minneapolis: University of Minnesota Press, 2006).

22. Breast cancer is a leading cause of mortality of women between the age of 40 and 50, an age at which the overall mortality of Western women is very low.

23. "National Cancer Institute's revision of its mammography guidelines," Hearings before the Human Resources and Intergovernmental Relations Subcommittee of the Committee on government operations, House of Representatives, 103rd Congress, 2nd sess., Mar. 8, 1994 (Washington, DC: U.S. Government Printing Office, 1994).

24. "Misused science: The National Cancer Institute's elimination of mammography guidelines for women in their forties." Sixteenth report by the Committee on Government Operations to the committee of the Whole House on the State of the Union, Oct. 20, 1994 (Washington, DC: U.S. Government Printing Office, 1994).

25. Susan Fletcher, "Whither scientific deliberation in health policy recommendations? Alice in the Wonderland of breast cancer screening," *New England Journal of*

Medicine 336 (1997): 1180–83. The screening controversy was studied by David Cantor. David Cantor, "When experts disagree: Public trust and the controversy over the screening of healthy women in their 40s," paper given at the conference "Sites and Styles: Exploring the comparative history of cancer," Manchester, England, Mar. 22–24, 2007. See also Robert A. Aronowitz, "Situating Health Risks: An Opportunity for Disease Prevention Policy," in *History and Health Policy in the United States: Putting the Past Back In*, ed. Charles Rosenberg, Rosemary Stevens, and Lawton R. Burns (New Brunswick, NJ: Rutgers University Press, 2006) 153–65.

26. Ismail Jatoi and Michael Baum, "American and European recommendations for screening mammography in younger women: A cultural divide?" *British Medical Journal* 307 (1993): 481–83.

27. Letter from the Medical Women Federation secretary, Dr. Jean Lawrie, to Mrs. Dorothy Leschinski, secretary of Public Affairs Subcommittee of the National Federation of Women's Institutes, Oct. 15, 1975, Documents of the Medical Women Federation, file F.13/5, Wellcome Archives, Wellcome Library, London, England (Wellcome Archives).

28. Statement by the British Breast Group of 9/8/75. Documents of the Medical Women Federation, file F.13/5, Wellcome Archives.

29. Patrick Forrest (chair), *Breast Cancer Screening: Report to the Health Ministers of England, Wales, Scotland and Northern Ireland* (London: Her Majesty's Stationery Office, 1986).

30. K. Gerard, J. Bron, and K. Johnston, "UK breast screening programme: How it reflects the Forrest recommendations," *Journal of Medical Screening* 4 (1997): 10–15; R. Smith Bindman, R. Ballard-Barbash, D. L. Migliorettin, et al., "Comparing the performance of mammography screening in the USA and the UK," *Journal of Medical Screening* 12 (2005): 50–54.

31. P. Schaffer, "Dépistage: Un acte médical déontologique et technique particulière," in *Dépistage des Cancers: De la Médecine à la Santé Publique*, ed. H. Sancho-Garner, C. Béraud, J. F. Doré, J. Pierret, and P. Schaffer (Paris: Editions INSERM, 1997), 17–28.

32. S. Wait, B. Schaffer, M. Séradou, et al., "Dépistage individuel du cancer du sein en France," *Bulletin du Cancer* 84 (1997): 619–24; Vincent Boissonat, "Un objet-réseau: Radiographie et dépistage du cancer de sein," in *Cooperations, Conflits et Concurences dans le Système de Santé*, ed. Genevieve Cresson (Rennes, France: Editions ENSP, 2003), 47–73.

33. C. Macia et al, "Quality control in mammography: An initiative in France," *The British Journal of Radiology* 67 (1994): 371–83.

34. http://sante-medecine.commentcamarche.net/cancer/13_le-cancer-du-sein .php3. Between 1995 and 2005, the introduction of regional and national mammography programs in France did not change mortality trends. Brigitte Séradour and R. Ancelle- Park, "Dépistage organisé des cancers du sein: Peut-on comparer les résultats du programme français aux résultats internationaux?" *Journal de Radiologie* 87 (2006): 1009–14.

35. Gardner, *Early Detection;* Barron Lerner, "When statistics provide unsatisfying

answers: Revisiting the breast self-examination controversy," *Canadian Medical Association Journal* 166 (2002): 199–201.

36. J. Wardle, A. Steptoe, H. Smith, et al., "Breast self examination: Attitudes and practices among young women in Europe," *European Journal of Cancer Prevention* 4 (1995): 61–68; François Eisinger, G. Geller, W. Burke, and N. A. Holtzman. "Cultural basis for differences between US and French clinical recommendations for women at increased risk of breast and ovarian cancer," *The Lancet* 353 (1999): 919–20.

37. Nancy Baxter, with the Canadian Task Force on Preventive Health Care, "Should women be routinely taught to screen for breast cancer?" *Canadian Medical Association Journal* 164 (2001), 1837–46; Beverly B. Green and Stephen H. Taplin, "Breast cancer screening controversies," *Journal of the American Board of Family Medicine* 16 (2003): 233–41; A. K. Hackshaw and E. A. Paul, "Breast self-examination and death from breast cancer: A meta-analysis," *British Journal of Cancer* 88 (2003): 1047–53.

38. Lerner, "When statistics provide unsatisfying answers."

39. Sarah Lochlann Jain, "Living in prognosis: Toward an elegiac politics," *Representations* 98 (2007): 77–92, on p. 88.

40. Philip Strax, "Control of breast cancer through mass screening: From research to action," *Cancer* 63 (1989): 1881–87.

41. Joanne G. Elmore, Mary B. Barton, Victoria M. Moeri, et al., "Ten year risk of false positive screening mammograms," *New England Journal of Medicine* 338 (1998): 1089–96.

42. Tibor Tot, "The limited prognostic value of measuring and grading small invasive breast carcinomas," *Medical Science Monitor* 12 (2006): 170–75.

43. Rose Kushner, intervention at National Cancer Institute conference on in situ cancers (undated, probably 1980), Kushner's papers, MC 453, box 3, folder 34, Schlesinger Library. See also Kushner's notes on this subject, box 2, folder 22.

44. Maurice S. Fox, "On the diagnosis and treatment of breast cancer," *JAMA* 241 (1979); 489–94. Fox analyzed survival of women treated for breast cancer in the United States from the 1940s to the 1970s. His call to take biological variability among tumors of the breast into account when interpreting results of treatment may be contrasted, e.g., with 2008 comments on an audit, conducted by the National Health Service (NHS) Breast Screening Programme (United Kingdom), on outcomes for women diagnosed with breast cancer through mammographic screening in 1990–1991 and 2000–2001. The audit had found that 61% of women whose cancers are detected by screening have the same life expectancy as women who never had cancer; this result was presented by NHS experts as a proof of efficacy of the screening program. It was greeted by press headlines such as "Breast cancer victims have normal lifespan—If it is detected early enough" (*The Times*, June 11, 2008); "Women's lifespan unchanged if cancer is seen early" (*Independent*, June 11, 2008); "Women with breast cancer can live as long as healthy women thanks to screening, says study" (*Daily Mail*, June 11, 2008).

45. Rose Kushner, ms of conference, "Early detection of cancer." Rose Kushner papers, box 2, folder 33, Schlesinger Library.

46. Rose Kushner, letter about planned TV program, of Apr. 11, 1978. Rose Kushner papers, box 2, folder 41, Schlesinger Library.

47. Lester Breslow, "The prevention of cancer," in *Cancer*, ed. Ronald W. Raven (London: Butterworth & Co, 1958), 6:464–493, on p. 479.

48. See, e.g., Indraneel Mitra, Michael Baum, Hazel Thronton, and Joan Hughton, "Is breast examination an acceptable alternative to mammographic screening?" *British Medical Journal* 321 (2000): 1071–73; Michael Baum, "Editorial: Breast cancer screening comes full circle," *Journal of the National Cancer Institute* 96 (2004): 1490–91.

49. Peter C. Gøtzsche and Ole Olsen, "Is screening for breast cancer from mammography justifiable," *The Lancet* 355 (2000): 129–34. Specialists agree that changes in breast cancer treatment contributed to the reduction of mortality from this disease in the 1970s and 1980s, when the clinical trials of mammography were conducted, but many contest Gøtzsche's and Olsen's affirmation that this was the only cause of the decrease in mortality from breast cancer. Henry de Koning, "Assessment of nationwide cancer-screening programs," *The Lancet* 355 (2000): 80–81; Donald A. Berry, Kathleen A. Cronin, Sylvia K. Piervritis, et al., "Effect of screening and adjuvant therapy on mortality from breast cancer," *New England Journal of Medicine* 353 (2005): 1784–92.

50. P. G. Gill, G. Farshid, C. G. Luke and D. M. Roder, "Detection by screening mammography is a powerful independent predictor of survival of women diagnosed with breast cancer," *The Breast*, 13 (2004): 15–22

51. Peggy L. Porter, A. Y. Bastawissi, M. T. Mandelson, et al., "Breast tumor characteristics as predictors of mammographic detection: comparison of interval- and screen-detected cancers." *Journal of the National Cancer Institute* 93 (2001): 151–52; Welch, *Should I Be Screened For Cancer*, 79–81.

52. See, for example, P. H. Zahl, B. H. Strand, and J. Maehlen, "Incidence of breast cancer in Norway and Sweden during introduction of nationwide screening: Prospective cohort study," *British Medical Journal* 328 (2004): 921–24. Some cancer specialists questioned the choice to fund screening for breast cancer rather than other public health interventions. Richard R. Love, Susan M. Love, and Adriano V. Laudico, "Breast cancer from a public health perspective," *The Breast Journal* 2 (2004): 136–40.

53. William C. Black, David A. Haggstrom, and H. Gilbert Welsh, "All-cause mortality in randomized trials of cancer screening," *Journal of the National Cancer Institute* 94 (2002): 167–73; Helen G. Juffs and Ian F. Tannock, "Editorial: Screening trials are even more difficult than we thought they were," *Journal of the National Cancer Institute* 94 (2002): 156–57.

54. George J. Cunningham, "The general pathology of malignant tumors," in *Cancer*, ed. Ronald W. Raven (London: Butterworth & Co, 1959), 2:1–27. Cunningham was a professor of pathology and responsible for pathological collections at the Royal College of Surgeons of England.

55. See, for example, Jehuda Folkman and Raghu Kalluri, "Cancer without disease," *Nature* 427 (2004): 787; J. E. Montie, D. P. Wood, E. Pontes, J. M. Boyett, and H. S. Levin, "Adenocarcinoma of the prostate in cyroprostatectomy specimen re-

moved for bladder cancer" *Cancer,* 63 (1989): 381–85. For a review of the cancer reservoir problem, see Welch, *Should I Be Tested for Cancer,* 59–89.

56. M. Nielsen, J. Jensen, and J. Andersen, "Precancerous and cancerous lesions during lifetime and at autopsy," *Cancer* 54 (1984): 612–15.

57. M. Nielsen, J. L. Thomsen, S. Primdahl, U. Dyreborg, and J. A. Andersen, "Breast cancer and atypia among young and middle aged women: A study of 110 medicolegal autopsies," *British Journal of Cancer* 56 (1987): 814–19.

58. P. S. Bhathat, R.W. Brown, C. G. Lesseur and I. S. Russel, "Frequency of benign and malignant breast lesions in 207 consecutive autopsies in Australian women," *British Journal of Cancer* 51 (1985): 271–78.

59. Gilbert Welch and William C. Black, "Using autopsy series to estimate the 'disease reservoir' for ductal carcinoma in situ of the breast: How much more cancer can we find?" *Annals of Internal Medicine* 127 (1997): 1023–28. Welch and Black point to important discrepancies between findings in autopsy studies. They attribute such discrepancies to differences in pathologists' definition of in situ carcinoma of the breast.

60. The correlation between number of analyzed slices of tissue and probability of uncovering cancerous or precancerous lesions was studied in prostate tumors. L. M. Franks, "Malignant tumors of the prostate," in *Cancer,* ed. Ronald W. Raven (London: Butterworth & Co, 1959), 2:253–268, on pp. 253–255. A study in which pathologists analyzed seven slices of amputated breast found fewer abnormalities than studies that analyzed fourteen and eighteen slices, respectively. N. Hoogerbrugge, P. Bult, J. J. Bonenkamp, M. J. L. Ligtenberg, L. A. Kiemeney, J. A. de Hullu, C. Boetes, M. F. Niermeijer, and H. G. Brunner, "Numerous high-risk epithelial lesions in familial breast cancer," *European Journal of Cancer* 42 (2006): 2492–98, on p. 2497.

61. M. Nielsen, J. Jensen, and J. Andersen, "Precancerous and cancerous lesions during lifetime and at autopsy," *Cancer* 54 (1984): 612–15; Nielsen, Thomsen, Primdahl, Dyreborg, and Andersen, "Breast cancer and atypia among young and middle aged women."

62. Editorial, "Carcinoma of the prostate," *The Lancet* 1 (1958): 1259–60. Quoted in Robert Sutherland, *Cancer: The Significance of Delay* (London: Butterworth & Co, 1960), 67. This issue was seldom discussed in the 1970s and 1980s.

63. On problems of overdiagnosis linked with the use of medical technology, see William C. Black and H. Gilbert Welch, "Advances in diagnostic imaging and overestimation of disease prevalence and the benefits of therapy," *New England Journal of Medicine* 328 (1993): 1237–43.

64. This opinion was contested later. Baines, "The Canadian National Breast Cancer Screening Study"; S. A. Narod, "On being the right size: A reappraisal of mammography trials in Canada and Sweden," *The Lancet* 349 (1997): 1846; O. Olsen and P. C. Gøtzsche, "Cochrane Review of screening for breast cancer with mammography," *The Lancet* 358 (2001): 1340–42.

65. Myles P. Cunningham, "Cancer detection demonstration project 25 years later," *CA: Cancer Journal for Clinicians* 47 (1997): 131–33.

66. Martin Kemp, "Mammary models," in M. Kemp, *Visualization: The Nature Book of Art and Science* (Oxford: Oxford University Press, 2000), 128.

67. Ralph Highnam and Michael J. Brady, "Mammographic image analysis" *Computational Imaging and Vision,* vol. 14 (Dordrecht: Kluwer, 1999).

68. Welch, *Should I Be Tested for Cancer?* 164.

69. Steven R. Pollei, Fred A. Mettler, Sue A. Bartow, Glenn Moradian, and Myron Moscowitz, "Occult breast cancer: Prevalence and radiographic detectability," *Radiology* 163 (1987): 459–62.

70. Daniel B. Kopans, Elisabeth Rafferty, Diane Georgian-Smith, Eren Yeh, Helen D'Alessandor, Richard Moore, Kevin Hughes, and Elkan Halpern, "A simple model for breast carcinoma growth may provide explanation for observation of apparently complex phenomena," *Cancer* 97 (2003) 2951–59; Welch, *Should I Be Tested for Cancer?* 86–89.

71. Karsten Juhl Jorgersen and Peter C. Gøtzsche, "Presentation of websites on possible benefits and harms from screening for breast cancer: Cross sectional study," *British Medical Journal* 328 (2004): 148–54. National Breast Cancer Coalition, Breast Cancer Action, and Center of Medical Consumers presented critical views of mammography on their websites. On history of these groups, see Batt, *Patient No More;* Altman, *Waking Up, Fighting Back;* Cassamayou, *The Politics of Breast Cancer;* Barbara Brenner, "Sister support: Women create a breast cancer movement," in *Breast Cancer: Society Shapes an Epidemic,* ed. Anne Kasper and Susan Ferguson (New York, St. Martin's Press, 2000), 325–53.

72. K. Mokbel, F. Lirosi, W. Al-Sarakbi, et al., "Women's views on the introduction of annual screening by mammography to those aged 40–49: A pilot study," *Current Medical Research Opinion* 17 (2001): 111–12; Larissa Nekhlyudov, Denis Ross-Degnant, and Susanne W. Fletcher, "Beliefs and expectations of women under 50 years old regarding screening mammography," *Journal of General Internal Medicine* 18 (2003): 182–89.

73. Claudia Z. Lee, "Comprehensive breast centers: Priorities and pitfalls," *The Breast Journal* 5 (1999): 319–24.

74. For example, the New York Weill Cornell Medical Center of the New York-Presbyterian Hospital established the Iris Cantor Women Health Center, which provides "health care for women at every stage of life." The center offers "one stop shopping" services such as mammography, blood testing, and bone density testing to detect osteoporosis and has a specific division on breast health. Advertisement for Iris Cantor Women Health Center, *The New York Times Magazine,* Apr. 28, 2002, 50.

75. Carol Weisman, *Women's Health Care: Activist Tradition and Institutional Change* (Baltimore: Johns Hopkins University Press, 1998).

76. Rose Kushner, "Breast cancer care," *The Cancer Letter* 12, no. 23 (June 6, 1986). Rose Kushner papers, box 3, folder 53, Schlesinger Library; Weisman, *Women's Health Care,* 175–82.

77. Mariamne H. Whatley and Nancy Worcester, "The role of technology in the cooptation of the Women's Health Movement: The case study of osteoporosis and

breast cancer screening," in *Healing Technology: Feminist Perspectives,* ed. Kathryn Strother Radcliff (Ann Arbor: University of Michigan Press, 1991), 199–220.

78. Kay Dickersin, "Breast screening in women aged 40–49: What next?" *The Lancet* 353 (1999): 1891–97. See also Michael Baum, "Patients' perception of risk and breast cancer awareness," *British Journal of Radiology* 77 (1997): 770–81.

79. Testimony of Jeanne, civil servant, Institut National du Cancer, "Bilan Plan Cancer 2003–2006: Dépistage: Des avantages quantitatives et qualitatives," 3.

80. Anthony B. Miller, "Screening for cancer," *Western Journal of Medicine* 149 (1988): 718–22.

81. Walter E. O'Donnell, "Cancer detection centers," in *Cancer,* ed. Ronald W. Raven. (London: Butterworth & Co, 1958), 3:425–444. In late 1950s, the recommended routine exams for cancer were incorporated into yearly checkups. They included stool examination for occult blood, clinical examination of breasts, Pap smear, and lung x-ray. Cytological examination of the sputum was optional.

82. Day, "Value of simple procedures in cancer examination," in *Cancer,* ed. Ronald W. Raven (London, Butterworth & Co, 1958), 3:445–457, on pp. 455–56.

83. Breslow, "The prevention of cancer," 483.

84. Circular of ACS, Apr. 27, 1954, Mary Lasker Papers, Box 97, Columbia University Health Sciences Library. ACS's statement on smoking from Feb. 24, 1954, explained that experts suspect that smoking increases the danger of lung cancer, but that there is no irrefutable proof that it is directly involved in the genesis of lung cancer. Ibid.

85. "Environmental cancer," *Cancer News* 10 (1956): 3–12.

86. Data from these studies are summed up in Henry Wagner and John C. Ruckdeschel, "Screening, early detection and early intervention strategies for lung cancer," *Cancer Control* 2 (1995): 493–502.

87. Gary Strauss and Lorenzo Dominioni, "Consensus statement: International conference on prevention and early diagnosis of lung cancer," *Cancer* 89 (2000): 2229–30; S. S. Biring and M. D. Peake, "Editorial: Symptoms and the early diagnosis of lung cancer," *Thorax* 60 (2005): 268–69; Gary M. Strauss, Lorenzo Dominioni, James R. Jett, Matthew Freedman, and Frederic W. Grannis, "Lung cancer screening for early diagnosis 5 years after the 1998 Varese conference," *Chest* 127 (2006): 1146–51; Claudia I. Hensheke, David F. Yankelevitz, Daniel M. Libby, et al., "Survival of patients with stage I lung cancer detected on CT screening,'" *New England Journal of Medicine* 355 (2006): 1763–71. Recent evaluations of this method question its efficacy in reducing mortality from lung cancer. Peter B. Bach, James R. Rett, Ugo Pastorino, Melvyn S. Tockman, Stephen J. Swensen, and Colin B. Begg, "Computed tomography screening and lung cancer outcomes, *JAMA* 297 (2007): 953–61; William C. Black and John A. Baron, "CT scanning for lung cancer: Spiraling into confusion?" *JAMA* 297 (2007): 995–97.

88. Aronowitz, "Situating health risks: An opportunity for disease prevention policy"; Carsten Timmerman, "As depressing as it was predictable? Lung cancer, clinical trials and the Medical Research Council in post-war Britain," *Bulletin of the History of Medicine* 81 (2007): 321–34. The strength of the link between lung cancer and tobacco

smoking, Timmerman argues, deflected attention from cancers in nonsmokers and those induced by environmental factors such as asbestos.

89. L. M. Franks "Malignant tumors of the prostate," in *Cancer,* ed. Ronald W. Raven (London: Butterworth & Co, 1958), 2:253–268, on p. 253.

90. R. J. Ablin, W. P. Bronson, and E. Witebsky, "Precipitating antigens of the normal human prostate," *Journal of Reproduction and Fertility* 22 (1970): 573–74. W. A. Soans, W. C. Wang, L. A. Venzuelle, G. P. Murphy, and T. M. Chu, "Purification of human prostate specific antigen," *Investigative Urology,* 1979, reproduced in *Journal of Urology* 167, no. 2 (2002): 960–64; W. J. Catalona, D. S. Smith, T. L. Radcliff, et al., "Measurement of prostate-specific antigen in serum as a screening for prostate cancer," *New England Journal of Medicine* 324 (1991): 1156–61.

91. For example, doctors were surprised to find out that a quarter of men who participated in clinical trial of chemoprevention of prostate cancer refused to undergo biopsy at the end of the trial, but as an ex-prostate patient noted, "Anyone who had endured this procedure will understand why." Stewart Justman, *Do No Harm: How a Magic Bullet for Prostate Cancer Became a Medical Quandary* (Chicago: Ivan R. Dee, 2008), 74.

92. Barnett S. Kramer, Martin Brown, Philip C. Prorok, Arnold L. Potosky, and John K. Gohagan, "Prostate cancer screening: What we know and what we need to know," *Annals of Internal Medicine* 119 (1993): 914–23; H. Ballentine Carter, "Editorial: Prostate cancer in men with low PSA levels—Must we find them?" *New England Journal of Medicine* 350 (2004): 2292–94.

93. S. Lilly Zheng, Jielin Sun, Fredrik Wiklund, et al., "Cumulative association of five genetic variants with prostate cancer," *New England Journal of Medicine* 358 (2008): 961–63; Edward P. Gelmann, "Complexities of prostate cancer risk," *New England Journal of Medicine* 358 (2008): 910–11; Gina Kolata, "$300 to Learn Risk of Cancer of the Prostate," *The New York Times,* Jan. 17, 2008.

94. Welch, *Should I Be Tested for Cancer?* 73–75.

95. J. I. Epstein, "What's new in prostate cancer assessment in 2006," *Current Opinion in Urology* 16 (2006): 146–51.

96. Christopher M. Coley, Michael J. Barry, Craig Fleming, Marianne C. Fahs, and Albert G. Mulley, "Early detection of prostate cancer: Clinical guidelines, part II," *Annals of Internal Medicine* 126 (1997): 468–79.

97. Steven Woloshin and Lisa M. Schwartz, "The U.S. Postal Service and cancer screening—Stamps of approval?" *New England Journal of Medicine* 340 (1999): 884–87.

98. Brena A. Sirovich, Lisa M. Schwartz, and Steven Woloshin, "Screening men for prostate and colorectal cancer in the United States: Does practice reflect the evidence?" *JAMA* 289 (2003): 1414–20; Grace Lu-Yao, Therese A. Stukel, and Siu-Long Yao, "Prostate specific antigen in elderly men," *Journal of the National Cancer Institute* 95 (2002): 1792–93.

99. Michael H. Farrell, Margaret Ann Murphy, and Carl E. Schneider, "How underlying patient beliefs can affect physician patient communication about prostate specific antigen testing," *Effective Clinical Practice* 5 (2002): 120–29; David R. Ransohoff, Mary McNaughton, and Floyd J. Flower, "Why is prostate testing so common

when the evidence is so uncertain? A system without a negative feedback," *The American Journal of Medicine* 113 (2002): 663–67.

100. D. E. Neal "Screening for prostate cancer," *Annals of Oncology* 9 (1998): 1289–92; M. Zappa, S. Ciatto, R. Bonardi, and A. Mazzotta, "Overdiagnosis of prostate carcinoma by screening: An estimate based on the results of Florence Screening Pilot Study," *Annals of Oncology* 9 (1998): 1297–1300. However, the French association of urologists did recommend in 2002 a systematic screening for prostate cancer, either through regular a clinical examination or PSA testing. C. Coulange, "Intérêt du dépistage du cancer de la prostate," *Mémoires de l'Académie Nationale de Chirurgie* 1 (2002): 4–5. Screening for this disease was not included, however, in the French cancer plan.

101. In a meeting on prostate cancer, the majority of U.S. experts favored PSA testing and opposed watchful monitoring of men with positive prostate biopsies, while the majority of European experts held the opposite opinion. Jerome Groopman, "The prostate paradox: Prostate cancer," *The New Yorker*, May 29, 2000.

102. S. Ciatto, M. Zappa, R. Bonardi, and G. Gervasi, "Prostate cancer screening: The problem of overdiagnosis and lessons to be learned from breast cancer screening," *European Journal of Cancer* 36 (2000): 1347–50.

103. See, e.g., age distribution data of cancer mortality in the United Kingdom in 2004 indicate that the great majority of deaths from prostate cancer (about 10,000 per year) occur over the age of 70; by contrast a sizable proportion of breast cancer deaths (about 14% of the approximately 15,000 deaths) occurred in women under 50. http://info.cancerresearchuk.org/cancerstats/mortality/ Similarly, the SEER data on cancer morbidity and mortality in the United States for 2003 estimated that each breast cancer death is equivalent to a loss of nineteen years of life, while prostate cancer death leads to an average loss of ten years of life. By consequence, while the difference in the number of deaths from these malignancies for that year is not very big (breast 40,200; prostate 28,900) the difference in cumulative years of life lost is much greater (breast 799,000 versus prostate 275,000). Reproduced in Welch, *Should I Be Tested For Cancer?* 191. Moreover, the media systematically presented breast cancer patients as young women, while they provided a more realistic image of prostate cancer patients. Karen M. Kedrowski and Marylin Stine Sarow, *Cancer Activism: Gender, Media and Public Policy* (Urbana and Chicago: University of Illinois Press, 2007), 93–123.

104. Kedrowski and Sarow, *Cancer Activism*, 184–99.

105. Jo Revill, "Both have cancer. But why can't one get the best care?" *The Observer*, July 9, 2006.

106. J. P. Lockhart-Mummery, "Cancer and heredity," *The Lancet* 1 (1925): 427–29.

107. Claude Emerson Welch, *Polypoid Lesions of the Gastrointestinal Tract* (Major Problems in Clinical Surgery Series, Philadelphia: Saunders, 1975); Robert Franklin and Barton McSwain, "Carcinoma of the colon, rectum and anus," *Annals of Surgery* 171 (1972): 811–28.

108. William I. Wolf and Hiromi Shinya, "A new approach to colonic polyps," *Annals of Surgery* 178 (1973), 367–76; William W. Wolf and Hiromi Shinya, "Definitive

treatment of 'malignant' polyps of the colon," *Annals of Surgery* 182 (1975): 516–25; Theodore Coustofides, Michael V. Sivak, Sanford Benjamin, and David Jagelman, "Colonoscopy and the management of polyps containing invasive carcinoma," *Annals of Surgery* 188 (1978): 638–41; William A. Webb, Linda McDaniel, and Leroy Jones, "Experience with 1000 colonoscopic polypectomies," *Annals of Surgery* 201 (1985): 626–30.

109. S. F. Miller and A. R. Knight, "The early detection of colorectal cancer," *Cancer* 40 (1997): 945–49; J. D. Hardcastle, T. W. Balfour, and S. S. Amar, "Screening for symptomless colorectal cancer by testing for occult blood in general practice, *The Lancet* 1 (1980): 791–93.

110. J. Hardcastle, J. Chamberlain, M. Robinson, et al., "Randomised controlled trial of faecal occult blood screening with faecal occult blood test," *The Lancet* 348 (1996): 1472–77; O. Kronborf, C. Fenger, J. Olsen, et al., "Randomised study of screening for colorectal cancer with faecal occult blood test," *The Lancet* 348 (1996): 1467–71.

111. Wendy Atkins, "Editorial: Implementing screening for colorectal cancer," *British Medical Journal* 319 (1999): 1212–13.

112. Document of the Commission sur les essais therapeutiques en hepato-enterologie, presented by M. Bellanger, July 6, 1976. file, documents on clinical trials 1973–1976, INSERM Archives.

113. M. A. Tazi, J. Faivre, F. Sassonville, et al., "Participation in faecal occult blood screening for colorectal cancer in a well defined French population," *Journal of Medical Screening* 4 (1997): 147–61; C. Herbert, G. Launoy, and M. Gignoux, "Factors affecting compliance with colorectal cancer screening in France," *European Journal of Cancer Prevention* 6 (1997), 44–52.

114. J. W. W. Coebergh, "Editorial: Colorectal cancer screening in Europe: First things first," *European Journal of Cancer* 40 (2004): 638–42.

115. Institut National du Cancer, "Bilan Plan Cancer 2003–2006: Dépistage: Des avantages quantitatives et qualitatives," 75–77; "Dépistage du cancer du colon," *Bulletin Epidemiologique Hebdomadaire* 2–3 (Jan. 13, 2009): 8; Jean-Pierre Grünefeldt, *Recommendations pour le Plan Cancer 2009–2013* (Paris: Editions Inca, 2009), 24.

116. R. C. J. Steele for U.K. Colorectal Cancer Screening Pilot Group, "Result of the first round of demonstration pilot of screening for colorectal cancer in the United Kingdom," *British Medical Journal* 329 (2004): 133–38.

117. J. E. Verne, R. Aubrey, S. B. Love, et al., "Population based randomised study of uptake and yield of screening by flexible sigmoidoscopy compared with screening by occult blood testing," *British Medical Journal* 317 (1998): 182–85.

118. Susan Mayor, "England to start national bowel cancer screening program," *British Medical Journal* 329 (2004): 1061. The plan started in 2006 and is scheduled to cover all of the United Kingdom in 2010. As of now (2009) there are no data on enrollment.

119. J. S. Mandel, T. R. Church, F. Ederer, and J. H. Bond, "Colorectal cancer mortality: Effectiveness of biennial screening for fecal occult blood," *Journal of the National Cancer Institute* 91 (1999): 434–37.

120. Michael Pignone, Melissa Rich, Steven M. Teutsch, et al., "Screening for col-

orectal cancer in adults at average risk: A summary of the evidence for the U.S. Preventive Services Task Force," *Annals of Internal Medicine* 137 (2002): 132–38.

121. Doctors often remove all the intestinal polyps found during a colonoscopy including those that have a very low probability of becoming malignant, putting patients at additional surgical risk. S. R. Odom, S. D. Duffy, J. E. Barone, V. Ghevariya, and S. J. McClane, "The rate of adenocarcinoma in endoscopically removed colorectal polyps," *The American Surgeon* 71 (2005): 1024–26.

122. Studies made in the United States also displayed a great variability in the quality of detection of premalignant polyps. David Lieberman, "Editorial: A call to action—Measuring the quality of colonoscopy," *New England Journal of Medicine* 355 (2006): 2588. In addition, not all colonoscopists remove flat lesions of the colon, considered more dangerous than polyps. David Lieberman, "Editorial: Nonpolypoid colorectal neoplasia in the United States: The parachute is open," *JAMA* 299 (2008): 1068–69.

123. S. Winawer, R. Fletcher, D. Rex et al., Gastrointestinal Consortium Panel: "Colorectal cancer screening and surveillance: Clinical guidelines and rationale—Update based on new evidence," *Gastroenterology* 124 (2003); 544–60; R. A. Smith, A. C. von Eschenbach, R. Wender, et al., "American Cancer Society guidelines for the early detection for prostate, colorectal and endometrial cancers," *CA: A Cancer Journal for Clinicians* 51 (2001): 38–75; S. J. Winawer and A. G. Zauber, "Colonoscopic polypectomy and the incidence of colorectal cancer," *Gut* 48 (2001): 753–54. The American College of Gastroenterology recognized the efficacy of alternative screening methods such as hemoccult or flexible sigmoidoscopy but stressed the superiority of colonoscopy.

124. "Increased use of colorectal cancer tests, United States, 2002 and 2004," *CDC-Morbidity and Mortality Weekly Report* (Mar. 24, 2006); Lu-Yao, Stukel, and Yao, "Prostate specific antigen in elderly men."

125. Denoix, professor of oncology at the Medical School of Paris University, headed one the biggest French cancer treating centers, Institut Gustave Roussy, in the years between 1956 and 1982 and between 1974 and 1978 was directeur général de la santé at the French Health Ministry (roughly the equivalent of surgeon general in the United Sates). He was also (1973–1978) the president of international coordination of oncology societies, Union Internationale Contre le Cancer.

126. Pierre Denoix, "Rapport du conseil permanent d'Hygiène sociale, commission du cancer" DGS, Ministre de la Santé. Meeting of May 14, 1976. Cancer commission file for 1974–1976, INSERM Archives.

127. Denoix's views are quoted in an internal document of BECC, "Cancer education: Investigation into the results of cancer education," of September 1957, box 90, BECC papers, Wellcome Archives.

128. Pierre Denoix, *Carcinologie Demain: Dictonnaire des Idées Non Reçues. Quelques Sujets de Reflexion pour Jeunes Medecins et pour les Autres*, undated manuscript, code U1116, BI4521, Bibliothèque de l'Institut des recherches scientifiques sur le cancer, Villejuif. The manuscript probably dates from 1982, because it is accompanied by a Denoix's handwritten note from June 18, 1982, probably destined to one of his co-

workers at the Villejuif hospital: "puisse ce 'dictonnaire' entretenir la contestation, source de vitalité" (I wish for this "dictionary" to keep critical thought, source of vitality alive). The subtitle "dictonnaire des idées non reçus" is an allusion to Flaubert's well-known satiric book: *Bouvard et Pécuchet: Dictionnaire des Idées Reçues* (Paris: A. Lemerre, 1881).

129. Denoix, *Carcinologie Demain,* 1–17. The word *lapalissade* is derived from a sentence, attributed to sixteenth-century French aristocrat Jacques II de Chabannes, lord of de La Palice, "s'il n'était pas mort, il serait encore en vie (if he were not dead, he would still be alive)—probably an erroneous transcription of, "s'il n'était pas mort, il ferait encore envie" (if he were not dead, he could have still made people envious).

130. Denoix, *Carcinologie Demain,* 19- 22.

131. Ibid., 133–36.

132. Ibid., 23.

133. Ibid., 29.

134. Ibid., 167.

135. Daren Schickle and Ruth Chadwick, "The ethics of screening; Is 'screenignitis' an incurable disease?," *Journal of Medical Ethics,* 29 (1994): 12–18; Gina Kolata, "New ability to find earlier cancers: A mixed blessing?" *New York Times,* Nov. 8, 1994; William C. Black, "Editorial: Overdiagnosis: An underrecognized cause of confusion and harm in cancer screening," *Journal of the National Cancer Institute* 92 (2000): 1280–82.

136. Jehuda Folkman and Raghu Kalluri, "Cancer without disease," *Nature* 427 (2004): 787.

137. J. M. G. Wilson, "Medical screening, from beginnings to benefits: A retrospective," *Journal of Medical Screening* 1 (1994): 121–23. Thoreau's quotation is from *Walden,* in C. Bode (ed.), *The Portable Thoreau* (London: Penguin Books, 1982), 328.

138. Lisa M. Schwartz, Steven Woloshin, Floyd J. Fowler, and H. Gilbert Welsh, "Enthusiasm for cancer screening in the United States," *Journal of the American Medical Association* 291 (2004): 71–78.

139. French philosopher Georges Canguilhem borrowed the expression "the silence of organs" from surgeon René Leriche to define health: "la santé, c'est la vie dans le silence des organes" (health is a life in the silence of organs). Georges Canguilhem, *Essai sur Quelques Problèmes Concernant le Normal et le Pathologique* (1943; reprinted Paris: Vrin, 1964).

140. Ulrich Beck, *Risk Society: Towards New Modernity* (London: Sage, 1992).

141. Nikolas Rose, "The politics of life itself," *Theory, Culture and Society* 18 (2001): 1–30; Nikolas Rose, "Introduction," in *The Politics of Life Itself: Biomedicine, Power and Subjectivity in the Twentieth-First Century,* ed. Nikolas Rose (Princeton: Princeton University Press, 2007).

142. French sociologist Patrice Pinell argues that education about cancer signs played a key role in the birth of the modern "homo medicus," trained to search hidden signs of disease in his or her body. Patrice Pinell, *Naissance d'un Fléau* (Paris: Anne Marie Metaillé, 1992; English version, *The Fight against Cancer: France 1890– 1940,* trans. David Maddell [London: Routledge, 2002]).

143. On the refusal of diagnostic tests by health care users who reject the risk of medical information, see Susan Markens, C. H. Browner, and Nancy Press, " 'Because of the risks': How US pregnant women account for refusing prenatal screening," *Social Sciences and Medicine* 49 (1999): 359–69.

144. Ann Robertson, "Biotechnology: Political rationality and discourses on health risk," *Health*, 5 (2001): 293–309. Robertson alludes to Foucault's use of the term *panopticon* (inspired by Jeremy Bentham's image of an ideal prison) to describe an intensive surveillance of people. Michel Foucault, *Surveiller et Punir, Naissance de la Prison* (Paris: Gallimard, 1975; English translation, *Discipline and Punish: The Birth of the Prison*, New York: Pantheon Books, 1977).

145. Robertson, "Biotechnology: Political rationality and discourses on health risk."

146. Cynthia Kraus, "On 'epistemic covetousness' in knowledge economies: The not nothing of social constructionism," *Social Epistemology* 19 (2005): 339–55.

147. I borrow this image from Graham Burnett's description of efforts to erase inscriptions on boundary stones. Graham D. Burnett, *Masters of All They Surveyed: Exploration, Geography, and a British El Dorado* (Chicago: University of Chicago Press, 2000).

148. Patricia Kaufert, "Women, resistance and the breast cancer movement," in *Pragmatic Women and Body Politics*, ed. Margaret Lock and Patricia Kaufert (Cambridge: Cambridge University Press, 1998), 287–309; Margaret Lock, "Breast cancer: Reading the omens," *Anthropology Today* 14 (1998): 7–16; Patricia A. Kaufert, "Screening the body: The pap smear and the mammogram," in *Living and Working with the New Medical Technologies;* Margaret Lock, Allan Young, and Alberto Cambrosio, eds. (Cambridge: Cambridge University Press, 2000).

149. Charles Rosenberg, "Managed Fear: Contemplating Sickness in an Era of Bureaucracy and Chronic Disease," American Osler Society Publication, 2008. In the United States, men became recently targets of similar strategies. Posters issued by the Utah department of health campaign to promote screening for prostate cancer ("be informed, be a man") explain that "because with a 1 in 6 chances of being diagnosed, men know it's important to get checked." Poster in the collection of National Library of Medicine, Bethesda.

Chapter Seven · Heredity

1. Frederick L. Hoffman, "Cancer in the North American Negro," *American Journal of Surgery and Gynecology* 22 (1908–9): 229–63, on p. 241.

2. Ilana Löwy and Jean-Paul Gaudillière, "Disciplining cancer: Mice and the practice of genetic purity," in *The Invisible Industrialist: Manufactures and the Production of Scientific Knowledge*, ed. J.-P. Gaudillière and I. Löwy (London: Macmillan, 1998), 209–249; Jean-Paul Gaudillière, "Circulating mice and viruses: The Jackson Memorial Laboratory, the National Cancer Institute and the genetics of breast cancer," in *The Practices of Human Genetics*, ed. Michael Frotrun and Everett Mendelsohn (Dordrecht: Kluwer, 1999), 89–124.

3. Alfredo Nicefore and Eugène Pittard, *Considerations Regarding the Possible Relationships of Cancer to Race, Based on Study of Anthropological and Medical Statistics of Certain European Countries* (Geneva: Publications de la Société des Nations, 1928). See also "La Société des Nations et la lutte contre le cancer," *La Lutte Contre le Cancer* 4 (Oct.–Dec. 1926), 110–15; "Enquête de la Ligue des Nations sur cancer et race, conduite par Prof. Nicefore et Pittard," *La Lutte Contre le Cancer* 4 (Jan.–Mar. 1927), 197–202.

4. Nicefore and Pittard, *Considerations Regarding the Possible Relationships of Cancer to Race*, 323–25.

5. E. E. Bashford, *The Influence of Heredity on Disease* (London: Longmans, Green & Co., 1909), 63–66; James Ewing, "Heredity and Cancer," *Bulletin of the American Society for the Control of Cancer* 24 (Aug. 1942): 4–7.

6. Such families, Janet Lane-Claypon affirmed, are rare, but their presence is very striking. Janet E. Lane-Claypon, *A Further Report on Cancer of the Breast with Special Reference to Its Associated Antecedent Conditions*, Reports on Public Health and Medical Subjects, Ministry of Health, publication no. 32 (London: His Majesty's Stationery Office, 1926).

7. J. Paterson MacLaren, *Medical Insurance Examination: Modern Methods and Rating of Lives* (New York: William Wood and Company, 1943), 530–31.

8. H. Cripps, "Two cases of disseminated cancer of the rectum," *Transactions of the Pathological Society* 33 (1882): 165.

9. John Percy Lockhart-Mummery, "The diagnosis of tumors in the upper rectum and sigmoid flexure by means of the electric sigmoscope," *The Lancet* 1 (1904): 1781–82. Lockhart-Mummery used a model of sigmoidoscope developed by Professor Strauss from Berlin and noted with satisfaction that the new method enables the doctor to explore the hitherto inaccessible portions of the human body. On the history of St. Mark's Hospital and specialized surgical treatment of rectum diseases, see Lindsay Graham, "Knowledge of bodies or bodies of knowledge: Surgeons, anatomists and rectal surgery, 1830–1985," in *Medical Theory, Surgical Knowledge: Studies in the History of Surgery*, ed. Christopher Lawrence (London: Routledge, 1992), 232–62.

10. John Percy Lockhart-Mummery, "Cancer and heredity," *The Lancet* 1 (1925): 427–29.

11. Lockhart-Mummery, "Cancer and heredity," 428. Cheatle's views on direct links between benign and malignant tumors of the breast (discussed in Chapter 3) were abandoned after World War II.

12. Lockhart-Mummery, "Cancer and heredity," 427. Italics mine, IL.

13. John Percy Lockhart-Mummery, leaflet, *Origins of Tumors* (London: John Bale Sons & Danielson, 1932). Archives of the British Empire Cancer Campaign, series SA/CRC: Clinics, pathology, research, box 52, file, E.3/12, papers of Sir John Percy Lockhart-Mummery (1875–1957), Wellcome Library, Archives and Manuscripts Department, London, England (Wellcome Archives).

14. John Percy Lockhart-Mummery, C. E. Dukes, and M. D. Edin, "Familiar adenomatosis of colon and rectum," *The Lancet* 2 (1939): 586–87.

15. Paolo Palladino, "Speculations on cancer-free babies: Surgery and genetics at

St. Mark Hospital, 1924–1995, in *Heredity and Infection: Historical Essays on the Transmission of Human Diseases*, ed. Jean-Paul Gaudillière and Ilana Löwy (London and New York: Routledge, 2001), 285–310, on p. 288.

16. Johannes Clemmesen, "On the etiology of some human cancers," *Journal of the National Cancer Institute* 12 (1952): 1–21, on p. 20.

17. See, for example, J. Rebulet, Influence de l'hérédité sur la frequence du cancer en Normandie (Paris: Maloine, 1898); A. Marmaduke Shield, *Clinical Treatise on Diseases of the Breast* (London: MacMillan, 1898), 308–11; Bashford, *The Influence of Heredity on Disease.*

18. William L. Rodman, *Diseases of the Breast, with Special Reference to Cancer* (London: Sidney Appleton, 1908), 181.

19. Lane-Claypon, *A Further Report on Cancer of the Breast.*

20. Olaf Jacobsen, *Heredity in Breast Cancer: A Genetic and Clinical Study of Two Hundred Probands* (London: H.K. Lewis, 1946).

21. Lionel Penrose, H. J. Mackenzie, and M. N. Karn, "A genetical study of human mammary cancer," *British Journal of Cancer* 2 (1948), 168–76. Penrose speculated about the possibility of a nongenetic transmission in family, e.g., through a virus in the mother's milk. At that time, a cancer-inducing virus was observed in mice (Bittner's "milk factor"). See also Pierre Denoix, M. Schwartzenberger, and G. Denoix, "Contribution à l'étude du rôle des facteurs héreditaires dans le cancer," *Bulletin de l'Institut National d'Hygiène* 8 (1953): 247–57.

22. V. Elving Anderson, Harold O. Goodman, and Sheldon C. Reed, *Variables Related to Human Breast Cancer* (Minneapolis: University of Minnesota Press, 1958).

23. See, e.g., Forum: "When primary cancer of the breast is treated, should the second breast be prophylactically removed," *Modern Medicine* 4 (Feb. 1966): 242–61.

24. Henry Patrick Leis, "Selective, elective prophylactic contralateral mastectomy," *Cancer* 28 (1971): 956–61; Charles E. Horton, Francis E. Rosato, Frank A. Scholer, and John McCraw, "Postmastectomy reconstruction," *Annals of Surgery* 188 (1978): 733–77.

25. David E. Anderson, "Familial susceptibility," in *Persons at High Risk of Cancer: An Approach to Cancer Etiology*, ed. Joseph F. Fraumeni (New York: Academic Press, 1975), 39–52.

26. Anderson, "Familial susceptibility," 42–45.

27. On the history of Lynch's studies in cancer genetics, see David Cantor, "The frustration of families: Henry Lynch and cancer control, 1962–1974," *Medical History* 50 (2006): 276–302, and on Lynch's involvement with studies of hereditary colon cancer, Rauo Antonio Necochea, "From cancer families to HNPCC: Henry Lynch and the transformation of hereditary cancer," *Bulletin of the History of Medicine* 81 (2007): 267–85.

28. Henry T. Lynch, "The surgeon, genetics and cancer control: The Cancer Family Syndrome," *Annals of Surgery* 185 (1977): 435–40; Henry T. Lynch, Jane Lynch, and Patrick Lynch, "Management and control of familiar cancer," in *Genetics of Human Cancer*, ed. John J. Mulvihill, Robert W. Miller, and Joseph F. Fraumeni (New York: Raven Press, 1977), 235–56.

29. Lynch, "The surgeon, genetics and cancer control," 435.

30. Joshua Lederberg, "Molecular biology, eugenic and euphenics," *Nature* 198 (1963): 428–29. On the 1960s hopes that organ transplantation would lead to revolution in medicine, see Ilana Löwy, "The impact of medical practice on biomedical research: The case of human leukocyte antigens studies," *Minerva* 25 (1987): 171–200.

31. Blake Cady, "Familial bilateral cancer of the breast," *Annals of Surgery* 172 (1970): 264–72; George G. Finney Jr., George G. Finney, Albert G. W. Montague, Geary L. Stonesifer, and Charles C. Brown, "Bilateral breast cancer, clinical and pathological review," *Annals of Surgery* 175 (1972): 635–42; D. E. Anderson, "Breast cancer in families," *Cancer* 40 (1977): 1855–60.

32. John J. Mulvhill, Andrew W. Safyer, and Jane K. Benning, "Prevention in breast cancer: Counseling and prophylactic mastectomy." *Preventive Medicine* 11 (1982): 500–511.

33. Henry T. Lynch, Randall E. Harris, Claude H. Organ, and Jane F. Lynch, "Management of familial breast cancer. II: Case reports, pedigrees, genetic counseling and team concept," *Archives of Surgery* 113 (1978): 1061–67. Lynch illustrates his argument with description of a case in which one identical twin developed a breast cancer and the other twin was not advised to undergo preventive mastectomy, in spite of a family history of breast malignancy.

34. Robert V. Hutter, "What is premalignant lesion?" in *Early Breast Cancer: Detection and Treatment*, ed. H. Stephan Gallagher (New York: John Willey and Sons, 1975), 165–69, on p. 165.

35. Robert M. Goldwyn, "Invited editorial comment," *Archives of Surgery* 113 (1978): 1067.

36. Walter F. Bodmer, "Cancer genetics," in *Inheritance of Susceptibility to Cancer in Man*, ed. Walter F. Bodmer (Oxford: Oxford University Press, 1982), 1–15, on p. 1.

37. Ilana Löwy, *Between Bench and Bedside: Science, Healing and Interleukin 2 in a Cancer Ward* (Cambridge, MA: Harvard University Press, 1996); Toine Peters, *Interferon: The Science and Selling of a Miracle Drug* (London and New York, Routledge, 2005).

38. First evaluations of cancer risk in carriers of *BRCA* mutations were made in families with especially high incidence of cancer. The estimates of such risk were lowered in 2008. Large-scale population studies indicated a 40% risk at the age of 70, with important variability among families, attributed either to presence of other, unknown, susceptibility genes, differences between effects of individual variants in the *BRCA1* and *BRCA2* genes, or lifestyle elements reproduced in families. Colin B. Begg, Robert W. Haile, Ake Borg, et al., "Variation of breast cancer risk among *BRCA1/2* carriers," *JAMA* 2999 (2008): 194–201.

39. Maurice Cassier and Jean-Paul Gaudillière, "Recherche, médecine et marché: La génétique du cancer du sein," *Sciences Sociales et Santé* 18 (2000): 29–49.

40. American Society of Clinical Oncology, "Genetic testing for cancer susceptibility," *Journal of Clinical Oncology* 14 (1996): 1730–36; Neil A. Holtzman and S. Watson, *Promoting Safe and Effective Genetic Testing in the United States: Final Report of the Task Force on Genetic Testing* (Baltimore: Johns Hopkins University Press, 1998).

41. According to Myriad Genetics, between 2001 and 2006 ten times as many Americans were tested for BRCA mutations as in the first period of marketing of the test for these mutations, 1996–2001. More than one hundred thousand Americans were tested during the first ten years of marketing of Myriad's BRCA test. Amy Harmon, "Couples cull embryos to halt heritage of cancer," The New York Times, Sept. 3, 2006.

42. Information about the lawsuit can be viewed on the Curie Institute's website: www.curie.net/actualites/myriad and information on the verdict can be found at www.curie.fr/home/presse/communiques-affaires.cfm/lang/_fr/affaire/3.htm (accessed Aug. 8, 2008).

43. In France and the United Kingdom, searching for BRCA mutations is fully reimbursed by the national health system. Searching for a known mutation is approximately ten times cheaper than for an unknown one.

44. In her moving book, Mapping Fate: A Memoir of Family, Risk and Genetic Research (New York: Random House, 1995), Alice Wexler describes a systematic denial of the presence of Huntington disease in her family. Wexler's mother, a biologist, refused to consider the possibility that she or her children might carry the Huntington gene in spite of the fact that Wexler's father and three brothers developed the disease.

45. The analysis of differences in uses of tests for BRCA mutations in France, the United Kingdom, and the United States relies on a research made in the framework of a collaborative project conducted by Maurice Cassier and Jean-Paul Gaudillière and myself. See Ilana Löwy, "Le risque héréditaire du cancer de sein et d'ovaire dans la clinique: Une approche comparative, France, Grande Bretagne, Etats Unis," in Prédisposition Génétique aux Cancers: Questions Psychologiques et Débats de Société, ed. Claire Julien Reynier, Janine Pierrert, and François Eisinger (Paris: John Libbey Eurotext, 2005), 33–44; Jean-Paul Gaudillière and Ilana Löwy, "Science, markets and public health: Contemporary testing for breast cancer predispositions," in Medicine, the Market and the Mass Media: Producing Health in the Twentieth Century, ed. Virginia Berridge and Kelly Loughin (London: Routledge, 2005), 266–87; Ilana Löwy and Jean-Paul Gaudillière, "Localizing the global: Testing for hereditary risks of breast cancer," Science, Technology and Human Values 33 (2008): 299–325. My part of this research, focused on clinical practices, was grounded in interviews conducted in the three countries. Interviewees included oncologists in charge of cancer genetic consultations and/or research units, and, in the United States, women health activists involved in public debates and regulation of testing practices. Interviews were prepared by reading the relevant scientific literature, by attending workshops and conferences on breast cancer genetics, and by collecting and analyzing the gray literature associated with the regulation of the field. The geographical distribution was the following: sixteen interviews in France, eighteen in the United States, and seven in the United Kingdom. In addition, I spent nine months observing oncogenetic consultations in a cancer hospital in Paris.

46. Andrew N. Freedman, Daniela Seminara, Mitchell H. Gail, et al., "Cancer risk prediction models: A workshop on development, evaluation and applications," Journal of the National Cancer Institute 97 (2005): 715–23, on p. 717.

47. INSERM, Expertise Collective: Risques Héréditaires des Cancers du Sein et

de l'Ovaire. Quelle Prise en Charge? (Paris: INSERM Editions, 1998); François Eisin-ger et al., "Recommendation for medical management of hereditary breast and ovarian cancer; The French National Ad Hoc Committee," *Annals of Oncology* 9 (1998), 939–50.

48. In the United States the method adopted by Myriad, the total sequencing of *BRCA* genes, is not specifically oriented toward the testing of people who have can-cer and their families. Nevertheless, in oncogenetic services affiliated with cancer hos-pitals, a significant proportion of women tested for *BRCA* mutations are currently being treated for cancer.

49. The introduction of *BRCA* testing to Britain was studied by Sahra Gibbon and Shobita Parthasarathy. Gihbon focused on changes in medical practice and their influence on women. Sahra Gibbon, *Breast Cancer Genes and the Gendering of Knowl-edge: Science and Citizenship in the Context of the "New" Genetics* (Basingstoke: Pal-grave Macmillan, 2007); Sahra Gibbon, "Charity, breast cancer and the iconic figure of the BRCA carrier," in *Biosocialities, Genetics and the Social Sciences,* ed. Sahra Gib-bon and Carlos Novas (London: Routledge, 2008), 19–37. Parthasarathy was espe-cially interested in differences between the United States and the United Kingdom and in the British resistance to Myriad strategy. Shobita Parthasarathy, "The patent is political: The consequences of patenting the BRCA genes in Britain," *Community Ge-netics* 8 (2005): 235–42; Shobita Parthasarathy, "Architectures of genetic medicine: Comparing genetic testing for breast cancer in the USA and the UK," *Social Studies of Science* 35 (2005): 5–40; Shobita Parthasarathy, *Building Genetic Medicine: Breast Cancer, Technology and the Comparative Politics of Breast Care* (Cambridge, MA: MIT Press, 2007).

50. James Mackay and Bruce A. J. Ponder, "The management of inherited breast cancer risk," in *Textbook of Breast Cancer,* ed. Gianni Bonadonna, Gabriel Nortobagui, and A. Massino-Gianni (London: Martin Dunitz, 2001), 85–97.

51. R. Harris, R. G. Elles, D. Crauford, et al., "Molecular genetics in the National Health Service in Britain, *Journal of Medical Genetics* 26 (1989): 219–25; Dan Donnai and Rob Elles, "Integrated regional genetic services: Current and future provision," *British Medical Journal* 322 (2001): 1048–52.

52. The risk is calculated at a given age. A sevenfold increase may look impressive, but it is not a very high risk for a women of 40 because at that age cancer risk of the general population is very low.

53. Eila Watson, Joan Austoker, and Anneke Lucassen, "A study of GP referrals to a family cancer clinics for breast/ovarian cancer, *Family Practice* 18 (2001): 131–34; An-nekee Lucassen, Eila Watson, and Diana Eccles, "Evidence based case report: Advice about mammography for a young woman with a family history of breast cancer," *British Medical Journal* 322 (2001): 1040–42; Geertruida de Bock, Christi van Asperen, Josephine de Vries, George Hageman, Michael Springer, and Job Kievit, "How women with a family history of breast cancer and their general practitioners act on genetic advice in general practice: Prospective longitudinal study," *British Medical Journal* 322 (2001): 26–27; Jon Emery and Susan Hayflick, "The challenge of integrating genetic medicine into primary care," *British Medical Journal* 322 (2001): 1027–30.

54. Lynch, Harris, Organ, and Lynch, "Management of familial breast cancer."

55. Victor G. Vogel, "Breast cancer prevention: A review of current evidence," *CA : Cancer Journal for Clincians*, 50 (2000): 156–70, on p. 156.

56. Decree (décret) no. 2000-570 of June 20, 2000, and Health Ministry decree (arrêté) of May 2, 2001.

57. Nearly all French centers for women at risk of cancer are situated in specialized cancer treatment institutions. These centers focus exclusively on genetic risk. Pascale Bourret, "BRCA patients and clinical collectives: New configurations of action in cancer genetic practices" *Social Studies of Science* 35 (2005): 41–68. Recently, however, the French general hospital system (AP-HP) opened a center for women at high risk of breast and ovarian cancer that also provides counseling for women at morphological risk of breast tumors. A information leaflet, distributed by this center, states that women with atypical breast hyperplasia or lobular carcinoma in situ "should benefit from supervision measures close to those proposed to women with identified BRCA mutations." Press Announcement of the French National Cancer Institute, May 9, 2006.

58. Health Department of the United Kingdom, Advisory Committee on Genetic Testing, *Report on Genetic Testing for Late Onset Disorders* (London: Her Majesty's Stationery Office, 1998).

59. Akin rejections of continuities in oncology were observed during the passage from "old" immunotherapies of cancer to the use of interleukins. Löwy, *Between Bench and Bedside*. On the tendency to stress technological novelty and forget continuities, see David Edgerton, *The Shock of the Old: Technology and Global History Since 1900* (Oxford: Oxford University Press, 2006).

60. C. R. Boland, "Familial colonic cancer syndromes," *The Western Journal of Medicine* 139 (1983): 351–59 ; D. M. Eccless, P. W. Lunt, Y. Wallins, et al., "An unusually severe phenotype for familiar adenomatous polyposis," *Archives of Disease in Childhood* 77 (1997): 431–35.

61. D. G. Jagelman, "Clinical management of familial adenomatous polyposis," *Cancer Surveys* 8 (1989): 159–67.

62. P. van Duijvendijk, J. F. Slors, C. W. Taat, P. Oosterverl, and H. F. Vasen, "Functional outcome after colestomy and ileeorectal anastomosis compared with protocolectomy and ileal pouch-anals anastomosis in familiar adenomatous polyposis," *Annals of Surgery* 230 (1999): 648–54.

63. T. G. Parks, H. J. R. Bussey, and H. E. Lockhart-Mummery, "Familial polyposis coli associated with extra-colonic abnormalities," *Gut* 11 (1970): 323–29.

64. Boland, "Familial colonic cancer syndromes"; Rodney J. Scott, Nicola J. Froggatt, Richard C. Trembath, et al., "Familiar infiltrative fibromatosis (desmoid tumors) caused by a recurrent 3@prime: APC gene mutation," *Human Molecular Genetics* 5 (1996): 1921–24; Yann Parc, Arnaud Piquard, Roger R. Sozois, Rolland Parc, and Emmanuel Tiret, "Long term outcome of familial adenomatous polyposis patients after restorative coloprotectomy," *Annals of Surgery* 239 (2004): 378–82.

65. J. M. Church, V. W. Fazion, I. C. Lavery, et al., "Quality of life after prophylactic colectomy and ilorectal anastomosis with family adenomatous polyposis," *Diseases of Colon and Rectum* 39 (1996): 1404–8.

66. Ellen Giarelli, "Self surveillance for genetic predisposition to cancer: Behaviors and emotions," *Oncology Nursing Forum* 33 (2006): 221–31.

67. H. T. Lynch, A. Krush, R.J. Thomas, et al., "Cancer family syndrome," in *Cancer Genetics*, ed. H. T. Lynch (Springfield, IL: Charles C. Thomas, 1976), 355–88.

68. Asad Umar, C. Richard Boland, Jonathan P. Terdiman, et al., "Revised Bethesda guidelines for hereditary nonpolyposis colorectal cancer (Lynch syndrome) and microsatellite instability, *Journal of the National Cancer Institute* 96 (2004): 261–68.

69. Doctors started also specific hereditary nonpolyposis colorectal cancer (HNPCC) registries, see, e.g., Torben Myrhoi, Igor Berenstein, Marie Louise Bisgard, et al., "The establishment of an HNPCC register," *Anticancer Research* 14 (1994): 1647–50; P. W. Rose, M. Murphy, M. Munafo, et al., "Improving the ascertainment of families at high risk of colorectal cancer: a prospective GP register study," *British Journal of General Practice* 54 (2004): 267–71.

70. I. Dove-Edwin, P. Sasieni, J. Adams, and H. J. Thomas, "Prevention of colorectal cancer by colonoscopic surveillance in individuals with a family history of colorectal cancer: 16 year, prospective, follow-up study," *British Medical Journal* 2 (2005): 1047–49; A. E. de Jong, Y. M. Hendriks, J. H. Kleibeuker, et al. "Decrease in mortality in Lynch syndrome families because of surveillance," *Gastroenterology* 130 (2006): 665–71.

71. J. M. Church, "Prophylactic colectomy in patients with hereditary nonpolyposis colorectal cancer," *Annals of Medicine* 28 (1996): 476–82.

72. Miguel Rodriguez-Bigas, Hans. A. Vasen, Jukka Pekka-Mecklin, et al., "Rectal cancer risk in hereditary non-polyposis colorectal cancer after abdominal colectomy," *Annals of Surgery* 225 (1997): 202–7.

73. Sapna Syngal, Jane C. Weeks, Deborah Schrag, Judy Garber, and Karen M. Kuntz, "Benefits of colonoscopic surveillance and prophylactic colectomy in patients with hereditary nonpolyposis colorectal cancer mutations," *Annals of Internal Medicine* 129 (1998): 787–96; Isis Dove Edwin, Peter Sasieni, Joanna Adams, and Huw J. W. Thomas, "Prevention of colorectal cancer by colonoscopic surveillance in individuals with a family history of colorectal cancer: 16 years, prospective follow up study," *British Medical Journal* 331 (2005): 1047–49; Sylvaine Olschwang, P. Laurent-Puig, F. Eisinger, and B. Millat, "An alternative to prophylactic colectomy for colon cancer prevention in HNPCC syndrome," *Gut* 54 (2005): 169–70.

74. Elisabeth Chow, Finley Macramé, and John Burn, "2005 survey of HNPCC management of responses from 18 international cancer centers," *Hereditary Cancer in Clinical Practice*, 3 (2005): 137–46. Surveillance of endometrial cancer risk by echography and biopsies is seen as efficient.

75. George T. Bateson, "On the treatment of inoperable case of carcinoma of the mamma: Suggestion for a new method of treatment with an illustrative case, *The Lancet* 2 (1896): 104–7; Michael J. Clarke, "Ovarian ablation in breast cancer, 1896–1998: Milestones along hierarchy of evidence from case report to Cochrane review," *British Medical Journal* 317 (1998): 1246–48.

76. Surgical Adjuvant Chemotherapy Breast Project was headed by Bernard Fisher, one of the main advocates of conservative treatment of breast cancer in the

United States. The finding of B-17 trials led to another trial, B-24, that tested use of ta-moxifen in women diagnosed with ductal carcinoma in situ (DCIS). B. Fisher, J. Dig-nam, N. Wolmark, D. L. Wickerham, et al., "Tamoxifen in treatment of intraductal breast cancer: National Surgical Adjuvant Breast and Bowel Project B-24 randomised controlled trial," *The Lancet* 353 (1999): 1993–2000.

77. Experts agree that DCIS can progress to fully invasive cancer but are not sure how frequently it happens. Harold J. Burstein, Kornelia Polyak, Julia S. Wong, et al., "Ductal carcinoma in situ of the breast," *New England Journal of Medicine* 350 (2004): 1430–41.

78. At the same time, the National Cancer Institute conducted a clinical trial of chemoprevention of prostate cancer. Finasterine—a drug of the family of alpha re-ductase inhibitors that contains molecules that prevent the conversion of testosterone into the more potent substance, dihydrotestosterone—was administered to men at higher than averge risk of prostate cancer. The trial, Prostate Cancer Prevention Trial (PCPT) had shown thar finasteride reduced rates of prostate cancer in the experi-mental group (30% reduction compared with the control group), but it induced sec-ondary effects, including higher percentage of high grade prostate tumors among the drug's users. Finasteride was therefore judged inappropriate for generalized prophy-lactic use. Ian M. Thompson, Phyllis J. Goodman, Catherine M. Tangen, et al., "The influence of finasteride on the development of prostate cancer," *New England Journal of Medicine* 349 (2003): 215–24, and for analysis, Stewart Justman, *Do No Harm: How a Magic Bullet for Prostate Cancer Became a Medical Quandary* (Chicago: Ivan R. Dee, 2008). During the seven years of PCPT, 18.4% of the men in the finasteride group and 24.4% of men in the control group were diagnosed with prostate cancer, a very high incidence rate, even taking into acount that these men had higher than average risk of developing prostate malignancies. Elevated rates of detection of prostate cancer among PCPT participants may be related to the close surveillance of this population.

79. For an internal history of NCI's B-14, B-17, and B-24 trials, see R. E. Smith and B. C. Good, "Chemoprevention of breast cancer and the trials of the National Surgi-cal Adjuvant Breast and Bowel Project and others," *Endocrine-Related Cancer* 10 (2003): 347–57, and for sociological analysis of these trials, Maren Klawiter, "Risk, prevention and the breast cancer continuum: The NCI, the FDA, health activism and the pharmaceutical industry," *History and Technology* 18 (2002): 309–53.

80. M. H. Gail, L. A. Brinton, D. P. Byar, et al., "Projecting individual probabilities of developing breast cancer for white females who are being examined annually," *Journal of the National Cancer Institute* 81 (1989): 1879–86. Sixty-year-old women with no additional risk factors and younger women with risk factors have an equal probability of getting breast cancer of 1.66%. Ibid. On the history of Gail model, see Klawiter, "Risk, prevention and the breast cancer continuum"; Jennifer Fosket, "Con-struction of "high risk women": The development and standardization of breast can-cer risk assessment tool," *Science, Technology and Human Values* 29 (2004): 291–313.

81. The Gail model included only variables seen as the most important. Other vari-ables, such as number of children, socioeconomic status, or weight, were neglected.

82. In the United States, the standard recommendation is an annual mammography between ages 40 and 75; in the United Kingdom, a triennial mammography between ages 50 and 70, and in France, a biennial mammography between the ages of 50 and 70. Consequently, women in the United States have a higher chance than women in the United Kingdom or in France to be diagnosed with a morphological risk of breast cancer (lobular carcinoma in situ, atypia), and, independently, to be classified as having a higher risk of breast cancer on the basis of past biopsies. U.S. specialists determined that 18% of women who have yearly mammographies for ten years will undergo biopsy at least once. Joanne G. Elmore, Mary B. Barton, Victoria M. Moeri et al., "Ten year risk of false positive screening mammograms," *New England Journal of Medicine* 338 (1998): 1089–96.

83. "Tamoxifen and breast cancer," Hearings before the subcommittee of the committee on appropriations, United States Senate, 105 Congress, 2nd sess., Apr. 21, 1998. (Washington, DC: U.S. Government Printing Office, 1998), 39–41.

84. B. Fisher, J. P. Constantino, D. L. Wickerham, et al., "Tamoxifen for prevention of breast cancer: Report of the National Surgical Adjuvant Breast and Bowel Project P-1 study," *Journal of the National Cancer Institute* 90 (1998): 1371–88; Trevor J. Powles, "Status of anti-estrogen breast cancer prevention trials," *Oncology* 12 (1998): 28–31. T. Powles, R. Eeles, S. Ashley, et al., "Interim analysis of the incidence of breast cancer in the Royal Mardsen Hospital Tamoxifen randomized chemoprevention trial," *The Lancet* 352 (1998): 98–101; U. Veronesi, P. Maisonneuve, A. Costa, et al., "Prevention of breast cancer with tamoxifen: Preliminary findings from the Italian randomized trial among hysteroctomized women," *The Lancet* 352 (1998): 93–97.

85. www.cancer.gov/star (accessed Aug. 8, 2008). On the background and organization of the STAR trial, see Jennifer Ruth Fosket, "Breast Cancer Risk and the Politics of Prevention: Analysis of a Clinical Trial," Ph.D. Thesis, University of California, San Francisco, 2002.

86. Victor G. Vogel, Joseph P. Costantino, D. Lawrence Wickham, and Walter M. Cronin, "Re- Tamoxifen for prevention of breast cancer," *Journal of the National Cancer Institute* 94 (2002): 1504.

87. Quoted by Christina Holmberg, "Participation in clinical trials: Societal aspirations, personal experience and healing—the meaning of participation," paper given at the conference, "Der Mensch in Experiment," ICI Kulturlabo, Berlin, May 22–24, 2008. I'm indebted to Christina Holmberg for sharing with me her unpublished text.

88. Holmberg, "Participation in clinical trials." Holmberg's data may indicate that, for some participants at least, aspirng to avoid cancer in the future was inseparatedly linked with attenuating the already existing consequences of a diagnosis of a precancerous condition.

89. www.cancer.gov/newscenter/pressreleases/STARresultsApr172006 (accessed Aug. 8, 2008).

90. www.dfci.harvard.edu/res/research/unveiling-of-star-trial-results-brings-kudos-to-participants.html (accessed Aug. 8, 2008).

91. The differences between secondary effects induced by tamoxifen and ralox-ifene were not statistically meaningful. Victor G. Vogel, Joseph P. Costantino, D. Law-rence Wickerham, et al., "Effect of Tamoxifen vs. Raloxifene on the risk of developing invasive breast cancer and other disease outcomes: The NSABP study of Tamoxifen and Ralxifene," *JAMA* 295 (2006): 2727–41; Stephanie R. Land, D. Lawrence Wicker-ham, Joseph P. Costantino, et al., "Patient-reported symptoms and quality of life dur-ing treatment with tamoxifen or raloxifene for breast cancer prevention," *JAMA* 295 (2006): 2742–51.

92. BCA, May 2006 E-mail alert, www.bcaction.org/Pages/GetInformed/Email Alerts/May2006EAlert.html (accessed Aug. 8, 2008).

93. Such direct-to-consumer publicity is increasingly popular in the United States while it is (as of now) illegal in Europe. Michael S. Wilkes, Robert A. Bell, and Rich-ard L. Kravitz, "Direct to consumer prescription drug advertising: Trends, impact and implications," *Health Affairs* 19 (2000): 110–28.

94. Elisa Rush Port, Leslie L. Montgomery, Alexander S. Heerd, and Patrick I. Bor-gen, "Patients' reluctance toward tamoxifen use for breast cancer primary preven-tion," *Annals of Surgical Oncology* 8 (2001): 580–85.

95. Rebecca Taylor and Kenneth Taguchi, "Tamoxifen for breast cancer preven-tion: Low uptake by high risk women after an evaluation of a breast lump," *Annals of Family Medicine* 3 (2005): 242–45.

96. Christine Gorman, "A better option?" *Time*, Apr. 24, 2006.

97. Julia Tchou, Nanjiang Hou, Alfred Rademaker, V. Craig Jordan, and Monica Morrow, "Acceptance of tamoxifen chemoprevention by physicians and women at risk," *Cancer* 100 (2004): 1800–1806, on p. 1805. See also Vogel, Costantino, Wickham, and Cronin, "Re- Tamoxifen for prevention of breast cancer." Apprehension induced by repeated biopsies and the physical deformation of the breast by biopsy scars may also favor the acceptance of preventive mastectomy.

98. Tchou, Hou, Rademaker, Jordan, and Morrow, "Acceptance of tamoxifen chemoprevention by physicians and women at risk," 1805.

99. This was for example the official position of American Cancer Society in Nov. 2006. www.cancer.org/docroot/CRI/content/CRI_2_6X_Tamoxifen_and_Raloxifene_ ; Questions_and_Answers_5.asp?sitearea= (accessed Aug. 8, 2008). European experts objected to a routine use of tamoxifen to prevent breast cancer and restricted its pro-phylactic uses to clinical trials. Veronesi, Maisonneuve, Costa, et al., "Prevention of Breast Cancer with Tamoxifen"; Powles, Eeles, Ashley, et al., "Interim Analysis of the Incidence of Breast Cancer."

100. See, for example, the statement of National Women Health Network on this subject at www.nwhn.org/alerts/alerts_details.php?aid=63 (accessed Aug. 8, 2008).

101. "Tamoxifen and breast cancer," Hearings before the subcommittee of the com-mittee on appropriations, United States Senate, 105th Congress, 2nd sess., Apr. 21, 1998 (Washington, DC: U.S. Government Printing Office, 1998), 13–14.

102. Rosalind A. Eeles and Trevor J. Powles, "Chemoprevention Options for *BRCA1* and *BRCA2* Mutation Carriers," *Journal of Clinical Oncology*, 18, 21S (2000): 93s–99s;

J. Cuzick, for International Breast Cancer Intervention Study, "A brief review of the International Breast Cancer Intervention Study (IBIS), the other current breast cancer prevention trials, and proposals for future trials," *Annals of the New York Academy of Sciences* 949 (2001): 123–33.

103. For a 2006 summary of available risk reducing options, see José G. Guillem, William C. Wood, Jeffrey F. Moley, Andrew Berchuck, et al., "ASCO/SSO Review of Current Role of Risk-Reducing Surgery in Common Hereditary Cancer Syndromes," *Journal of Clinical Oncology* 24 (2006): 4642–60. Preventive surgery reduces, but does not totally eliminate cancer risk, and some experts recommend the continuation of intensive surveillance of women who underwent such surgery. Dawn Allain, Kevin Sweet, and Doreen M. Agnese, "Management options after prophylactic surgeries in women with BRCA mutations," *Cancer Control* 14 (2007): 330–37.

104. Janet E. Lane-Claypon, *A Further Report on Cancer of the Breast*, 4.

105. P. Weir and Clarence C. Little, "The incidence of uterine cancer in Jews and Gentiles," *Bulletin of the American Society for the Control of Cancer* 16 (1934): 6–8.

106. W. Sampson Handley, "The prevention of cancer," *The Lancet* 1 (1936): 987–91, on p. 990.

107. Georg Wolff, "Cancer and race with specific reference to the Jews," *The American Journal of Hygiene* 29 (1939): 121–37, on p. 136.

108. Weir and Little, "The incidence of uterine cancer in Jews and Gentiles."

109. Troy Duster, *Backdoor to Eugenics* (New York: Routledge, 1990).

110. J. Ekstein and H. Katzenstein, "The Dor Ysharim story: Community based screening for Tay Sachs disease," *Advances in Genetics* 44 (2001): 297–310; Barbara Prainsack and Gil Siegal, "The rise of genetic couplehood? A comparative view of premarital genetic testing," *BioSocieties* 1 (2006): 17–36; Keith Wailoo and Stephen Pemberton, *The Troubled Dream of Genetic Medicine: Ethnicity and Innovation in Tay-Sachs, Cystic Fibrosis, and Sickle Cell Disease* (Baltimore: Johns Hopkins University Press, 2006).

111. Jeffrey P. Steruving et al., "The carrier frequency of the *BRCA 1* del185 mutation is approximately 1% in Ashkenazi Jewish individuals," *Nature Genetics* 11 (1995): 198–99.

112. Karen H. Rothenberg, "Breast cancer, the genetic 'quick fix' and the Jewish community: Ethical, legal and social challenges," *Health Matrix* 7 (1997): 97–124.

113. Rothenberg, "Breast cancer, the genetic 'quick fix' and the Jewish community," 101–2.

114. The prevalence of these mutations among Ashkenazi women is approximately 2.5% (one in forty women). E. Levy-Lahad, R. Catane, S. Eisenberg, et al. "Founder BRCA1 and BRCA2 Mutations in Ashkenazi Jews in Israel: Frequency and differential penetrance in ovarian cancer and in breast-ovarian cancer families," *American Journal of Human Genetics* 60 (1997): 1059–67. Estimates on prevalence of *BRCA* mutation in the population vary, however, according to the method of sampling used. Kenneth Offit, "Editorial: BRCA mutation frequency and penetrance: New data, old debate," *Journal of the National Cancer Institute* 98 (2006): 1675–77.

115. Rose Kushner had argued that lifestyle elements, such as sedentary urban lifestyle and late childbirth, may explain the seemingly higher global prevalence of breast cancer among Jewish women in the United States. Rose Kushner, "Cancer risks in Jewish women: Nutrition and lifestyle, not genetics may determine the differences in incidence rates," Kushner's papers, MC 453, box 2, Arthur and Elizabeth Schlesinger Library on the History of Women in America, Radcliffe Institute of Advanced Study, Harvard University (Schlesinger Library).

116. www.sharsheret.org/index.php (accessed Aug. 8, 2008).

117. Marie Claire King, J. H. Marks, J. B. Mandell, and New York Breast Cancer Study Group, "Breast and ovarian cancer risk due to inherited mutations in *BRCA1* and BRCA2," *Science* 302 (2003): 643–46.

118. Many American women elect not to inform their insurer about *BRCA* testing, fearing discrimination, which may change as a result of 2008 legislation barring discrimination on the basis of genetic information. An affordable price of a test is therefore an especially interesting advantage.

119. Troy Duster, "Buried alive: The concept of race in science," in *Genetic Nature/Culture,* Ian Goodman, Deborah Heath and Susan Lindee, eds. (Berkeley and Los Angeles: University of California Press, 2003), 258–77, esp. p. 273. French reluctance to use racial categories may be related to the use of an official "fichier des juifs" by the Vichy government to send Jews to Nazi extermination camps during the Second World War.

120. Some specialists became interested in the legal "right for ignorance," e.g., Graeme T. Laurie, "In defense of ignorance: Genetic information and the right not to know," *European Journal of Health and Law* 6 (1999): 119–32. Legal issues are, however, only one among many dilemmas surrounding testing for hereditary risk of cancer. On difficulties of resisting a genetic or molecular interpretation of disease, see Michel Callon and Vololona Rhaberisoa, "Gino's lesson on humanity: Genetic, mutual entanglement and the sociologist's role," *Economy and Society* 33 (2004): 1–27.

121. In this regard, breast cancer seems to occupy an intermediary place between colon cancer (both FAP and HNPCC), a pathology in which early detection is seen as an efficient way to limit morbidity and mortality and a refusal of surveillance is seen as irrational and prostate cancer, a pathology in which the value of early detection remains controversial and a refusal of surveillance is viewed by many doctors as a reasonable choice.

122. Mary-Jo Delveccio Good, "Cultural studies of biomedicine: An agenda for research," *Social Studies of Medicine* 41 (1995): 461–73.

123. Victor G. Vogel, "Tools for evaluating a patient's 5 year and lifetime probabilities," *Postgraduate Medicine* 105 (1999): 49–61. On critique of this view, see Ann Robertson, "Biotechnology: Political rationality and discourses on health risk," *Health* 5 (2001): 293–309; Jessica Poltzer and Ann Robertson, "From familial diseases to 'genetic risk': Harnessing women's labour in the (co)production of scientific knowledge about breast cancer," in *Gendered Risks,* ed. Kelly Hannah-Moffat and Pat O'Malloy (London : Routledge, 2007), 31–53.

124. K. Phillips, K. Kerlikowske, L. Baker, et al., "Factors associated with women's

adherence to mammography screening guidelines," *Health Services Research* 33 (1998): 29–53; Aldeswars and Sachs, "Risk discourse," 207.

125. See, e.g., Deborah Lupton, "Femininity, responsibility and the technological imperative: Discourses on breast cancer in the Australian press," *International Journal of Health Services* 24 (1994): 73–89.

126. Sarah Wainberg and Janice Husted, "Utilization of screening and preventive surgery among unaffected carriers of a BRCA1 or BRCA2 gene mutation," *Cancer Epidemiology Biomarkers and Prevention*, 13 (2004): 1989–95: Michael Fatouros, Georgios Baltoyiannis, and Dimitrios H. Roukos, "The predominant role of sugery in the prevention and new trends in surgical treatment of women with BRCA1/ 2 mutations," *Annals of Surgical Oncology*, 15 (2008): 21–33. Fatouros, Baltoyiannis, and Roukos present surveillance with medication as an alternative to prophylactic surgery, but at the same time they explain that this approach is linked with high risk of a late diagnosis of cancer. Ibid., 27.

127. Lederberg, "Molecular biology, eugenic and euphenics."

128. Diane Paul, *The Politics of Heredity: Essays on Eugenics, Biomedicine, and the Nature-Nurture Debate* (Albany: State University of New York Press, 1998); Ruth Schwartz Cowan, *Heredity and Hope: The Case for Genetic Screening* (Cambridge, MA: Harvard University Press, 2008).

129. On the replacement of old eugenics by new, individual-focused trends, see Deborah Wertz, "Eugenics is alive and well: Survey of genetic professionals around the world," *Science in Context* 11 (1998): 493–510; Merryn Ekberg, "The old eugenics and the new genetics compared," *Social History of Medicine* 20 (2007): 581–93; Ruth Cowan strongly rejects this view. Cowan, *Heredity and Hope*, 223–45. On the individualization of mangement of risks, see Robert Aronowitz, "Situating Health Risks: An Opportunity for Disease Prevention Policy," in *American Health Care, History and Policy,* ed. Charles Rosenberg, Rosemary Stevens, and R. Burns (Berkeley and Los Angeles: University of California Press, 2006), 153–65.

130. Robert Aronowitz, *Making Sense of Illness: Science, Society and Disease* (Cambridge: Cambridge University Press, 1998); Elodie Giroux, "An epidemiological perspective into the philosophical debate on the definition of health and disease," seminar paper, Max Planck Institute for the History of Science, March 2006.

131. On the role of drug companies in this development, see Jeremy A. Greene, *Prescribing by Numbers: Drugs and the Definition of Disease* (Baltimore: Johns Hopkins University Press, 2007).

132. Rothenberg, "Breast cancer, the genetic 'quick fix' and the Jewish community," 124.

133. On the difficulty of escaping the internalization of the state of "being at risk" and its transformation into a status of the "pre-symptomatic ill," see Margaret Lock, "Breast cancer: Reading the omens," *Anthropology Today* 14 (1998): 7–16, and on the "choice of no choice" introduced by new medical technologies, see Marylin Strathern, *After Nature: English Kinship in the Late Twentieth Century* (Cambridge: Cambridge University Press, 1992).

Chapter Eight · The New Surgical Radicalism

1. Ilana Löwy, *Between Bench and Bedside: Science, Healing and Inerleukin-2 in a Cancer Ward* (Harvard: Harvard University Press, 1996); Toine Pieters, *Interferon: The Science and Selling of a Miracle Drug* (London: Routledge, 2005).

2. On the role of patients' activism in promoting a more conservative surgery for breast cancer, see, e.g., Barron H. Lerner, *The Breast Cancer Wars* (New York: Oxford University Press, 2001); Nancy K. Bristlow, "Battling breast cancer," *Reviews in American History* 30 (2002): 114–23, and on the role of shift in expert's perception of natural history of breast cancer in the abandonment of radical mastectomy, Pamela Sanders Goebel, "Crisis and controversy: Historical patters in breast cancer surgery," *Canadian Bulletin of the History of Medicine* 8 (1991): 77–90.

3. Bernard Fisher, "The changing role of surgery in the treatment of cancer," in *Cancer: A Comprehensive Treatise,* ed. Frederick F. Becker (New York: Plenum Press, 1977), 401–21, on p. 404. On Fisher's role in initiating clinical trials of conservative treatment of breast cancer in the United States, see Lerner, *The Breast Cancer Wars,* 226–31, and on his career, Kate Travis, "Bernard Fisher reflects on a half-century worth of breast cancer research," *Journal of the National Cancer Institute* 97 (2005): 1636–37.

4. Bernard Fisher, "Personal contributions to progress in breast cancer research and treatment," *Seminars in Oncology* 23 (1996): 414–27.

5. Bernard Fisher, "From Halsted to prevention and beyond: Advances in the management of breast cancer during the twentieth century," *European Journal of Cancer* 3 (1999): 1963–73, on p. 1971.

6. Anne-Marie de Grazia, "The Amazon choice: One woman's radical attempt to avoid breast cancer," www.grazian-archive.com/quiddity/preventive%20mastectomy .htm (accessed Mar. 10, 2008).

7. Susan Ferraro, "Peace of mind, but at a price. Removing healthy breast may prevent cancer in some women. It can be an agonizing choice," *Daily News,* June 30, 1997. For a discussion of this episode, see Kathleen Woodward, "Statistic panic," *Differences: A Journal of Feminist Cultural Studies* 11 (1999): 177–203, on p. 186. Prophylactic mastectomy was discussed in episode 21, season 3, of the CBS drama series *Chicago Hope.* The late 1990s were a transition period. At that time numerous American and British doctors had already adopted preventive mastectomy for women at high hereditary risk of breast cancer.

8. http://mayoclinic.org/patientstories/janetvittone.html (accessed Mar. 10, 2008).

9. Salynn Boyels, "Preventive mastectomy satisfying," WebMed, Mar. 17, 2006, www .webmd.com/content/article/120/113654.htm (accessed Mar. 10, 2008).

10. Jerome Groopman, "Decoding destiny: Genetic testing," *The New Yorker,* Feb. 9, 1998. In the introduction to his collection of essays, *Second Opinion* (New York: Viking, 2000), Groopman reveals that his wife—a physician whose opinion he respects greatly—disagreed with his recommendation of preventive surgery. This information does not appear, however, in his widely read *New Yorker* article.

11. Karen explains her decision by her wish to see her children grow up, a view that

equates hereditary breast cancer risk with a quasi-certainty of an early death. On a systematic identification of presence of a hereditary risk with the worse possible outcome, see Margaret Lock, "Breast cancer: Reading the omens," *Anthropology Today* 14 (1998): 7–16.

12. B. Cutuli, P. H. Cottu, J. P. Guastalle, et al., "A French national survey on infiltrating breast cancer," *Breast Cancer Research and Treatment* 95 (2006): 55–64.

13. The results are published in Ilana Löwy, "Le risque héréditaire du cancer de sein et d'ovaire dans la clinique: Une approche comparative, France, Grande Bretagne, Etats Unis," in *Prédisposition Génétique aux Cancers: Questions Psychologiques et Débats de Societé,* ed. Claire Julien Reynier, Janine Pierrert, and François Eisinger (Paris: John Libbey Eurotext, 2005), 33–44; Jean-Paul Gaudillière and Ilana Löwy, "Science, markets and public health: Contemporary testing for breast cancer predispositions," in *Medicine, the Market and the Mass Media: Producing Health in the Twentieth Century,* ed. Virginia Berridge and Kelly Loughin (London: Routledge, 2005), 266–87; Ilana Löwy and Jean-Paul Gaudillière, "Localizing the global: Testing for hereditary risks of breast cancer," *Science, Technology and Human Values* 33 (2008): 299–325.

14. François Eisinger, Nicole Alby, et al. "Recommendation for medical management of hereditary breast and ovarian cancer: The French National Ad Hoc Committee," *Annals of Oncology* 9 (1998): 939–50.

15. French oncogeneticists discussed in 1999 the advantages and the disadvantages of preventive mastectomy, but as far as I know, they saw such a debate mainly as a rhetorical exercise. Oncogeneticists I observed believed that women can enjoy their breasts as long as they are cancer free. Nicolas Janin, "Pour quels raisons devrait-on s'abstenir de conseiller une mastectomie prophylactique chez les femmes à risque?" *Bulletin du Cancer* 86 (1999): 760–66; Dominique Stoppa-Lyonnet, "Pour quelles raisons pourrait-on conseiller une mastectomie prophylactique à une femme à risque?" *Bulletin du Cancer* 86 (1999): 754–59.

16. L.C. Hartman, "Prophylactic mastectomy: Preliminary retrospective cohort analysis," *Proceeding of the American Association for Cancer Research* 38 (1997): 168. Data on prophylactic mastectomy in France are anecdotal. A register of such data was established the in late 1990s, but in 2008, these data were not (as yet) published.

17. François Eisinger, G. Geller, W. Burke, and N. A. Holtzman, "Cultural basis for differences between US and French clinical recommendations for women at increased risk of breast and ovarian cancer," *The Lancet* 353 (1999): 919–20.

18. François Eisinger, Dominique Stoppa-Lyonnet, Christine Lasset, et al. "Comparison of physician' and cancer prone women's attitudes about breast/ ovarian prophylactic surgery: Results from two national surveys" *Familial Cancer* 1 (2001): 157–62: Claire Julian Reynier, Louise Bouchard, Garret Evans, et al., "Women's attitudes towards preventive strategies for hereditary breast or ovarian carcinoma differ from one country to another: Differences among English, French and Canadian women," *Cancer* 92 (2001): 959–68; Laura Newman, "French national ad hoc committee strongly resists prophylactic mastectomy," *Journal of the National Cancer Institute* 93 (2001): 339–40.

19. Sara Wainberg and Janice Husted, "Utilization of screening and preventive surgery among unaffected carriers of a *BRCA1* or *BRCA2* gene mutation," *Cancer Epidemiology, Biomarkers and Prevention* 13 (2004): 1989–95; Yolanda Antill, John Reynolds, Mary-Anne Young, et al., "Risk reducing surgery in women with familial susceptibility for breast and ovarian cancer," *European Journal of Cancer* 42 (2006): 621–28.

20. Wainberg and Husted, "Utilization of screening and preventive surgery."

21. G. Geller, B. A. Berhanrdt, T. Doksum, et al., "Decision making about breast cancer susceptibility testing: How similar are the attitudes of physicians, nurse practitioners and at risk women," *Journal of Clinical Oncology* 16 (1998): 2868–76.

22. Louise Bouchard, Isabelle Blancquaert, François Eisinger, et al., "Prevention and testing for breast cancer: Variations in medical decisions," *Social Sciences and Medicine* 58 (2004): 1085–96.

23. Sue Fisher, *In the Patient's Best Interest: Women and the Politics of Medical Decision* (New Brunswick: Rutgers University Press, 1986), 32–35; George Weisz, *Divide and Conquer: A Comparative History of Medical Specialization* (Oxford: Oxford University Press, 2005), 208–9; Cutuli, Cottu, Guastalle, et al., "A French national survey on infiltrating breast cancer."

24. T. K. F. Hoskins, J. E. Stopfer, K. A. Calzone, et al., "Assessment and counseling for women with a family history of breast cancer," *JAMA* 273 (1995): 577–85.

25. L. C. Hartman, T. A. Sellers, D. J. Schaid, et al., "Efficacy of Bilateral Prophylactic Mastectomy in *BRCA1* and *BRCA2* Gene Mutation Carriers," *Journal of National Cancer Institute* 93 (2001): 1586–87; Meijers Heijboer, H. B. van Geel, W. L. van Putten, et al., "Breast cancer after prophylactic bilateral mastectomy in women with *BRCA1* or *BRCA2* mutation," *New England Journal of Medicine* 345 (2001): 159–64.

26. Timothy R. Rebbeck, Tara Friebel, Henry T. Lynch, et al., "Bilateral prophylactic mastectomy reduces breast cancer risk in *BRCA1* and *BRCA2* mutation carriers: The PROSE study group," *Journal of Clinical Oncology* 22 (2004): 1055–62.

27. K. Anderson, J. S. Jacobson, D. F. Heitjan, J. G. Zivin, et al., "Cost-effectiveness of preventive strategies for women with a *BRCA1* or a *BRCA2* mutation," *Annals of Internal Medicine* 144 (2006): 397–406; Dawn Allain, Kevin Sweet, and Doreen M. Agnese, "Management options after prophylactic surgeries in women with *BRCA* mutations," *Cancer Control* 14 (2007): 330–37; Michael Fatouros, Georgios Baltoyiannis, and Dimitrios H. Roukos, "The predominant role of surgery in the prevention and new trends in surgical treatment of women with *BRCA1/ 2* mutations," *Annals of Surgical Oncology,* 15 (2008): 21–33.

28. François Eisinger, B. Bressac, D. Castaigne, et al., "Identification and management of hereditary predisposition to cancer of the breast and the ovary (update 2004)," *Bulletin du Cancer* 91 (2004): 655–56. The 2004 text adds, however, that this conclusion, based on small samples and short-term surveys, is temporary only.

29. "Forum: Cancer du sein et hérédité": www.essentielles.net/communaute/public/forums/forumdetail.asp?s=500&fid=73 (accessed Mar. 10, 2008). This forum is probably not very representative. Its "core participants" strongly support preventive surgery and try to convince other correspondents that this is the best possible choice.

30. In spite of a larger consensus in favor of this intervention, rates of preventive oophorectomy are also highly variable. A 2004 survey that identified data on preventive surgeries in *BRCA* mutation carriers from seven centers (five American and two Dutch) had found that rates of preventive mastectomy varied between 0% and 54%, and those of preventive oophorectomy, between 13% and 53%. Wainberg and Husted, "Utilization of screening and preventive surgery."

31. Timothy Rebbeck, H. T. Lynch, S. L. Neuhasen, et al., "Prophylactic oophorectomy in carriers of *BRCA1* and *BRCA2* mutations," *New England Journal of Medicine* 346 (2002): 1616–22.

32. Michael J. Clarke, "Ovarian ablation in breast cancer, 1896 to 1998," *British Medical Journal* 17 (1998): 1246–48. Women's readiness to undergo surgical castration as part of treatment of breast cancer may be contrasted with men's reluctance to undergo castration to treat prostate cancer. Letter from developer of silbesterol (DES) Charles Dodds on its uses in the therapy of cancer of the prostate. British Empire Cancer Campaign (BECC), series SA/CRC: Clinics, pathology, research Box 50, File E/6: Papers of Sir Charles Dodds (1899–1973), Wellcome Archives, Wellcome Library, London, England (Wellcome Archives).

33. A. Eisen, J. Lubinski, J. Klijn, et al., "Breast cancer risk following bilateral oophorectomy in *BRCA1* and *BRCA2* mutation carriers: An international case-control study," *Journal of Clinical Oncology* 23 (2005): 7491–96. Women with *BRCA2* mutations seem to be less protected by oophorectomy. Noah D. Kauff, Susan M. Domchek, Tara M. Friebel, et al., "Risk reducing sapingo-oophorectomy for the prevention of *BRCA1* and *BRCA2* associated breast and gynecological cancer: A multicenter, prospective study," *Journal of Clinical Oncology* 26 (2008): 1331–37.

34. Timothy R. Rebbeck, T. Friebel, T. Wagner, et al., "Effect of short-term hormone replacement therapy on breast cancer risk reduction after bilateral prophylactic oophorectomy in *BRCA1* and *BRCA2* mutation carriers," *Journal of Clinical Oncology* 23 (2005): 7804–10. Oophorectomy is seen by many women as a more acceptable prophylactic treatment than mastectomy: for example, in an Israeli sample, 78% of *BRCA*-mutation carriers underwent preventive oophorectomy and only 18% preventive mastectomy. Vardit Kram, Tamar Perez, and Michal Sagi, "Acceptance of preventive surgeries by Israeli women who had undergone *BRCA* testing," *Familial Cancer* 5 (2006): 327–35.

35. Some U.S. oncologists also systematically propose such a test for women of Ashkenazi Jewish origins diagnosed with a breast tumor.

36. Amy Harmon reports a story of a woman who elected to undergo preventive oophorectomy without genetic testing, fearing that if she tested positive she would never be able to buy health insurance. Amy Harmon, "Fear of Insurance Trouble Leads Many to Shun or Hide DNA Tests," *New York Times,* Feb. 24, 2008.

37. In 2000, 68% of U.S. genetic counselors questioned affirmed that they would not notify their insurer if they had to be tested themselves for *BRCA* mutations. Ellen T. Matloff, Heather Shapell, Karina Brierly, et al., "What would you do? Specialists' perspective on cancer genetic testing, prophylactic surgery and insurance discrimination, *Journal of Clinical Oncology* 181 (2000): 2484–92.

38. Some specialists claim that breast cancer in *BRCA*-positive women does not need to be treated more aggressively than does a similar tumor in a *BRCA*-negative patient. This is, however, a minority view. B. G. Haffty, and D. Lannin, "Is breast conserving therapy in the genetically predisposed breast cancer patients a reasonable and appropriate option?" *European Journal of Cancer* 40 (2004): 1105–8; François Eisinger, L. Huiart, and Hagai Sobol, "The choice of bilateral prophylactic mastectomy," *Journal of Clinical Oncology* 23 (2005): 1330–31; François Eisinger, "Editorial: It's not for me. . . . It's for my daughter," *European Journal of Cancer* 43 (2007): 226–27.

39. Mark D. Schwartz, Caryn Lerman, Barbara Brogan, et al., "Impact of *BRCA1/BRCA2* counseling and testing on newly diagnosed breast cancer patient," *Journal of Clinical Oncology* 22 (2004): 1823–29; Marc D. Schwarts, Beth N. Peshkin, and Claudine Isaacs, "The choice of bilateral prophylactic mastectomy," *Journal of Clinical Oncology* 23 (2005): 1331.

40. Kelly A. Metcalfe, Jan Lubinski, Parviz Ghadirian, et al., "Predictors of contralateral prophylactic mastectomy in women with a *BRCA1* or *BRCA2* mutation: The hereditary breast cancer clinical study group," *Journal of Clinical Oncology* 26 (2008): 1093–97.

41. Kelly A. Metcalfe, Daphna Birenbaum-Carmeli, Jan Lubinski, et al., "International variations in rates of uptake of preventive options in *BRCA1* and *BRCA2* mutation carriers," *International Journal of Cancer* 122 (2008): 2017–22. Choices of *BRCA*-positive women in the United States may reflect a general increase in more aggressive surgery for breast cancer. Between 1998 and 2003, the number of American women operated for breast cancer who elected a prophylactic ablation of the contralateral breast increased from 4.2% to 11%. Todd M. Tuttle, Elisabeth B. Habermann, Erin H. Grund, Todd J. Morris, and Beth A. Virnig, "Increasing use of contralateral prophylactic mastectomy for breast cancer patients: A trend toward more aggressive surgical treatment," *Journal of Clinical Oncology* 25 (2007): 5203–9; Fisher, "From Halsted to prevention and beyond."

42. Margaret Lock, "Biomedical technologies, cultural horizons and contested boundaries," in *The Handbook of Science and Technology Studies,* ed. Edward J. Hackett, Olga Amsterdamska, Michael Lynch, and Judy Wajtzman (Cambridge, MA: MIT Press, 2007), 875–900.

43. Schwartz, Lerman, Brogan, et al., "Impact of *BRCA1/BRCA2* counseling and testing," 1826.

44. Eisinger, Huiart, and Hagai Sobol, "The choice of bilateral prophylactic mastectomy."

45. K. K. Khurana, A. Losmann, P. J. Numann, and S. A. Khan, "Prophylactic mastectomy: Pathological findings in high risk patients," *Archives of Pathology and Laboratory Medicine* 124 (2000): 378–81; N. Hoogerbrugge, P. Bult, L. M. de Widt-Levert, et al., "High prevalence of premalignant lesion in prophylactically removed breasts from women at hereditary risk for breast cancer," *Journal of Clinical Oncology* 21 (2003): 41–45; N. D. Kauf, E. Brogi, L. Scheurer, et al., "Epithelial lesions in prophylactic mastectomy specimens from women with *BRCA* mutations," *Cancer* 97 (2003): 1601–8; C. Adem, C. Reynolds, C. L. Soderberg et al., "Pathological characteristics of

breast parenchyma in patients with hereditary breast carcinoma, including *BRCA1* and *BRCA2* mutation carriers," *Cancer* 97 (2003): 1–11.

46. R. Kerner, E. Sabo, R. Gershoni-Baruch, D. Beck, and O. Ben-Izhak, "Expression of cell cycle regulatory proteins in ovaries prophylactically removed from Jewish Ashkenazi *BRCA1* and *BRCA2* mutation carriers: Correlations with histopathology," *Gynecology and Oncology* 99 (2005): 367–75; Brena B. J. Hermsen, Paul J. Van Diest, Johannes Berkhof, et al., "Low prevalence of (pre) malignant lesions in the breast and high prevalence in the ovary and Fallopian tubes in women at hereditary risk of breast and ovarian cancer," *International Journal of Cancer* 119 (2006): 1412–18. The "low" prevalence in the title of the latter article may be misleading, since the authors' conclusion is that the hereditary risk of breast/ovarian cancer was associated with a high risk of premalignant lesions in the ovary and Fallopian tubes.

47. Women with strong family history of breast cancer but no *BRCA1* or *BRCA2* mutations have even higher rates of proliferative lesions of the breast than they have mutation carriers. N. Hoogerbrugge, P. Bult, J. J. Bonenkamp, M. J. L. Ligtenberg, et al., "Numerous high-risk epithelial lesions in familial breast cancer," *European Journal of Cancer* 42 (2006): 2492–98.

48. Jessica Queller, *Pretty Is What Changes: Impossible Choices, the Breast Cancer Gene, and How I Changed My Destiny* (New York: Spiegel and Grau, 2008), 205.

49. Masha Gessen, *Blood Matters: From Inherited Illness to Designer Babies: How the World and I Found Ourselves in the Future of the Gene* (Orlando, FL: Harcourt, 2008), 195.

50. I. Dove-Edwin, P. Sasieni, J. Adams, and H. J. Thomas, "Prevention of colorectal cancer by colonoscopic surveillance in individuals with a family history of colorectal cancer: 16 year, prospective, follow-up study," *British Medical Journal* 331 (2005): 1033–34; A. E. de Jong, Y. M. Hendriks, J. H. Kleibeuker, et al., "Decrease in mortality in Lynch syndrome families because of surveillance," *Gastroenterology* 30 (2006): 665–71.

51. People diagnosed with predisposition for nonpolypous forms of colon cancer (mutations in genes *MSH2*, *MLH1*, and several others) undergo a preventive ablation of colon polyps during colonoscopy.

52. The term *pathography* was proposed by Anne Hunsaker Hawkins. Anne Hunsaker Hawkins, *Reconstructing Illness: Studies in Pathography* (West Lafayette, IN: Purdue University Press, 1993).

53. On bias in the presentation of breast cancer as a disease that affects above all young women, see Gerd Gigerenzer, *Calculated Risks: How to Know When Numbers Deceive You* (New York: Simon and Schuster, 2002), 80–81. Maureen Casamayou explains that in its lobbying activity National Breast Cancer Coalition (NBCC) deliberately had chosen to bring to the foreground younger women, preferably mothers of young children, in order to maximize emotional impact and enrol politicians' support. Maureen Hogan Casamayou, *The Politics of Breast Cancer* (Washington, DC: Georgetown University Press, 2001).

54. "My breast cancer story," Cancer Crusade On Line, 1999. www.avoncompany.com/women/avoncrusade/bbsindex.htm (accessed July 3, 2008).

55. www.susanlovemd.org/breastcancer/content.asp?L2=7&L3=3&SID=358 (accessed July 3, 2008).

56. Ibid.

57. Ibid.

58. Joanna L. Yesk, "Breast cancer in the family," *Plus Magazine*, Mar. 2004, 38–39.

59. www.susanlovemd.org/breastcancer/content.asp?L2=7&L3=3&SID=358 (accessed July 3, 2008); some experts criticize an aggressive treatment of the majority of women diagnosed with ductal carcinoma in situ (DCIS). The risk of such treatment, they propose, may be greater than that of the disease itself. DCIS-related mortality rates are very low, while radiotherapy may increase the long-term risk of cardiovascular diseases. Tamoxifen was also linked with an increased risk of cardiovascular disease and stroke; see, e.g., M. A. Thorat, V. Parmar, M. S. Nadkarni, and R. A. Badwen, "Radiation therapy for ductal carcinoma in situ: Is it really worth it?" *Journal of Clinical Oncology* 25 (2007): 461–62; T. Powles, R. Eccles, S. Ashley, et al., "Interim analysis of the incidence of breast cancer in the Royal Mardsen Hospital Tamoxifen randomised chemoprevention trial," *The Lancet* 352 (1998), 98–101. If one follows critics of aggressive treatment of in situ breast lesions, one can propose an alternative scenario, in which ten years after her therapy Beth Evans is sitting in a wheelchair, a victim of iatrogenic complications of an overtreatment of her DCIS.

60. Silja Samerski, "The 'decision trap': How genetic counseling transforms pregnant women into managers of fetal risk profiles," in *Gendered Risks*, ed. Pat O'Malley and Kelly Hannah-Moffat (New York: Routledge-Cavendish, 2007).

61. For example, when offered a choice by nondirective genetic counselors whether to undergo prenatal testing or not, practically all the German women elected to be tested. Barbara Duden, "The euro and the gene—perceived by a historian of the unborn," Lecture at the Robert Schuman Centre for Advanced Studies, European University Institute, Florence, May 7, 2002.

62. People aware of their cancer risk have a great difficulty viewing themselves as healthy and perceive themselves as "presymptomatically ill" instead. Lock, "Breast cancer: Reading the omens." Probably the most efficient way to avoid the internalization of dread of the future is to deny hereditary risk, an attitude that favors escape from an overwhelming medical surveillance. However, women who chose this attitude seldom write pathoblogs or participate in web discussions on genetic risk.

63. On the contradiction between optimistic discourse of cancer and the way this disease is seen by relatives of people with cancer, see James T. Patterson, *The Dread Disease: Cancer and the Modern American Culture* (Cambridge, MA: Harvard University Press, 1987).

64. Ann M. Geiger, Carmen N. West, Larissa Nekhlyudov, et al., "Contentment with quality of life among breast cancer survivors with and without contralateral prophylactic surgery," *Journal of Clinical Oncology* 24 (2006): 1350–56. A previous study had reached similar conclusions. Marc D. Schwartz, "Contralateral prophylactic mastectomy: Efficacy, satisfaction and regret," *Journal of Clinical Oncology* 23 (2005): 7777–79.

65. www.healthfinder.gov/news/newsstory.asp?docID=531628 (accessed Mar. 10, 2008).

66. Jonathan Rees, Michael G. Clarke, Dympna Wardron, Ciaran O'Boyle, Paul Ewings, and Ruaraidth MacDonagh, "The measurement of response shift in patients with advanced prostate cancer and their partners," *Health and Quality of Life Outcomes* 3 (2005): 21.

67. Y. R. B. M. van Gestel, A. C. Voogd, A. J. J. M. Vingerhoets, et al., "A comparison of quality of life, disease impact and risk perception in women with invasive breast cancer and ductal carcinoma in situ," *European Journal of Cancer* 43 (2007): 549–56.

68. Roberta Altman, *Waking Up, Fighting Back: The Politics of Breast Cancer* (Boston: Little, Brown and Company, 1996); Barbara Brenner, "Sister support: Women create a breast cancer movement," in *Breast Cancer: Society Shapes an Epidemics*, ed. Anne Kasper and Susan Feergunson (New York: St. Martin Press, 2000), 325–53; Casamayou, *The Politics of Breast Cancer.*

69. Mette Nordhal Svensen, "Pursuing knowledge about a genetic risk of cancer," in *Managing Uncertainty: Ethnographic Studies of Illness, Risk and the Struggle for Control*, ed. Vibeke Steffen, Richard Jenkins and Hanne Jensen (Copenhagen; University of Copenhagen—Museum Tucsulanum Press, 2005), 93–121, on pp. 113–114.

70. For a similar argument, see Nikolas Rose, *The Politics of Life Itself* (Princeton: Princeton University Press, 2007), 106–29.

71. Svensen, "Pursuing knowledge about a genetic risk of cancer," 115–16. Svensen describes pressures within the family to persuade people to get tested. She frames such pressures in terms of people's moral duty to understand themselves, move toward certainty, and take a personal responsibility for their health. On more problematic aspects of a pressure "to know," see Michel Callon and Vololona Rabeharisoa, "Gino's lesson on humanity: Genetics, mutual entanglement and the sociologist's role," *Economy and Society* 33 (2003): 1–27.

72. http://bebrightpink.org/forum/read.php?3,235. (accessed Mar. 10, 2008). However, the majority of women diagnosed with *BRCA* mutations in the United States (2006 data) elect surveillance, not preventive surgery. José G. Guillem, William C. Wood, Jeffrey F. Moley, Andrew Berchuck, et al., "ASCO/SSO review of current role of risk-reducing surgery in common hereditary cancer syndromes," *Journal of Clinical Oncology* 24 (2006): 2642–60, on p. 2644.

73. www.facingourrisk.org/publications/newsletter.html (accessed Mar. 10, 2008).

74. Dixie A. King, "Women's perspective on breast and ovarian cancer genetic testing," Genetics and IVF, Institute, 1997. www.givf.com/womens_perspectivesv.cfm (accessed Mar. 10, 2008).

75. http://oncolink.org/coping/article.cfm?c=6&s=31&ss=76&id=236 (accessed Mar. 10, 2008).

76. http://bebrightpink.org/forum/read.php?3,259 (accessed Mar. 10, 2008). This message illustrates the role of display of suspicious changes in breast tissues (a "cystic growth") in reinforcing the conviction that prophylactic mastectomy was the right decision.

77. www.susanlovemd.org/community/sharing/donna2003.html (accessed Mar. 10, 2008).

78. Avon Breast Cancer Crusade; testimony of Feb. 4, 2004, http://134.65.5.228/discus/messages/2580/2580.html?1148323314 (accessed Mar. 10, 2008).

79. Messages (from 2005 and 2006) on "Forum: Cancer du sein et hérédité": www.essentielles.net/communaute/public/forums/forumdetail.asp?s=500&fid=73 (accessed Mar. 10, 2008). Message of Caro59, Feb. 28, 2006; message of "Marie Barcelona," Jan. 30, 2006.

80. Gessen published online a description of the process of informing herself about the meaning of being positive for *BRCA* mutation and then deciding what to do next: www.slate.com/id/2102171/entry/2102173/ (accessed Mar. 10, 2008). She then included some of this material in her book, *Blood Matters,* which was published in 2008.

81. Gessen, *Blood Matters,* 74. Italics in the original.

82. Ibid., 196.

83. http://bluegalinaredstate.blogspot.com/2006/04/news-was-goodi-went-shopping.html (accessed Mar. 10, 2008). This is only example of a feminist critique of preventive mastectomy for high risk women I found among breast cancer blogs.

84. Ibid.

85. Posted on Bright Pink site, January 2008; http://bebrightpink.org/forum/read.php?3,237.

86. www.slate.com/id/2102171/ entry/2102179/ (accessed Mar. 10, 2008).

87. Hearing before the subcommittee on health care of the committee on finance of the U.S. Senate, 105th Congress, 1st sess., on Women Health and Cancer Right Act of 1997, S-249, Nov. 5, 1997. (Washington, DC: U.S. Government Printing Office, 1997).

88. www.slate.com/id/2102171/entry/2102179/ (accessed Mar. 10, 2008).

89. Marcia Angel, *Science on Trial: The Clash of Medical Evidence and the Law in Breast Implants Case* (New York: W.W. Norton Company, 1996). Angel, a former editor of *New England Journal of Medicine,* strongly criticized the treatment of implant controversy by U.S. courts, and the attribution of damages to women without adequate scientific evidence on links between implants and autoimmune disease.

90. Angel, *Science on Trial,* 38–46.

91. www.susanlovemd.org/community/sharing/donna2003.html (accessed Mar. 10, 2008).

92. M. Salgarello and E. Farallo, "Immediate breast reconstruction with definitive anatomical implants after skin-sparing mastectomy," *British Journal of Plastic Surgery* 58 (2005): 216–22; C. De Greef, "Reconstruction mammaire par le lambeau DIEP: A propos de 100 cas," *Annales de Chirurugie Plastique Esthetique* 50 (2005): 56–61. Studies made by plastic surgeons seldom mention psychological effects of preventive mastectomy, such as a decrease in libido.

93. K. B. Clough, I. Sarfati, A. Fitousi, and P. Leblanc-Talent, "Reconstruction mammaire par prothèse: Vieillissement et resultats tardifs," *Annales de Chirurugie Plastique Esthetique* 50 (2005): 560–74.

94. W. M. Jacobsen, N. B. Meland, and J. E. Woods, "Autologous breast reconstruc-

tion with the use of transverse rectus abdminis musclocoutaneus flap: Mayo Clinic's experience with 147 cases," *Mayo Clinics Proceedings* 69 (1994): 635–40; S. E. Gabriel, J. E. Woods, W. M. Fallon, et al., "Complications leading to surgery after breast implantation," *New England Journal of Medicine* 336 (1997): 677–82.

95. Mary B. Barton, Carmen N. West, et al., "Complications following bilateral prophylactic mastectomy," *Journal of the National Cancer Institute Monographs,* 35 (2005): 61–66. This paper, attuned to women's experiences, was written by a group of eleven women.

96. C. M. Contant, M. B. Menke-Pluimers, C. Seynave, et al., "Clinical experience of prophylactic mastectomy followed by immediate breast reconstruction in women at hereditary risk of breast cancer or a proven *BRCA1* and *BRCA2* germ-line mutation," *European Journal of Surgical Oncology* 28 (2002): 627–32; Rebbeck, Friebel, Lynch, et al., "Bilateral prophylactic mastectomy reduces breast cancer risk in *BRCA1* and *BRCA2* mutation carriers."

97. Margaret L. Polinsky, "Functional status of long term breast cancer survivors: demonstrating chronicity," *Health and Social Work* 19 (1994): 165–72. W. C. S. Smith, D. Bourne, J. Squair, et al., "A retrospective cohorts study of post-mastectomy pain syndrome," *Pain* 83 (1999): 91–95; L. MacDonald, J. Bruce, N. W. Scott, W. C. S. Smith, and W. A. Chambers, "Long term follow-up of breast cancer survivors with post-mastectomy pain syndrome," *British Journal of Cancer* 92 (2005): 225–30.

98. Ellen Leopold, "Barbie meets breast cancer," *Breast Cancer Action Newsletter,* Sept. 2005, 3–4.

99. Rose Kushner to Michael Baum, London, July 29, 1986. Kushner's papers, MC 453, box 2, folder 31, Arthur and Elizabeth Schlesinger Library on the History of Women in America, Radcliffe Institute of Advanced Study, Harvard University (Schlesinger Library); Kushner's testimony before the Committee on Aging of the House of Representatives, Oct. 23, 1985. Kushner's papers, MC 453, box 6, folder 97, Schleslinger Library. Kushner's testimony before the advisory committee on medical devices and radiological health, FDA, Nov. 22, 1988. Kushner's papers, MC 453, box 6, folder 99, Schlesinger Library.

100. R. Eeles, T. Cole, R. Taylor, P. Lunt, and M. Baum, "Prophylactic mastectomy for genetic predispositions to breast cancer: The proband story," *Clinical Oncology* 8 (1996): 222–25, on p. 225.

101. Eeles, Cole, Taylor, Lunt and Baum, "Prophylactic mastecomy."

102. Testimony on Susan Love breast cancer site (mastectomy): www.susanlove md.com/community/sharing/index.html (accessed Mar. 10, 2008).

103. Testimony on Susan Love breast cancer site: www.susanlovemd.org/community/library/cancer_survivors/ (accessed Mar. 10, 2008).

104. Ibid.

105. Fabienne Rubert, *La Vie Est Là, Simplement* (Paris: Albin Michel, 2006), 96

106. Ibid., 145.

107. Rees, Clarke, Wardron, O'Boyle, Ewings, and MacDonagh, "The measurement of response shift in patients."

108. Women who expressed satisfaction with prophylactic surgeries answered stand-

ardized questionnaires. Schwartz, "Contralateral prophylactic mastectomy: Efficacy, satisfaction and regret"; Geiger, West, Nekhlyudov, et al., "Contentment with quality of life among breast cancer survivors."

109. In this study, 684 American women who underwent prophylactic mastectomy answered the open-ended questionnaire. Andrea Altschuler, Larissa Nekhlyudov, Sharon J. Rolnick, at al., "Positive, negative, and disparate—Women's differing long-term psychosocial experiences of bilateral or contralateral prophylactic mastectomy" *Breast Journal* 14 (2008): 25–32.

110. Sandra M. Gillford, "The meaning of lumps: A case study of the ambiguities of risk," in *Anthropology and Epidemiology: Interdisciplinary Approaches to the Study of Health and Disease,* ed. Craig R. Janes, Ron Stall, and Sandra Gillford (Dordrecht: Reidel, 1986), 213–46, on p. 236.

111. Lucy Grealy, *Autobiography of a Face* (New York: Perennial, 1994); Ann Patchett, *Truth and Beauty: A Friendship* (New York: HarperCollins, 2004).

112. I observed such account of the unavoidable consequences of prophylactic surgery in an oncology consultation in a French hospital and during two conferences on the management of patients at a hereditary risk of cancer. A survey of professional literature reveals similar attitudes in the United States and the United Kingdom.

113. Harry T. Lynch, Jane F. Lynch, and Wendy S. Rubinstein, "Editorial: Prophylactic mastectomy: Obstacles and Benefits," *Journal of the National Cancer Institute* 93 (2001): 1586–86. Italics mine, IL.

114. On the role of new biomedical technology in producing of "choice of no choice," see Marylin Strathern, *After Nature: English Kinship in the Late Twentieth Century* (Cambridge: Cambridge University Press, 1992).

115. Masha Gessen, Medical Quest, www.slate.com/id/2102171/entry/2102173/ (accessed Mar. 10, 2008).

Conclusion

1. Ludwik Fleck, *Genesis and Development of a Scientific Fact,* trans. Fred Bradley and Thaddeus J. Trenn (1935; reprinted Chicago: University of Chicago Press, 1979).

2. Experts estimated thus that in some populations, between 50% and 70% of positive Wasserman results were "true false positives." J. E. Moore and E. F. Mohr, "Biologically false positive serological tests for syphilis, *JAMA* 150 (1952): 467–73; C. Carpenter, R. A. Clair, and R. A. Brook, "Tests for syphilis: Increasing incidence of false positive reactions as measured by Treponema pallidum immobilization," *California Medical Journal* 103 (1965): 13–15.

3. Numerous pathologies, from autoimmune diseases to heart or liver dysfunctions, induce a positive result of the Wassermann test. This effect eluded earlier investigators because they tested only people already strongly suspected to be infected with *Treponema,* thus subpopulations with high incidence of syphilis. In such subpopulations the number of people with a positive Wassermann test induced by a different disease was negligible. This was not the case, however, in the general population. Among nonselected people, pathologies such as heart or liver diseases were often more frequent

than was syphilis. Ilana Löwy, "Testing for a sexually transmissible disease, 1907–1970: The history of the Wassermann reaction," in *AIDS and Contemporary History*, ed. Virginia Berridge and Philip Strong (Cambridge University Press, 1993), 74–92.

4. "Un ensemble résolument hétérogène, comportant des discours, des institutions, des aménagements architecturaux, des décisions réglementaires, des lois, des mesures administratives, des énoncés scientifiques, des propositions philosophiques, morales, philanthropiques, bref: Du dit, aussi bien que du non-dit, voilà les éléments du dispositif. Le dispositif lui-même, c'est le réseau qu'on peut établir entre ces éléments," Michel Foucault, "Le jeu de Michel Foucault," in M. Foucault, *Dits et Ecrits 1954–1988*, Daniel Deferet and François Evald, eds. (Paris: PUF, 1994), 298–329, on p. 299. I'm indebted to Christiane Sinding for this reference.

5. I'm following Bruno Latour's description of the emergence of new scientific findings. Bruno Latour, *Science in Action* (Cambridge, MA: Harvard University Press, 1987), 87–88.

6. I use the term *stable* to describe classificatory categories that are adopted by the majority of stakeholders, not those that have a single, well-defined meaning. Boundary concepts that have a stringent definition in a single site use and a looser definition in intersite use facilitate collaborations across heterogeneous sites and help consolidate practices. Such concepts or categories are, however, open-ended, not controversial or ambivalent. Coronary heart disease is an open-ended diagnostic category, fibromyalgia is a contested one. See, e.g., Ilana Löwy, "The strength of loose concepts: Boundary concepts, federal experimental strategies and disciplinary growth. The case of immunology," *History of Science* 30 (1992): 373–96.

7. Charles Rosenberg, "The tyranny of diagnosis: Specific entities and individual experience," *The Milbank Quarterly* 80 (2002): 237–60.

8. For examples of dilemmas produced by unstable diagnostic categories, see Keith Wailoo, *Drawing Blood: Technology and Disease Identity in Twentieth-Century America* (Baltimore: Johns Hopkins University Press, 1997); Robert Aronowitz, *Making Sense of Illness: Science, Society and Disease* (Cambridge: Cambridge University Press, 1998).

9. Mass screening campaigns for syphilis conducted in the late 1930s were followed by administration of antisyphilis drugs to people who tested positive. These drugs, usually variants of arsephenamine (Ehrlich's compound 606), induced numerous side effects. In the 1940s, the development of penicillin, a much more efficient and less toxic therapy of syphilis, greatly reduced the danger of overtreatment of this disease. In parallel, the Wassermann test was gradually replaced by more specific tests that revealed the presence of *Treponema pallidum*. Löwy, "Testing for a sexually transmissible disease, 1907–1970."

10. A book about pathology is dedicated to "all those who helped us to understand the primal patient—the cell." Guido Majno and Isabelle Joris, *Cells, Tissues and Diseases: Principles of General Pathology* (Oxford: Blackwell Science, 1996).

11. The role of "traces" in science was discussed by Hans Jörg Rheinberger. Hans Jörg Rheinberger, *Toward a History of Epistemic Things: Synthesizing Proteins in the Test Tube* (Palo Alto, CA: Stanford University Press, 1997), 110–11.

12. For an early criticism of such suppositions, see Goustave Roussy, *Le Cancer* (Paris, Armand Collin, 1929), 71–72.

13. For example, gender was described as incorrigible proposal. The "sex/gender system" presupposes that humanity is divided into two distinct, mutually exclusive groups, "men" and "women." The observation that some people combine traits of both sexes does not undermine that validity of this binary division, because these exceptions are presented as intermediary forms: "masculinized women" or "feminized men." Susan J. Kessler and Wendy McKenna, *Gender: An Ethnomethodological Approach* (New York: John Wiley & Sons, 1978).

14. The low level of visibility of head and neck tumors may be related not only to the fact that the disease itself and its treatments may produce frightening mutilations, difficult to sanitize and make presentable, but also to the difficulty of linking these pathologies with the "do not delay" principle. Early detection of these tumors does not always improve outcomes.

15. A third exemplary malignancy, lung cancer, played a key role in the understanding of epidemiology of cancer but not in debates on clinical fate of malignancies.

16. Sarah Franklin, "Stem cells R us: Emergent life forms and the global biological," in *Global Assemblages*, ed. A. Ong and S. Collier (Malden, MA: Blackwell, 2005), 59–78.

17. In absence of such pressures, pathologists may opt for a binary distinction between cancerous and noncancerous tissues.

18. Robert Aronowitz, *Unnatural History: Breast Cancer and American Society* (Cambridge: Cambridge University Press, 2007).

19. Fleck, *Genesis and Development of a Scientific Fact*, 43. Fleck added that a tendency to transform scientific terms into slogans was not limited to lay people but affected scientists as well: "this magical power of slogans, with 'vitalism' in biology, 'specificity' in immunology and 'bacterial transformation' in bacteriology, clearly extend to the very depth of specialist research." Ibid.

20. Susan Sontag, *Illness as Metaphor* (New York: Farrar, Strauss & Giroux, 1978).

21. While less fashionable today, this concept of "cancer personality" did not disappear, perhaps because some individuals elect to blame themselves for their cancer—and therefore to give meaning to their suffering—rather than to view their disease as a random event.

22. Charles Rosenberg, *The Care of Strangers: The Rise of American Hospital System* (New York: Basic Books, 1987); Joel Howell, *Technology in the Hospital: Transforming Patient Care in the Early Twentieth Century* (Baltimore: Johns Hopkins University Press, 1995); George Weisz, *Divide and Conquer: A Comparative History of Medical Specialization* (Oxford: Oxford University Press, 2006).

23. Pierre Rosanvallon made a similar argument about the rise of capitalism. According to Rosanvallon, Adam Smith's *The Wealth of Nations* was published in 1776, before the popularization of inventions, such as steam-powered machines and trains, that shaped modern capitalism. Pierre Rosanvallon, *Le Capitalisme Utopique: Critique de l'Idéologie Economique* (Paris: Point Essais, 1999).

24. One can point nevertheless to important advances in treatment of selected, relatively rare, malignant tumors such as testicular cancer or Hodgkin's lymphoma, cures of many of childhood tumors, the increase of survival of people with disseminated malignancies thanks to perfection of radiotherapy and chemotherapy, and the reduction of incidence of lung cancer in men (in developed countries) thanks to the demonstration of links between this tumor and cigarette smoking.

25. Other medical specialties, such as endocrinology or neurology, also successfully articulated laboratory investigations and clinical practices, but these domains have a lower public visibility. On the centralization of cancer therapies in the interwar era, see Patrice Pinell, *Naissance d'un Fléau* (Paris: Anne Marie Metaillé, 1992; English version, *The Fight against Cancer: France 1890–1940*, trans. David Maddell [London: Routledge, 2002]), and on role of cancer treatment in reorganization of medical work after the Second World War, Alberto Cambrosio and Peter Keating, *Biomedical Platforms* (Cambridge, MA: MIT Press, 2003).

26. For example, recently some authors have claimed that a delay in diagnosis of cancer, including in the exemplary female malignancies (breast, cervix, endometrium), has only a limited effect on prognosis. Richard Sansbury, "Effect on survival of delays in referral of patients with breast cancer symptoms: A retrospective analysis," *The Lancet* 353 (1999): 1132–35; P. Symonds, B. Bolger, D. Hole, and T. Cooke, "Advanced stage cervix cancer: Rapid tumor growth rather than late diagnosis," *British Journal of Cancer*, 83 (2000): 566–68; Simon C. Crawford, Jonathan A. Davis, Nadeem A. Siddiqui, Linda de Caestecker, Charles R. Gillis, and David Hole, "The waiting time paradox: Population based retrospective study of treatment delay and survival of women with endometrial cancer in Scotland," *British Medical Journal* 325 (2002): 196–99; R. Paul Symonds, "Cancer biology may be more important than diagnostic delay," *British Medical Journal* 325 (2002): 774 ; Cheslea Hardin, SuEllen Pommier, and Rodney F. Pommier, "The relationships among clinician delay of diagnosis of breast cancer and tumor size, nodal status and stage," *The American Journal of Surgery* 192 (2006): 506–8, and for discussion, see Alan S. Coates, "Commentary. Breast cancer: delays, dilemmas and delusions," *The Lancet* 353 (1999): 1112–13.

27. Edmund Biernacki, Istota i granice wiedzy lekarskej (Warsaw: Biblioteka Dziel Wyborowych, 1899; English translation of excerpts in Ilana Löwy, *The Polish School of Philosophy of Medicine: From Tutus Chalubinski to Ludwik Fleck* (Dordrecht: Kluwer, 1990), 30–67.

28. Lester King, *Medical Thinking: A Historical Preface* (Princeton: Princeton University Press, 1982).

29. King, *Medical Thinking*, 309.

30. Robert Aronowitz, "To screen or not to screen: What is the question," *Journal of General Internal Medicine* 10 (1995): 295–97; Charles E. Rosenberg, "Managed fear: Contemplating sickness in an era of bureaucracy and chronic disease," American Osler Society, 2008; Charles E. Rosenberg, "Managed fear," *Lancet* 373 (2009): 802–3; Aronowitz, *Unnatural History*.

31. One may draw a parallel between early twentieth-century physicians' ability to use the newly developed bacteriological tests to diagnose infectious diseases and their

limited capacity to cure these diseases and the early twentieth-first-century physicians' ability to use newly elaborated molecular biology techniques to display changes in genes or gene expression and their limited capacity to prevent negative consequences of such changes.

32. Sandra M. Gifford, "The meaning of lumps: A case study of the ambiguities of risk," in *Anthropology and Epidemiology: Interdisciplinary Approaches to the Study of Health and Disease,* ed. Craig R. Janes, Ron Staff, and Sandra Gifford (Dordrecht: Reidel, 1986), 213–46.

33. On the risk of medical information, see Susan Markens, C. H. Browner, and Nancy Press, "'Because of the risks': How US pregnant women account for refusing prenatal screening," *Social Sciences and Medicine* 49 (1999): 359–69.

34. For a rare example of a physician explicitly acknowledging the risk for professionals, see Dr. Power's statement in *Early Breast Cancer: Detection and Treatment,* ed. H. Stephen Gallagher (New York: John Wiley & Sons), 175.

35. The argument about rise of "suspicion-based" policies was developed by Ron Suskind in his discussion of the ways the "preventive war" in Iraq was justified by conservative U.S. politicians. Ron Suskind, *The One Percent Doctrine: Deep Inside America's Pursuit of Its Enemies Since 9/11* (New York: Simon & Schuster, 2006).

36. "Il ne faut savoir ne pas ouvrir une armoire, sans avoir prevu ce qu'on fera du squelette qu'elle continent peut être. Il faut savoir ne pas laisser une squelette dans un armoire où l'on a trouvé un homme bien portant." This warning against excesses of preventive approaches in oncology ends Denoix's unpublished manuscript *Carcinologie Demain: Dictonnaire des Idées Non Reçues. Quelques Sujets de Reflexion pour Jeunes Médecins et pour les Autres* (undated. code U1116, BI4521, Bibliothèque de l'Institut des recherches scientifiques sur le cancer, Villejuif), 168.

37. Lorraine Daston and Peter Galison, "The image of objectivity," *Representations* 40 (1992): 81–128.

38. Ludwik Fleck, "Some specific features of the medical way of thinking," *Archiwum Historji i Filozofji Medecyny* 6 (1927): 55–64. English translation in *Cognition and Fact: Materials on Ludwik Fleck,* ed. Robert Cohen and Thomas Schnelle (Dordrecht: Reidel, 1986) 39–46.

39. Paul Edwards, "The army and the Microword: Computers and the politics of gender identity," *Signs,* 16 (1990): 102–27.

40. Gaston Bachelard, *Le Nouvel Esprit Scientifique* (1934; reprinted Paris: PUF, 1968), quoted by Rheinberger, *Towards the History of Epistemic Things,* 28.

41. Rheinberger, *Towards the History of Epistemic Things,* 181.

42. Bruno Latour aptly proposed calling such aggregates of practices "worknets," rather than networks, to bring to the foreground the labor necessary to construct and maintain these arrangements. Bruno Latour, "A dialog on actor-network theory," in *The Social Study of Information and Communication Technology: Innovation, Actors and Contexts,* ed. Chrisanthi Avgerou, Claudio U. Ciborra and Frank F. Land (Oxford: Oxford University Press, 2004), 65–79.

43. Fleck, *Genesis and Development of a Scientific Fact;* Löwy, "The strength of loose concepts," Rheinberger, *Towards the History of Epistemic Things.*